Complementary & Alternative Therapies in Nursing

Sixth Edition

Mariah Snyder, PhD, RN, is Professor Emeritus at the University of Minnesota School of Nursing. Her professional career has included teaching courses on complementary therapies, conducting research on the use of complementary therapies in persons with dementia and on managing stress in persons with chronic illnesses, and assisting international nurses in incorporating complementary therapies in practice and education. Dr. Snyder was a founding member of the Center for Spirituality and Healing in the Academic Health Center at the University of Minnesota and was a primary contributor to the development of its interdisciplinary minor—the first such minor in the United States. Her retirement activities include using complementary therapies in women with addictions who are imprisoned. She is also assisting in the development of the library at Cristo Rey Jesuit High School in Minneapolis, a college preparatory school for students from economically poor families.

Ruth Lindquist, PhD, RN, ACNS-BC, FAAN, FAHA, is a Professor in the School of Nursing and faculty member of the Center for Spirituality and Healing in the Academic Health Center of the University of Minnesota. She is a research consultant for the Women's Heart Health Program of the Minneapolis Heart Institute at Abbott Northwestern Hospital. Her research as a Densford Scholar in the Katharine J. Densford International Center for Nursing Leadership focused on critical care nurses' attitudes toward and use of complementary/alternative therapies. Her recent research focuses on cardiovascular patient response to the use of therapies in the context of hospitalization with acute cardiac conditions, and the use of complementary therapies, exercise, and cardiac support groups to reduce stress and improve quality of life in women with heart disease.

Complementary & Alternative Therapies in Nursing

Sixth Edition

MARIAH SNYDER, PhD, RN

RUTH LINDQUIST, PhD, RN, ACNS-BC, FAAN, FAHA

Editors

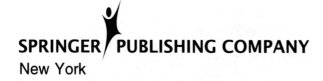

SPRINGER PUBLISHING COMPANY
New York

Springer Publishing Company, LLC
11 West 42nd Street
New York, NY 10036
www.springerpub.com

Acquisitions Editor: Margaret Zuccarini
Project Manager: Pamela Lankas
Cover Design: Steve Pisano
Composition: International Graphic Services

E-book ISBN: 978-0-8261-2429-6

13/ 5 4 3 2

The author and the publisher of this Work have made every effort to use sources believed to be reliable to provide information that is accurate and compatible with the standards generally accepted at the time of publication. Because medical science is continually advancing, our knowledge base continues to expand. Therefore, as new information becomes available, changes in procedures become necessary. We recommend that the reader always consult current research and specific institutional policies before performing any clinical procedure. The author and publisher shall not be liable for any special, consequential, or exemplary damages resulting, in whole or in part, from the readers' use of, or reliance on, the information contained in this book. The publisher has no responsibility for the persistence or accuracy of URLs for external or third-party Internet Web sites referred to in this publication and does not guarantee that any content on such Web sites is, or will remain, accurate or appropriate.

Library of Congress Cataloging-in-Publication Data

Complementary & alternative therapies in nursing / [edited by] Mariah Snyder, Ruth Lindquist.--6th ed.
   p. ; cm.
   Rev. ed. of: Complementary/alternative therapies in nursing / Mariah Snyder, Ruth Lindquist, editors. 5th ed. c2006.
   Includes bibliographical references and index.
   ISBN 978-0-8261-2428-9 (alk. paper)
   1. Holistic nursing. 2. Nurse and patient. 3. Alternative medicine. I. Snyder, Mariah.
II. Lindquist, Ruth. III. Complementary/alternative therapies in nursing. IV. Title:
Complementary and alternative therapies in nursing.
   [DNLM: 1. Complementary Therapies—nursing. 2. Holistic Nursing. WY 86.5 C7375 2009]
   RT41.I53 2009
   610.73—dc22
                                  2009036392

Printed in the United States of America by Gasch Printing.

To nurses around the world who incorporate complementary therapies into their care of patients so as to provide holistic quality care.

Contents

Contributors

Susan M. Bee, RN, MSN, CNS
Clinical Nurse Specialist
Pain Rehabilitation Center
Mayo Clinic
Rochester, MN

Carie A. Braun, PhD, RN
Associate Professor of Nursing
College of Saint Benedict/Saint
John's University
Saint Joseph, MN

Ulf G. Bronäs, PhD, MS, ATC, ATR
Clinical Assistant Professor
School of Nursing
University of Minnesota
Minneapolis, MN

Miriam E. Cameron, PhD, MS, MA, RN
Faculty, Center for Spirituality
and Healing
University of Minnesota
Minneapolis, MN

Kuei-Min Chen, PhD, RN
Professor and Dean
School of Nursing
Fooyin University
Kaoshiung, Taiwan

Corjena K. Cheung, PhD, RN
Assistant Professor
St. Catherine University
St. Paul, MN

Linda L. Chlan, PhD, RN
Associate Professor
School of Nursing, Center for
Spirituality and Healing
University of Minnesota
Minneapolis, MN

Suzanne M. Cutshall, MS, RN, ACNS-BC, AHN-BC
Integrative Health Specialist
Mayo Clinic
Rochester, MN

Michele M. Evans, RN, MS, MSN, CNS
Clinical Nurse Specialist
Pain Rehabilitation Center
Mayo Clinic
Rochester, MN

Maura Fitzgerald, MS, RN, MA, CNS
Clinical Nurse Specialist
Children's Hospital and Clinics
of Minnesota
Integrative Medicine Project
St. Paul, MN

Melissa Frisvold, MS, RN, CNM
Doctoral Candidate,
School of Nursing
University of Minnesota
Minneapolis, MN

Marion Good, PhD, RN, FAAN
Arline H. and Curtis F. Garvin
Professor of Nursing Excellence
Frances Payne Bolton School of
Nursing
Case Western Reserve University
Cleveland, OH

**Thora Jenny Gunnarsdottir, PhD,
RN**
Assistant Professor
University of Iceland
Rekjavik, Iceland

**Niloufar Hadidi, PhD, RN, ACNS-
BC, FAHA**
Assistant Professor
University of Minnesota
School of Nursing

Linda L. Halcón, PhD, MPH, RN
Associate Professor and Coopera-
tive Head
School of Nursing
University of Minnesota
Minneapolis, MN

Mary Jo Kreitzer, PhD, RN
Director, Center for Spirituality
and Healing,
Professor, School of Nursing
University of Minnesota
Minneapolis, MN

**Mary Langevin, RN, MSN, CPON,
HN-BC**
Family Nurse Practitioner
Advanced Practice Nurse-
Hematology/Oncology
Children's Hospitals and Clinic
of Minnesota
Minneapolis, MN

Barbara Leonard, PhD, RN, FAAN
Professor
Director, Children with Special
Health Care Needs
School of Nursing University of
Minnesota
Minneapolis, MN

Daniel L. Mark, MD, ABMS
Medical Orthopedics
St. Mary's/Duluth Clinic Health
System
Duluth, MN

**Margaret P. Moss, PhD, JD, RN,
FAAN**
2008–2009 Robert Wood John-
son Health Policy Fellow
Senate Special Committee on
Aging, Washington DC
Associate Professor, University of
Minnesota
Minneapolis, MN

Kathleen Niska, PhD, RN
Associate Professor
Department of Nursing
College of St. Scholastica
Duluth, MN

(or field of consciousness) that promotes the healing potential and an experience of well-being of the patient.

Complementary & Alternative Therapies in Nursing is organized around the recognized National Center for Complementary and Alternative Medicine (NCCAM, 2007) fields of practice, which are nursing interventions—mind–body therapies, energy and biofield therapies, manual therapies, and biologically based therapies. The authors of this text advocate a "both/and" instead of an "either/or" approach in interfacing these complementary/alternative therapies with contemporary medical and surgical therapies. It is crucial that nurses continue to become more informed about complementary/alternative therapies so they may safely and appropriately become integrated into current nursing practice, education, and research.

These complementary/alternative therapies are not used in a mechanical manner. Each nurse must be sensitive to where these modalities may lead. As the nurse leads a patient into a relaxed state, the individual may touch different levels of her/his story and the suffering around the story that is often unknown to the nurse. Suffering is an individual's story around pain in which the signs of suffering may be physical, mental, emotional, social, behavioral, and/or spiritual; it is anguish experienced—internal and external—as a threat to one's composure, integrity, and the fulfillment of intentions.

As nurses blend the art and science of evidence-based practice with each therapy, they recognize the use of intention. Intention is the conscious awareness of being in the present moment to help facilitate the healing process and a volitional act of love. Nurses also incorporate the use of intuition, the perceived knowing of things and events without the conscious use of rational processes, which may engage many of the senses to receive information.

With the use of these complementary/alternative therapies, human caring is experienced. This is the moral state in which the nurse brings her or his whole self into relationship with the whole self of significant beings that reinforces the meaning and experience of oneness and unity. Working with patients to choose and implement these therapies is a privilege and a responsibility. It is beneficial for each nurse to have experienced each therapy before using it so as to anticipate various emotions that may manifest during and after a session. Nurses that integrate complementary/alternative therapies are demonstrating their leadership capacities to inspire others to act to transform health care that can lead to healthy people and a healthy world (Nightingale Initiative for Global Health, 2009). To transform health care to include practice that is patient centered and involves relationship care that also blends complementary/alternative therapies is crucial in the twenty-first century. These therapies lead to the development of the healing of individuals, organizations, and societies. Transformational leadership is a way of leading in which the leader is a learner, a mentor, and a teacher. She/he is a trailblazer and mapmaker. She/he is concerned not only with improving conditions within existing frameworks and mind-sets, but with going one step further to design and lead processes that shift the frameworks and mind-sets themselves.

Starting in the 1880s, Nightingale began to write that it would take 100 or 150 years to have nurses educated to transform hospitals and health care. *Complementary & Alternative Therapies in Nursing* is a guide for nurses today to be twenty-first century Nightingales; this is what Nightingale knew would occur in the future (Dossey, 2010; Dossey, Selanders, Beck, & Attewell, 2005). The message in this book is the essence for all that nursing can be and to which we must continue to aspire.

Barbara Dossey, PhD, RN, AHN-BC, FAAN
International Co-Director, Nightingale Initiative for Global Health
Arlington, Virginia and Ottawa, Ontario, and
Director, Holistic Nursing Consultants, Santa Fe, New Mexico

REFERENCES

American Holistic Nurses Association and American Nurses Association. (2007). *Holistic nursing: Scope and standards of practice.* Silver Spring, MD: Nursesbooks.Org

Dossey, B. M. (2010). *Florence Nightingale: Mystic, visionary, healer, Commemorative edition.* Philadelphia: F. A. Davis.

Dossey, B. M., & Keegan, L. (2008). *Holistic nursing: A handbook for practice* (5th ed.). Sudbury, MA: Jones and Bartlett.

Dossey, B. M., Selanders, L. C., Beck, D. M., & Attewell, A. (2005). *Florence Nightingale today: Healing, leadership, global action.* Silver Spring, MD: Nursesbooks.Org

National Center for Complementary and Alternative Medicine. (2007). Available at http://www.nccam.nih.gov

Nightingale Initiative for Global Health. Retrieved August 14, 2009, from http://www.nightingaledeclaration.net

Preface

We are so pleased to introduce the sixth edition of *Complementary & Alternative Therapies in Nursing*. The format and organization, practice applications, examples, and evidence-based approach of the book have sustained its appeal and popularity over time. Indeed, the book is unique in its field, and we have carefully worked to carry forward all of the book's well-recognized strengths. Its up-to-date, easy-to-retrieve, authoritative information has become a valued asset for busy professionals, hence the book has been popular amongst nursing faculty, nursing students, and practicing nurses alike. This new edition is timely and the content even more essential than ever before. Never has there been a greater desire for complementary and alternative therapies on the part of our patients and the public. Indeed, the majority of the public is already using these therapies, and the demand only continues to grow.

It is essential for nurses to have a readily available resource that provides current information on complementary and alternative medicine (CAM). We need such a resource to provide our patients with basic information on as well as answers to their questions about CAM therapies, including questions of safety and efficacy. We, in our professional capacity, need to be informed about potential contraindications for these therapies as well as their potential interactions with concurrently prescribed conventional medical therapies. We also need to be knowledgeable about these therapies ourselves so that we may offer them to our patients as expanded options for comfort and relief. We are hopeful that this book goes a long way toward meeting these essential needs. The usefulness of the book is extended by the inclusion of links to various Web sites, where further details and current and updated information may be sought.

So one might ask, "What's new" in the sixth edition? In a world teeming with change, we have worked to provide cutting-edge information from the available evidence base as well as from the experience of the numerous experts who have authored the chapters of this book, many of whom regularly use these therapies in practice. There are rich new chapters, including one on light therapy and another on creating optimal healing environments. We have also separated out material on practice, education, and research into separate chapters in their own right, to provide greater depth in those areas. The references are fresh and current. There are new authors, as we continue to draw upon the expertise of authors from around the world, including Korea, Sweden, Iceland, Iran, Taiwan, and Japan. There is a healthy mix of experience and expertise among the authors in terms of their basis in research, practice, teaching, and practice settings, encompassing a broad range of health care institutions, schools, academic health centers, public health settings, and private practice. Today there is strong interest in including effective healing therapies and practices from countries and cultures around the world in the provision of health care. The world is becoming increasingly smaller; hence, we need to understand the use of CAM therapies and practices indigenous to various cultures and populations. Thus, besides the expanded emphasis on culture in chapter 1, perhaps the most exciting and pervasive change in (and strength of) the sixth edition is the inclusion of cultural applications in each chapter. These changes can serve to broaden and deepen our understanding of the basis for and use of complementary therapies.

Complementary therapies assume a key role in the promotion of healing, comfort, and care. More than 1,800 complementary/alternative therapies and systems of care have been identified. Many of these therapies have been used by nurses for centuries, and now an increasing number of such therapies that have been a part of systems of care across the world are receiving attention in the United States. The increasing mobility of society, whether through immigration, travel, or attendance at international conferences, requires that nurses be knowledgeable about ancient therapies used by many persons around the world. Throughout this book, attention is paid to health care practices of other cultures, so that nurses may acquire knowledge about and respect for these practices and therapies and, if possible, accommodate them into the plan of care. Thus, this book is needed more than ever to help prepare students and practitioners for the broad range of complementary and alternative therapies that they will encounter in their practice. It is imperative that nurses not miss opportunities to employ a therapy that could benefit a patient in pain or that could relieve or prevent anxiety; likewise, it is important for nurses to identify therapies that may be misapplied or having adverse effects on the user.

All of the chapters describing therapies have sections that include background, definitions, scientific basis, intervention(s), and one or more techniques that can be used to implement a therapy, along with precautions to be aware of in applications, conditions, and patient populations in which these therapies have been used, as well as cultural applications, and suggestions for research. The new inclusion in this edition of cultural applications can broaden the understanding of the basis and use of a therapy. The uniform format is a structure that provides a clear way to organize knowledge and educate patients. The information provided is practical. The holistic and caring aspects of these therapies have been and continue to be valued both by nurses and by those to whom care is provided in the United States and in countries around the world. Nursing roles continue to evolve, but within all of these varied roles and settings in which nurses practice, concern for the comfort and healing of patients remains uppermost in their minds.

This actively developing frontier of science is generating important and much-needed evidence to support our informed use of complementary and alternative therapies. Various groups, including the National Academy of Science, have proposed goals to expand research on complementary therapies. There is a concomitant increase in the number of journals focusing on these therapies. We trust that we have captured the most current evidence for the therapies in the sixth edition of this text. Conducting and disseminating the research-based evidence for the use of complementary therapies is an endeavor in which nurses can be integrally involved. Many nurses have provided leadership in research, education, and practice applications of these therapies.

As the consumer demand for and use of complementary therapies continue to increase, it is critical that nurses gain knowledge about complementary therapies, so that they can select and include them in their practice, provide patients with information about them, be informed about research and practice guidelines related to complementary therapies, alert patients to possible contraindications and even incorporate some of these therapies into their own self-care.

We wish to thank the many nurses and students who across the years have used our text and who have encouraged us to continue updating the information in this edition. The interest they have shown in the use of complementary therapies for practice and self care has prompted us to continue our quest to obtain new information about complementary therapies that can be used by nurses. We appreciate and thank the authors—some new, many returning—who have spent countless hours in writing or revising the chapters to bring you the most useful and updated information. We thank our colleagues at the School of Nursing and the Center for Spirituality and Healing at the University of Minnesota for their ongoing efforts to develop the knowledge base for complementary therapies through research, and to educate students about these therapies for their future practice, to the benefit of countless patients whom they have yet to encounter.

Mariah Snyder, PhD, RN
Ruth Lindquist, PhD, RN, ACNS-BC, FAAN, FAHA

Complementary & Alternative Therapies in Nursing

Sixth Edition

Foundations for Practice

OVERVIEW

Complementary therapies have become widely known and used in Western health care. However, the therapies included in many of the surveys that have been done about the use of complementary therapies are rather limited in scope and number. As Thomas Friedman (2005) puts it, our world is becoming flat. Expanding the perspectives on complementary medicine so that nurses become more knowledgeable about therapies that are practiced by persons in multiple cultures across the globe is critical to competent health care. In chapter 1 and in subsequent chapters throughout this book, the authors have taken a new tack: to note therapies that are not routinely considered part of the "Western" complementary therapy armamentarium. Yet, this effort reveals only the tip of the iceberg in terms of therapies that many of the patients seeking health care are already using. Thus, it is imperative for nurses and other health care professionals to do a holistic assessment of their patients to determine which from a broad array of healing practices they will use. This is true not only for recent immigrants, but for all patients.

Modeling the holistic, caring philosophy that underlies many of the complementary therapies typically used is an important aspect of care. Taking care of oneself is even more important in the increasingly pressure-filled health care settings in which nurses and other health professionals practice today. In chapter 2, therapies and practices that nurses can use to lessen stress and focus on the patient and his/her family are discussed.

Two therapies—presence and communication—are critical elements in the implementation of any of the complementary therapies. Many patients and families comment about a nurse who was "really present to us." Presence is difficult to define, but, as an old adage says, "You know it when you see it." The multiple facets of communication, both verbal and nonverbal, are likewise important keys to providing the holistic care that is part of the philosophy underlying the use of complementary therapies. Nonverbal communication becomes more important when interacting with persons who are not from Western cultures. Several years ago, Madeline Leininger (1991) stressed the importance of gaining knowledge about other cultures. This knowledge is even more important today, with our increasing cultural diversity in every health care system. The knowledge of customs as basic as whether it is acceptable to shake the hand of the patient and family or touch someone of another gender is foundational in establishing the kind of therapeutic relationship that is integral to the success of complementary therapies. Discussions in chapters 3 and 4 seek to heighten the nurse's awareness of the importance of presence and communication skills in building such relationships.

REFERENCES

Friedman, T. (2005). *The world is flat: A brief history of the twenty-first century.* New York: Farrar, Straus, & Giroux.

Leininger, M. M. (1991). *Cultural care diversity and universality: A theory of nursing.* New York: National League of Nursing.

1 Complementary/Alternative Therapies and Cultural Aspects of Care

MARIAH SNYDER
KATHLEEN NISKA
RUTH LINDQUIST

Complementary and alternative therapies have become an important part of health care in the United States and other countries. Although the term *complementary therapies* will be used primarily in this book, numerous other designations have been used for such therapies that are not a part of the traditional Western system of medical care. The term *complementary* is preferred by some because it conveys that a therapy is used as an adjunct to Western therapies, whereas *alternative* indicates a therapy that is used in place of a Western approach to medicine. Both terms are used by the National Center for Complementary and Alternative Medicine (NCCAM) of the National Institutes of Health (NIH). More recently, the term *integrative medicine* is being used to convey that the care provided is a blend of Western medicine, complementary therapies, and therapies from other systems of health care. A growing body of research to support use of these therapies is emerging.

DEFINITION AND CLASSIFICATION

A number of definitions of complementary therapies are currently in use. Nursing and other health professions frequently call the area com-

3

plementary *therapies* while NCCAM refers to them as complementary *medicine*. The broad scope of these therapies and the many health professionals and therapists who are involved in delivering them create challenges for finding a definition that captures the breadth of this field.

The definition of complementary/alternative therapies put forth by NCCAM is:

> Complementary and alternative medicine is a group of diverse medical and health care systems, practices, and products that are not presently considered to be part of conventional medicine. (NCCAM, 2008, p. 1)

In this definition, conventional refers to Western biomedicine. The NCCAM definition acknowledges that other systems of health care exist and are used.

The ambiguity in the definition of complementary therapies poses challenges when comparing findings across surveys that have been conducted on the use of complementary therapies. Some surveys have included multiple therapies while others have limited the number. For example, in the NCCAM/National Center for Health Statistics survey (NCCAM, 2008), adding prayer for health reasons to the analyses increased the percent of use of complementary therapies from 36 to 62%.

According to Kreitzer and Jensen (2000), more than 1,800 therapies have been identified as being complementary. NCCAM has classified these multiple therapies and systems of care into five categories. The NCCAM categories and examples of the types of therapies in each category are shown in Exhibit 1.1. Some of these therapies have been used widely and researched while others are relatively unknown in the United States. A number of the therapies noted in Exhibit 1.1 have been a part of nursing for many years.

Health care professionals are becoming increasingly aware of culture-specific medical practices of immigrants that may be used by persons in health care facilities. These practices or therapies may be ones carried out by shamans, healers, family members, or the patient him/herself. Knowledge about common practices in various ethnic groups will assist nurses in providing culturally sensitive care.

USE OF COMPLEMENTARY THERAPIES

Interest and use of complementary/alternative therapies has increased exponentially during the past quarter century. Surveys have addressed

Exhibit 1.1

NCCAM Classification for Complementary Therapies and Examples of Therapies

Mind–Body Therapies
Interventions use a variety of techniques to enhance the mind's ability to affect body functions and symptoms. Examples: imagery, meditation, yoga, music therapy, prayer, journaling, biofeedback, humor, tai chi, art therapy.

Biologically Based Therapies
Therapies use substances found in nature. Examples: plant-derived preparations (herbs and essential oils), special diets, orthomolecular medicine (nutritional and food supplements), other products such as cartilage.

Manipulative and Body-Based Therapies
Therapies are based on manipulation or movement of one or more parts of the body. Examples: chiropractic medicine, massage, body work such as rolfing.

Energy Therapies
Therapies focus on the use of energy fields, such as magnetic and biofields that are believed to surround and permeate the body. Examples: healing touch, therapeutic touch, Reiki, external qi gong, magnets.

Systems of Care
Whole systems of care are built upon theory and practice and often evolved apart from and earlier than Western medicine. Therapies noted above may be from these systems of care.

use within English-speaking and largely Caucasian groups (Barnes, Powell-Griner, McFann, & Nahin, 2004; Rhee, Barg, & Hershey, 2004; Rosen, Azzam, Levi, Braun, & Krivoy, 2003). Recently surveys have explored complementary therapy use within minority groups: African American and Hispanic (Bazargan et al., 2008); Hispanic adolescents (Feldmann, Wiemann, Sever, & Hergenroeder, 2008); Whites, Blacks, Mexican Americans, and Chinese Americans (Chao & Wade, 2008); and Chinese Americans (Fang & Schinke, 2007). Interest in the use of complementary therapies is a phenomenon found not only in the United States; as surveys on the use of these therapies have been conducted in many countries, including Saudi Arabia (Al-Faris et al., 2008), Germany (Ernst, 2008), Japan (Hori, Mihaylov, Vasconcelos, & McCoubrie, 2008), and Turkey (Erci, 2007). The number of persons using complementary therapies varied, but incidence of use was often 40 to 50%.

Numerous studies have explored the use of complementary therapies in specific health conditions, including obesity (Bertisch, Wee, &

McCarthy, 2008), multiple sclerosis (Esmonde & Long, 2008), cancer (Hok, Tishelman, Ploner, Forss, & Falkenberg, 2008), stroke survivors (Shah, Engelhardt, & Ovbiagele, 2009), and arthritis (Strois, 2008). In most studies, not only the percent of persons using therapies but the specific therapies used were identified. These therapies varied across the groups.

Some researchers have attempted to identify characteristics of users of complementary therapies. Rosen and colleagues (2003) found that more females than males used these therapies. Also, a higher percentage of persons using complementary therapies had academic degrees as compared with a non-user group. These findings were further validated in the national survey conducted by the NCCAM and the National Center for Health Statistics (NCCAM, 2008). Struthers and Nichols (2004) reviewed studies on the use of complementary therapies in racial and ethnic minority populations; in seven studies, persons in minority groups did not use complementary therapies more than persons in other groups.

Currently, third-party payers such as insurance companies pay for a limited number of complementary therapies. The therapies most frequently covered are chiropractic, acupuncture, and biofeedback. In most instances, physician referral is required for reimbursement. Some states, such as Washington, require the inclusion of complementary therapists in private, commercial insurance products (Lafferty et al., 2004). According to NCCAM (2008), Americans spent between $36 billion and $47 billion on complementary therapies in 1997, $12 billion to $20 billion of which was paid for directly by the consumer. Obviously, people must feel that complementary therapies produce positive results if they continue to personally pay for these therapies.

What has prompted this rapidly growing interest in complementary therapies? First, the holistic philosophy underlying complementary therapies differs significantly from the dualistic or Cartesian philosophy that for several centuries has permeated Western medicine. In the administration of complementary therapies, the total person is considered: physical, emotional, mental, and spiritual. The goal is to bring harmony or balance within the person. Persons are seeking care from complementary therapists or facilities because they want to be treated as a whole person and not as a heart attack or fractured hip.

Another reason is that they want to be involved in the decision making: They want to be empowered. In a study by Mitzdorf and colleagues (1999), 64% of patients stated that they had minimal time to discuss their health concerns with their physicians, and 42% noted that they were not afforded time to ask questions. The increasing pressure of cost containment in health care has reduced the amount of time physicians and nurses spend with their patients. People heal themselves; physicians, nurses, and others provide assistance in this process, but true healing can only come from within the patient.

A third reason cited for seeking care from complementary therapists relates to quality of life. Patients have reported they do not want the treatment for a health problem to be worse than the initial problem itself. The focus of Western medicine largely has been on curing problems, whereas the philosophy underlying complementary therapies is focused on harmony within the person and promotion of health. Mitzdorf et al. (1997) found that 82% of patients cited the side effects of medications as a reason for using complementary therapies.

The personal qualities of the complementary therapist (whether a nurse, physician, or other therapist) are key in the healing process. Caring, which has been integral to the nursing profession across the years, is also a key component in the administration of complementary therapies. Two aspects of such therapies that will be covered in subsequent chapters, presence and active listening, convey caring. Remen (2000), a physician who is involved in cancer care, has stated:

> I know that if I listen attentively to someone, to their essential self, their soul, as it were, I often find that at the deepest, most unconscious level, they can sense the direction of their own healing and wholeness. If I can remain open to that, without expectations of what the someone is supposed to do, how they are supposed to change in order to be better, or even what their wholeness looks like, what can happen is magical. By that I mean that it has a certain coherency or integrity about it, far beyond any way of fixing their situation or easing their pain that I can devise on my own. (p. 90)

The heightened interest in complementary therapies prompted the NIH to establish the Office of Alternative Medicine in 1992, which was renamed the National Center for Complementary/Alternative Medicine in 1998. What was significant about the establishment of this NIH office was that consumers rather than health professionals lobbied for it. The purposes of the NCCAM are fourfold:

1. To facilitate the evaluation of therapies
2. To investigate and evaluate the efficacy of therapies
3. To serve as an information clearinghouse on complementary therapies
4. To support research training.

NCCAM has funded research for individual researchers and for centers that explore the efficacy of a number of specific complementary therapies such as acupuncture and Saint John's wort. Other centers explore the use of complementary therapies in the treatment of specific conditions such as addictive disorders, arthritis, cardiovascular disease, and neurological disorders.

IMPLICATIONS FOR NURSING

Complementary therapies (under a different name) and their basic philosophies have been a part of the nursing profession since its beginnings. In *Notes on Nursing* (1936/1992), Florence Nightingale stressed the importance of creating the environment in which healing could occur and the importance of therapies such as music in the healing process. Complementary therapies today simply provide yet another opportunity for nurses to demonstrate caring for patients.

Although it is indeed gratifying to see that medicine and other health professions are recognizing the importance of listening and presence in the healing process, nurses need to assert that many of these therapies have been taught in nursing programs and have been practiced by nurses for centuries. Therapies such as meditation, imagery, support groups, music therapy, humor, journaling, reminiscence, caring-based approaches, massage, touch, healing touch, active listening, and presence have been practiced by nurses throughout time.

Complementary therapies are receiving increasing attention within nursing. Journals, such as the *Journal of Holistic Nursing* and *Complementary Therapies in Nursing & Midwifery*, are devoted almost exclusively to complementary therapies. Many journals have devoted entire issues to exploring the use of complementary therapies. Articles inform nurses about complementary therapies and how specific therapies can be used in providing care.

Because of the increasing use of complementary therapies by patients to whom nurses provide care, it is critical that nurses possess knowledge about these therapies. Patients expect health professionals to know about complementary therapies; nurses need such knowledge so that they can:

- provide guidance in obtaining health histories and assessing patients;
- answer basic questions about use of complementary therapies and refer patients to reliable sources of information;
- refer patients to competent therapists; and
- administer a selected number of complementary therapies.

Obtaining a complete health history requires that questions about the use of complementary therapies be an integral part of the information obtained. Many patients may not volunteer information about using complementary therapies unless they are specifically asked; others may be reluctant to share this information unless the practitioner displays an acceptance of complementary therapies. Although information about all complementary therapies is needed, obtaining information about use of herbal preparations is critical because interactions between certain prescription drugs and certain herbal preparations may pose a threat to health.

The vast number of complementary therapies makes it impossible for nurses to be knowledgeable about all of them, but knowledge about the more common ones will assist nurses in answering basic questions. Many organizations, professional associations, individuals, and groups have excellent Web sites that provide information about specific therapies. Caution is needed, however, in accepting information from any Web site. NCCAM (2008) urges that the following questions be posed:

- What group/organization operates the site and funds it?
- What is the purpose of the site?
- Where does the information originate and what guides the content presented?
- Who selects the information contained on the site, such as an editorial board?
- How often is the content updated?
- Do links to other sites exist?

■ Is information about the user of the site collected and can the user contact someone if questions arise?

Web sites for specific therapies are identified throughout this book.

Referring patients to competent therapists or helping patients to identify competent therapists is another role for nurses, and this is not an easy task. Because many complementary therapists are not members of a health profession, licensure and regulations often do not apply to them, and regulations vary greatly from state to state. Minnesota has legislation that places unlicensed complementary and alternative therapies under the auspices of the Department of Health. Notably, the legislation provides for a patient bill of rights. If clients have concerns, they can make these known to the commissioner for complementary and alternative therapies. This law is a first step.

CULTURE-RELATED ASPECTS OF COMPLEMENTARY THERAPIES

Culture refers to the shared way of life of a group of people. Medical anthropologists McElroy and Townsend (2004) specified that "the culture of a group is an information system transmitted from one generation to another through non-genetic mechanisms" (p. 110). The use of symbols, categories, rules, rituals, and other learned behaviors enhance the adaptation of the group, enabling them to survive within their ecological setting. People transform their healing systems in this process of adaptation, yet also maintain fidelity to long-standing traditions (Rogoff, 2003).

Four traditional healing systems that have persisted over thousands of years and are still alive today are (1) Hmong medicine, (2) Samoan medicine, (3) the healing traditions of Somali nomads of East Africa, and (4) native medicine of aboriginal peoples of the Americas (see Table 1.1). Although differences exist among these systems, a common theme is that health is based on harmony within the self and between the self and the universe. The healing systems of these four cultures in which traditional healers enact a range of therapies for members of their culture are described in the text that follows. Knowledge about traditional healers and healing practices of other cultures will help nurses to be aware of practices persons may be using from their respec-

Table 1.1

TRADITIONAL THERAPIES WITHIN SELECTED CULTURAL SYSTEMS

HMONG THERAPIES	SAMOAN THERAPIES	SOMALI THERAPIES	MEXICAN AMERICAN THERAPIES	NATIVE AMERICAN THERAPIES
Herbal medicine	Herbal medicine	Herbal medicine	Herbal medicine	Herbal medicine
Massage therapy	Massage therapy	Isolation	Massage therapy	Massage therapy
Shamanic ritual	Prayer	Religious acts	Prayer	Prayer
Cupping and coining	Simple surgery	Dancing	Divination	Storytelling
Diet therapy	Incantation	Burning with needles		Singing
Magical healing		Scarification		Talking circle
				Drum circle
				Sweat lodge purification

tive cultures as well as help determine whether these practices are congruent with the prescribed therapies and overall health plan.

Hmong Medicine

The Hmong lived in China for four thousand years prior to their migration in the 19th century to Laos, Vietnam, and Thailand. After assisting the United States Central Intelligence Agency during the Vietnam War, the Hmong were persecuted and fled to Thailand, occupying refugee camps. From the refugee camps, Hmong migrated primarily to California, Minnesota, and Wisconsin.

Hmong Americans are organized into 18 clans. After marriage, a woman joins her husband's clan. Within a clan, the oldest male is the leader of the multigenerational, extended family. Pfeifer and Lee (2005) estimated that 70% of Hmong Americans adhere to traditional practices of animism and ancestor worship. Hmong animism consists of an unseen world of spirits and visible world of persons. Each person has at least three souls. A cycle of life exists in which, upon death, one soul journeys to join the ancestors, another soul is incarnated, becoming a new individual, and the third soul protects the body in the grave. If during life a soul is snatched by a spirit from the unseen world, the person becomes ill. A shaman is called upon to travel to the unseen world and negotiate with the spirit(s) to recover the soul (Gerdner, Cha, Vang, & Tripp-Reimer, 2007).

Whereas spiritual forces that create disease require a shaman for cure, natural forces that cause diseases require an herbalist, practitioner of massage, or magic healer for a cure. Herbalists prepare teas or light soups and fashion poultices to treat illnesses such as infertility, headaches, and intestinal problems. Practitioners of massage relieve fevers, colds, and muscle aches. Having tight muscles, numbness, and tingling in the hands is caused by built-up air or pressure when the blood is circulating improperly. Massage, followed by cupping and coining (a technique in which oil is placed on the skin and rubbed with a coin) relieves the pressure of trapped air (Culhane-Pera, Her, & Her, 2007). Magic healers use incense and chanting to heal burns, wounds, and rashes (Her & Culhane-Pera, 2004). Dietary prescriptions to restore balance would encourage eating of bland food. Activity proscriptions would limit heavy work and encourage rest. Illness caused by socially stressful situations is treated using a forgiveness ceremony.

Health care providers working with Hmong patients would benefit from listening to the Hmong shaman for insight about the patient's distress, or, if the shaman is not present, from asking the patient what the Hmong shaman has explained and done to lessen the patient's distress. Health care providers need to respect social taboos, such as not talking openly about death without using euphemisms such as "last breath" or "living to 120 years." At death, autopsy and embalming are prohibited. Traditionally, the family grooms the body of the deceased and dresses the body with funeral attire. Funeral duration of an elder is 3 to 4 days, usually, but may be as long as 9 days.

Samoan Medicine

Ancient Samoans taught that all humans were descendants of gods, known as *atua* and *aitu*. Illnesses were the result of the gods' anger at the lack of respect by individuals and families (Macpherson & Macpherson,

2003). Traditional Samoan medicine consisted of prayers, incantations, herbal medicine, massage with scented oils, and simple surgery.

Samoans contracted new illnesses brought to them by contact with European explorers and merchants who introduced influenza, measles, mumps, whooping cough, and syphilis. Botanical fieldworkers found 336 medicinal plants in Samoa in 1868, even though the Samoans were using nine such plants at the time. With education, Samoans learned how to use many more native plants for medicinal purposes (Macpherson & Macpherson, 2003). When Margaret Mead (1928/2001) lived among the Samoans, she noted:

> There is no specialization among women, except in medicine and midwifery, both the prerogatives of very old women who teach their arts to their middle-aged daughters and nieces. The only other vocation is that of the wife of an official orator, and no girl will prepare herself for this one type of marriage which demands special knowledge, for she has no guarantee that she will marry a man of this class. (p. 25)

Folk remedies that Samoan women employed were restricted to herbal medicines and massage. From contact with Western visitors, a hybrid healing system emerged. Samoan healers continued to diagnose and treat intrinsically Samoan illnesses that had their root cause in social or spiritual imbalance related to pre-Christian gods (Ishida, Toomata-Mayer, & Mayer, 1996). Samoan healers diagnosed and treated illnesses caused by trauma, effects of the ecosystem, and germs using Western diagnostic categories and biomedicine for treatment. In a recent study using a systematic, random sampling of 1,834 Samoans living in American Samoa ($n = 609$), Hawaii ($n = 610$), and Los Angeles ($n = 615$), 752 (41% of the sample) used Samoan healers for 58 different illnesses (Mishra, Hess, & Luce, 2003). This hybrid system of traditional medicine alongside of biomedicine persists for many Samoan Americans.

When treating Samoan patients, health care providers ought to inquire whether a patient is concurrently seeing a Samoan healer, consider culture-specific health beliefs requiring the intervention of a Samoan healer, and acknowledge the multifactorial etiology of disease and the contributions of indigenous Samoan healers.

Somali Medicine

Traditional medicine in Somalia emerged from thousands of years of oral tradition and over a thousand years of Islamic written tradition

(Abdullahi, 2001). Somalis are Muslim. A *wadaad* is a Somali priest and ritual leader who travels from community to community to teach. If a wadaad becomes the caretaker of a mosque, he is an imam. Some wadaads are appointed as judges to enforce family law. In rural areas, the wadaad performs rites of passage. A wadaad may be an expert in traditional medicine, an herbalist, and a bonesetter, but some experts in traditional medicine are not a wadaad. Yusuf et al. (1984) found that traditional healers in four communities around Mogadishu learned healing arts from their fathers and grandfathers and then were selected for the role by a community elder. The traditional healers commonly treated psychosomatic disorders, sexually transmitted diseases, respiratory illnesses, digestive complaints, snake bites, injuries, and skin diseases. The role for women in healing is that of the midwife who cares for pregnant women and for infants.

An Italian physician who worked for decades in East Africa wrote, "To the Muslim the physician is Allah's instrument, and it is Allah who allows him to cure a patient when he, Allah, has decided that he shall recover" (Pirajno, 1955/1985, p. 21). Pirajno learned that disease is sent by Allah for expiation of sins. Allah works to send disease through the stars, people, or spirits. Itinerant spirits (*jinns*) cause epidemics; stationary jinns cause endemic disease; and personal jinns cause individual disease (p. 22). An ethnographer in the 1950s, after decades of work, detected a willingness to accept European medicine, stating, "This skeptical, or at best ambiguous, attitude toward mystical power is characteristic of the Somalis who, while acknowledging that God is the ultimate causal force in the universe, prudently also seek more immediate causes and remedies. There is thus no contradiction in employing modern medicines alongside traditional remedies with an Islamic base" (Lewis, 2008, p. 22).

Somali medical students examined the types of traditional medical practices used in four communities around Mogadishu (Yusuf et al., 1984). The foremost practice was isolation (>50%), followed by religious rituals (28%), dancing (28%), herbs (21%), burning with needles (11%), scarification (7%), and reduction of fractures (5%). Isolation was used for patients with tuberculosis, leprosy, or chicken pox. Religious rituals were performed for psychosomatic symptoms. Dancing was recommended for mental illness. Herbal medicines were administered for respiratory conditions, abdominal ailments, and snake bites.

Political turmoil and civil war in Somalia in the mid 1980s was followed by the collapse of the Republic in 1991, prompting many Somalis to flee to refugee camps and eventually settle in Europe, Canada, and the United States (Bradbury, 2008; Lewis, 2008). Upon arrival at these destinations, premigration infectious diseases were initially treated to alleviate the spread of tuberculosis, malaria, and intestinal parasites (Palinkas et al., 2003). Health care providers responded to stress-induced mental distress by listening to Somalis and constructing explanatory models that accounted for the cause, course, short- and long-term consequences, and expected ways of being treated. Health care providers worked on confidence building with the Somali community and identified culturally appropriate idioms expressing Somali "wisdom" well-recognized among Somalis and used these idioms in their health teaching and counseling.

Health care providers have learned that Somalis prefer to be treated by health care providers of the same sex. Somali women have been humiliated by wearing examination gowns that violate religious rules of modesty. Using two drapes is preferred for optimum modesty, unwrapping only the part needed for each step of the examination. Somali women communicated pain using body language and quiet speech; they are expected to deal with pain by reading the Koran, resting, and using red hot needles (Finnstrom & Soderhamn, 2005). Somali women giving birth appreciated the support of *doulas* during labor and delivery (Dundek, 2006).

Somali men shake hands with other Somali men using only the right hand; Somali men do not shake hands with women health care providers. Similarly, food taken at meals is eaten only with the right hand. The left hand is regarded as unclean.

As Somalis have adopted facets of lifestyles within host countries, risk factors for diabetes, cardiovascular diseases, and cancer have been noted, requiring patient education to diminish the new risk. Jackson and Skinner (2007) improved retention of information offered during clinic visits by giving Somali interpreters hand-held recorders. After the office visit, the interpreter recorded the content in the patient's language. Patients kept the recording and were reminded about advice given, instructions for medication use, and the need for follow-up appointments. Heath care providers have become more culturally competent working with Somali Americans by recognizing the foundation of Islamic spirituality underlying health practices, understanding the role of traditional wadaadic healers and midwives, and accommodating biomedical practice using idiomatic Somali expressions in counseling and health education, while teaching patients to manage new types of illness prevalent within the host country.

Native Traditions of the Americas

Broadly speaking, Mehl-Medrona (2003) observed of North American native healing that:

> Traditional Native American cultures perceive health as a state of balance of spirit, mind, and body; illness is the result of disharmony or imbalance. Illness requires treatment at the many levels, including personal, family, community, and spiritual. Traditional medicine includes herbalists, shamans, purification ceremonies, healing rituals, emotional therapies, manipulative medicine, teas, herbs, and special foods. (p. 211)

Similarly, of Mesoamerican and South American healing, Mendoza (2003) stated:

> Mexica Aztec, Inca or Quechua, Aymara or Kalawaya, and other American Indian doctors and physicians were required to balance herbal and surgical treatments with interpretive models of causation ranging from the supernatural and magical to the natural and physical. (p. 234)

Botanists have documented the native use of more than 1500 species of medicinal plants, among which the Indians especially valued coca, mescaline, curare, quinine, belladonna, and dopamine (Stark, 1981).

Native Americans

In the context of North America, the land has been a source of healing. The first step for an Indian doctor was to learn to walk in balance with the Earth Mother, then to seek the power that came from the Great Spirit (Steiger, 1984). Indian doctors organized the power to heal through songs, stories, and ritual acts (McMaster & Trafzer, 2004). Lame Deer and Erdoes (1992) describe the typical medicine man among the Lakota as knowing the right songs to go with every medicine he used in every ceremony he performed. Ritual acts among the First

Nations of Canada were the talking circle, the drum circle, smudging, and the sweat lodge ceremony (Hunter, Logan, Barton, & Goulet, 2004). Massage was a healing procedure among the Cherokees and Pawnees (Vogel, 1970). The Cree healing ceremony had five parts, beginning with ritual to purify and open the door to the spiritual world, petition of the patient and the healer, treatment with herbal medicine and a sweat lodge ceremony, education of the patient, and closure of the ceremony emphasizing that the Great Spirit would continue the healing already underway (Morse, Young, & Swartz, 1991). Among the Ojibway, Johnston (1976) noted:

> Initially, healers were herbalists—Eventually herbalists became medicine men; and the medicine men became philosophers concerned not only with preserving life and mitigating pain, but also with offering guidance and principles for living the good life whose end was to secure general well being. (p. 71)

Peacock and Wisuri (2002) affirmed:

> [M]edicine people sometime still come all the way from Canada to visit Ojibwe communities. They travel throughout Ojibwe country via an informal network of traditional people, who let each other know when the medicine person will be in town....They are among the most highly respected members of our communities because they are the purveyors and keepers of ancient sacred knowledge. (p. 102)

Native Americans were found to have the highest use (29%) of herbal medicine compared with Asian (26%), Latino (23%), Black (19%), and White (12%) Americans in a national probability survey (Mackenzie, Taylor, Bloom, Hufford, & Johnson, 2003). In using herbal remedies, Native American healers celebrate sacred earth, selecting particular herbs from their sacred landscape (Cohen, 2003a). Medicine bags are sacred and private for the individual carrying them and remain with the body of the person after death (Cohen, 2003b).

Mexican Americans

In Mesoamerican traditional medicine, Lipp (2001) clarified, "illnesses are signs of natural disequilibrium or disorder, and therapeutic treatment is fundamentally concerned with restoring harmonious relations between internal body processes and the physical, social, and cosmological order" (p. 109). When a family member became ill, household remedies consisted of medicinal plants, fright-illness rituals, massage, and sweat baths. If no relief resulted, the shaman joined the family and relatives for a curing ceremony of prayer, sacrificial offerings, ritual meals, and a pilgrimage to local shrines. In Nahuatl, the classical idiom of northern Mesoamerica, the main medical goddess was Tzapotlateman. Divine intervention was the rule that pervaded all facets of life. Health, recovery from illness, and effective use of medicine depended upon divine assistance for healing (Viesca, 2003). In colonial Mexico, the Moorish influence in Spanish medicine blended into indigenous healing practices, creating a strong herbal base, an emphasis on balance between light/dark and hot/cold, and Christian belief that healing came from the power of God using prayer and ritual (Torres, 1984).

In the mid-twentieth century, good health in the Mexican American family was associated with the ability to work (Baca, 1969), whereas illness was associated with sadness, because illness prevented members from working in ways that sustained the family (Ulibarri, 1978). Samora (1978) identified a conceptualization of health in which being healthy was attributed to the beneficence of God.

By the late-twentieth century, Hayes-Bautista (1998) noted that for Latinos, the strong emotions of fright, shame, sorrow, rejection, and disillusionment were perceived as triggers for illness. For instance, strong emotions of fright, anger, and sadness were believed to cause Type 2 diabetes by Mexican Americans (Coronado, Thompson, Tejeda, & Godina, 2004). Herbal treatments for diabetes included prickly pear cactus pulp and aloe vera pulp. Folk medicine use among Mexican American immigrant women ($N = 70$) included 39% having visited a massage therapist (*sobador*), 26% having consulted a folk healer (*curandero*), and 20% having used an herbalist (*yerbero*) (Lopez, 2006). Herbal medicine use was explored in El Paso, Texas, and across the border in Ciudad Juarez, Mexico, among surgical patients (Rivera, Chaudhuri, Gonzalez-Stuart, Tyroch, & Chaudhuri, 2005). Among samples in El Paso ($n = 115$) and Ciudad Juarez ($n = 112$), 92% of patients in El Paso and 93% of patients in Ciudad Juarez did not inform their surgeons that they had used herbal medicines within the last 30 days before surgery. In El Paso, these products were chamomile, garlic, chaparral, ginseng, ginko biloba, noni, and hawthorn. In Ciudad Juarez, chamomile and garlic were used. Chamomile, garlic, Ginko biloba, and hawthorn are anticoagulants. Ginseng increases blood pressure and heart rate. Chaparral causes liver toxicity.

When working with Mexican American patients, compassionate listening conveys respect. Problem solving can be facilitated by the use of analogies, wisdom sayings, and stories. Health care providers will want to assess recent use of herbal medicines and treatments provided by traditional healers.

Implications for Nurses and the Health Care Team

Entire systems of health care have survived for thousands of years among cultures around the globe, whose immigrants have come to live within the United States and have shared healing traditions with health care workers in this country. Patients from other cultures may be visiting traditional healers in their locality and seeing biomedical health care providers for the same concerns. These different ways of healing can work well together. The spiritual worldview of the patient is foundational for the patient's understanding of health and disease, the patient should continue to incorporate traditional healing and follow treatments recommended by traditional therapies while reaching out to biomedical providers of care. Biomedical providers of care will want to investigate other therapies the patient is receiving so as to assure safe care for the patient from a biomedical perspective.

Although nurses may not know minute details of ancient healing traditions, it is helpful for nurses to be familiar with the worldviews of these traditions. When nurses are familiar with the patient's worldview, nurses can ask patients and family members about specific needs and preferences that are a natural part of the individual's or family's healing tradition.

REFERENCES

Abdullahi, M. D. (2001). *Culture and customs of Somalia.* Westport, CT: Greenwood Press.

Al-Faris, E. A., Al-Rowais, N., Mohamed, A. G., Al-Rukban, M. O., Al-Kurdi, A., Aalla Al-Noor, M. A., et al. (2008). Prevalence and pattern of alternative medicine use: The results of a household survey. *Annals of Saudi Medicine, 28,* 4–10

Baca, J. (1969). Some health beliefs of the Spanish speaking. *American Journal of Nursing, 69,* 2172–2176.

Barnes, P. M., Powell-Griner, E., McFann, K., & Nahin, R. L. (2004, May 27). Complementary and alternative medicine use among adults: United States, 2002. *Advance Data, 343,* 1–19.

Bazargan, M., Ani, C. O., Hindman, D. W., Bazargan-Hejazi, S., Baker, R. S., Bell, D., et al. (2008). Correlates of complementary and alternative medicine utilization in depressed, underserved African-American and Hispanic patients in primary care setting. *Journal of Complementary & Alternative Medicince, 14,* 537–544.

Bertisch, S. M., Wee, C. C., & McCarthy, E. P. (2008). Use of complementary and alternative therapies by overweight and obese adults. *Obesity, 16,* 1610–1615.

Bradbury, M. (2008). *Becoming Somaliland.* London: Progressio.

Chao, M. T., & Wade, C. M. (2008). Socioeconomic factors and women's use of complementary and alternative medicine in four racial/ethnic groups. *Ethnicity & Disease, 18,* 65–71.

Cohen, K. (2003a). Where healing dwells: The importance of sacred space. *Alternative Therapies in Health and Medicine, 9*(4), 68–72.

Cohen, K. (2003b). *Honoring the medicine: The essential guide to Native American healing.* New York: Random House.

Coronado, G., Thompson, B., Tejeda, S., & Godina, R. (2004). Attitudes and beliefs among Mexican Americans about type 2 Diabetes. *Journal of Health Care for the Poor and Underserved, 15,* 576–588.

Culhane-Pera, K., Her, C., & Her, B. (2007). "We are out of balance here": A Hmong cultural model of diabetes. *Journal of Minority Health, 9,* 179–190.

Dundek, L. (2006). Establishment of a Somali doula program at a large metropolitan hospital. *Journal of Perinatal & Neonatal Nursing, 20,* 128–137.

Erci, B. (2007). Attitudes towards holistic complementary and alternative medicine: A sample of healthy people in Turkey. *Journal of Clinical Nursing, 16,* 761–768.

Ernst, E. (2008). Complementary medicine in Germany. *Climacteric, 11,* 91–92.

Esmonde, L., & Long, A. F. (2008). Complementary therapy use by persons with multiple sclerosis: Benefits and research priorities. *Complementary Therapies in Clinical Practice, 14,* 176–184.

Fang, L., & Schinke, S. P. (2007). Complementary alternative medicine use among Chinese Americans: Findings among a community mental health service population. *Psychiatric Services, 58,* 402–404.

Feldman, J. M., Wiemann, C. M., Sever, L., & Hergenroeder, A. C. (2008). Folk and traditional medicine use by a subset of Hispanic adolescents. *International Journal of Adolescent Medicine & Health, 20,* 41–51.

Finnstrom, B., & Soderhamn, O. (2005). Conceptions of pain among Somali women. *Journal of Advanced Nursing, 54,* 418–425.

Gerdner, L., Cha, D., Yang, D., & Tripp-Reimer, T. (2007). The circle of life: End-of-life care and death rituals for Hmong-American elders. *Journal of Gerontological Nursing, 33*(5), 20–29.

Hayes-Bautista, D., & Chiput, R. (1998). *Healing Latinas: Reslidad y fantasia.* Los Angeles: Cedars-Sinai Health System.

Her, C., & Culhane-Pera, K. (2004). Culturally responsive care for Hmong patients. *Postgraduate Medicine, 116*(6), 39–43.

Hok, J., Tishelman, C., Ploner, A., Forss, A., & Falkenberg, T. (2008). Mapping patterns of complementary and alternative medicine use in cancer: An explorative cross-sectional study of individuals with reported positive "exceptional" experiences. *BMC Complementary & Alternative Medicine, 8,* 48.

Hori, S., Mihaylov, I., Vasconcelos, J. C., & McCoubrie, M. (2008). Patterns of complementary and alternative medicine use amongst outpatients in Tokyo, Japan. *BMC Complementary & Alternative Medicine, 8,* 14.

Hunter, L., Logan, J., Barton, S., & Goulet, J. (2004). Linking aboriginal healing traditions to holistic nursing practice. *Journal of Holistic Nursing, 22,* 267–285.

Ishida, D., Toomata-Mayer, T., & Mayer, J. (1996). Samoans. In J. Lipson, S. Dibble, & P. Minarik (Eds.), *Culture & nursing care* (pp. 250–263). San Francisco, CA: UCSF Nursing Press.

Jackson, A., & Skinner, J. (2007). Improving consultations in general practice for Somali patients: A qualitative study. *Diversity in Health & Social Care, 4,* 61–67.

Johnston, B. (1976). *Ojibway heritage.* Lincoln, NE: University of Nebraska Press.

Kreitzer, M. J., & Jensen, D. (2000). Healing practices: Trends, challenges, and opportunities for nurses in acute and critical care. *AACN Clinical Issues, 11,* 7–16.

Lafferty, W. E., Bellas, A., Corage Baden, A., Tyree, P. T., Standish, L. J., & Patterson, R. (2004). The use of complementary and alternative medical providers by insured cancer patients in Washington state. *Cancer, 100,* 1522–1530.

Lame Deer, A., & Erdoes, R. (1992). *Gift of power: The life and teaching of a Lakota medicine man.* Santa Fe, NM: Bear & Company Publishing.

Lewis, I. (2008). *Understanding Somalia and Somaliland.* New York: Columbia University Press.

Lipp, F. (2001). *Southern Mexican and Guatamalan shamans.* In B. Huber & A. Sandstrom (Eds.), *Mesoamerican healers* (pp. 95–116). Austin, TX: University of Texas Press.

Lopez, R. (2006). Use of alternative folk medicine by Mexican American women. *Journal of Immigrant Health, 7,* 23–31.

Mackenzie, E., Taylor, L., Bloom, B., Hufford, D., & Johnson, J. (2003). Ethnic minority use of complementary and alternative medicine (CAM): A national probability survey of CAM utilizers. *Alternative Therapies in Health and Medicine, 9*(4), 50–56.

Macpherson, C., & Macpherson, L. (2003). When healing cultures collide: A case from the Pacific. In H. Selin (Ed.), *Medicine across cultures* (pp. 191–207). Boston: Kluwer Academic Publishers.

McElroy, A., & Townsend, P. (2004). *Medical anthropology in ecological perspective.* Boulder, CO: Westview Press.

McMaster, G., & Trafzer, C. (Eds.), (2004). *Native universe: Voices of Indian America.* Washington, DC: The Smithsonian Institution.

Mead, M. (1928/2001). *Coming of age in Samoa.* New York: HarperCollins.

Mehl-Madrona, L. (2003). Native American medicine: Herbal pharmacology, therapies, and eldercare. In H. Selin (Ed.), *Medicine across cultures* (pp. 209–224). Boston: Kluwer Academic Publishers.

Mendoza, R. (2003). Lords of the medicine bag: Medical science and traditional practice in ancient Peru and South America. In H. Selin (Ed.), *Medicine across cultures* (pp. 225–257). Boston: Kluwer Academic Publishers.

Mishra, S., Hess, J., & Luce, P. (2003). Predictors of indigenous healer use among Samoans. *Alternative Therapies in Health and Medicine, 9*(6), 64–70.

Mitzdorf, U., Beck, K., Horton-Hausknecht, J., Weidenhammer, W., Kindemrmann, A., Takaxc, M., et al. (1999). Why do patients seek treatment in hospitals of complementary medicine? *Journal of Complementary & Alternative Medicine, 5*, 463–473.

Morse, J., Young, D., & Swartz, L. (1991). Cree Indian healing practices and Western health care: A comparative analysis. *Social Science & Medicine, 32*, 1361–1366.

National Center for Complementary and Alternative Therapies. (2008). *The uses of complementary and alternative medicine in the United States.* Retrieved November 17, 2008, from http://nccam.nih.gov/news/camsurvey_fs1.htm

National Center for Complementary and Alternative Medicine. (2008). *What 10 things to know about evaluating medical resources on the web?* Available at: http://nccam.nih.gov/health/webresources

Nightingale, F. (1992). *Notes on nursing.* Philadelphia: Lippincott. (Original work published 1935)

Palinkas, L., Pickwell, S., Brandstein, K., Clark, T., Hill, L., Moser, R., et al. (2003). The journey to wellness: Stages of refugee health promotion and disease prevention. *Journal of Immigrant Health, 5*, 19–28.

Peacock, T., & Wisuri, M. (2002). *Ojibwe waasa inaabidaa—We look in all directions.* Afton, MN: Afton Historical Society Press.

Pfeifer, M., & Lee, T. (2005). Hmong religion. *Hmong Today, 2*(16), 24.

Pirajno, A. (1955/1985). *A cure for serpents.* London: Eland Publishing.

Remen, R. N. (2000). *My grandfather's blessings.* New York: Riverhead Books.

Rhee, S. M., Barg, V. K., & Hershey, C. O. (2004). Use of complementary and alternative medicines by ambulatory patients. *Archives of Internal Medicine, 164*, 1004–1009.

Rivera, J., Chaudhuri, K., Gonzalez-Stuart, A., Tyroch, A., & Chaudhuri, S. (2005). Herbal product use by Hispanic surgical patients. *American Surgeon, 71*, 71–76.

Rogoff, B. (2003). *The cultural nature of human development.* New York: Oxford University Press.

Rosen, I., Azzam, A. S., Levi, T., Braun, E., & Krivoy, N. (2003). Patient approach and experience regarding complementary medicine: survey among hospitalized patients in a university hospital. *Pharmocoepidemiology & Drug Safety, 12*, 679–685.

Samora, J. (1978). Conceptions of health and disease among Spanish-Americans. In R. Martinez (Ed.), *Hispanic culture and health care* (pp. 65–74). St. Louis, MO: Mosby.

Shah, S. H., Englelhardt, R., & Ovbiagele, B. (2009). Patterns of complementary and alternative medicine use among United States stroke survivors. *Journal of Neurological Science, 27*, 18–185.

Stark, R. (1981). *Guide to Indian herbs.* Blaine, WA: Hancock House.

Steiger, B. (1984). *Indian medicine power.* Gloucester, MA: Para Press.

Strois, F. M. (2008). Provider-based complementary and alternative medicine use among three chronic illness groups: Associations with psychosocial factors and concurrent use of conventional health-care services. *Complementary Therapies in Medicine, 16*, 73–80.

Struthers, R., & Nichols, L. A. (2004). Utilization of complementary and alternative medicine among racial and ethnic minority populations. Implications for reducing health care disparities. In *Annual review of nursing research* (Vol. 2, pp. 285–313). New York: Springer Publishing Company.

Torres, E. (1984). *The folkhealer: The Mexican-American tradition of curanderismo.* Kingsville, TX: Nieves Press.

Torres, E. (1983). *Green medicine.* Kingsville, TX: Nieves Press.

Ulibarri, H. (1978). Social and attitudinal characteristics of Spanish-speaking migrant and ex-migrant workers in the Southwest. In N. Wagner & M. Haug (Eds.), *Chicanos: Social and psychological perspectives* (pp. 164–170). St. Louis, MO: Mosby.

Viesca, C. (2003). Medicine in ancient Mesoamerica. In H. Selin (Ed.), *Medicine across cultures* (pp. 259–283). Boston: Kluwer Academic Publishers.

Vogel, V. (1970). *American Indian medicine.* Norman, OK: University of Oklahoma Press.

Yusuf, H., Adan, A., Egal, K., Omer, A., Ibrahim, M., & Elmi, A. (1984). Traditional medical practices in some Somali communities. *Journal of Tropical Pediatrics, 30*(2), 87–92.

2

Self As Healer

BARBARA LEONARD
SUE TOWEY

For nursing students and practitioners of complementary and alternative therapies, the process of developing an authentic self is as integral to practice as learning the technical skills for administering these therapies. An individual's explorations into self-knowledge, self-awareness, consciousness, and spiritual development are an ongoing dialogue between the inner and outer parts of one's being. A nurse must be in-the-moment and fully present to a patient while also embarking on his/her own self-healing journey. Living an undivided life facilitates the journey toward wholeness (Palmer, 2004). Kabat-Zinn (2005) describes healing as a process of recognizing our wholeness "even when we are terrified or broken apart in life" (p. 336). Nurses integrating complementary therapies into their practice need to pursue a path of personal inner and outer development as part of their professional journey. The student and the practitioner must be aware that they need to care for the self.

Self-awareness and self-care are an integral part of reflective holistic nursing practice. In its Code of Ethics, the American Holistic Nurses Association (AHNA) states that "the nurse has a responsibility to model healthy behaviors. Holistic nurses strive to achieve harmony in their own lives and assist others striving to do the same" (AHNA, 2009, p. 2). Each nurse needs to do her or his own work so as to become a conduit of healing energy for patients. They need to become whole persons and live authentic lives. The physical, emotional, and spiritual health of practitioners is experienced in their relationship with patients. A nurse's commitment to the use of self as an instrument of healing and understanding is the focus of this chapter.

A metaphor from the reductionistic biomedical health care system may help us to understand issues associated with self as healer. Just as surgical instruments are washed and sterilized before being used for another procedure, professionals who are instruments of healing must identify therapies that will ensure the cleansing of self so as to provide a personal energy field and space that facilitates healing for self and patients.

In the literature on energy-healing therapies, Brennan (1987) describes the human energy field as the "manifestation of universal energy that is intimately involved with human life" (p. 41). Energetic healing is a term for healing that occurs at the bioelectromagnetic level of a person (AHNA, 2009). How do we care for ourselves as "instruments of healing" in our work with patients? Barbara Dossey, a leader in holistic nursing, stated that self-care includes activities that promote an awareness of self that facilitates being an instrument of healing (Horrigan, 1999).

SELF-CARE

Becoming a healer is a very individual process, one that grows from the inside. Each person is unique and must assess his or her individual strengths and talents so as to move toward wholeness. There are many ways to create a plan for self-care and intentional personal healing. Therapies that will help a person to increase self-knowledge, become more aware of transpersonal experiences, and accept the paradoxical mysteries in life need to be explored.

Several concepts and techniques that are widely accepted as important in self-care are:

- A balanced diet appropriate to current health needs
- Exercise appropriate to the individual
- Adequate sleep and rest
- Social support systems

- Stress-management skills
- Meditation and prayer
- An active sense of humor (Towey, 1995, p. 11).

Many of the therapies included in this book may be used singly or in combination to heal the self. Santorelli (2000) suggested use of mindfulness meditation, a mind–body intervention, to heal the self. Nature is another therapy frequently used in self-healing (Gunnarsdottir & Peden-McAlpine, 2004). Spending time outdoors is innately renewing, restorative, and healing. According to Lewis (1996), "as we garden, tramp through field or forest, we may come to an unexpected door that opens inward to self" (p. xix). Two other interventions that can be used in the healing of self, namely, spiritual direction and dreams, will be discussed later in this chapter.

TRANSFORMATIONAL JOURNEY

Healing is a key element of the transformational journey. Dossey defines holistic healing as the integration of the whole person, in body, mind, and spirit—not just for the patient, but for the nurse healer as well (Horrigan, 1999). The healer is one who is capable of producing and catalyzing integration within self and patients. The spiritual journey involves the process an individual undergoes in search of the meaning and purpose of life. Florence Nightingale's life was an exquisite spiritual journey of transformation in her work as a visionary nurse healer (Dossey, 2000).

The healer's self-care journey is described in two recent books on holistic prevention and management of depression by psychiatrists Henry Emmons (2006) and James Gordon (2008). Their personal stories reflect their lived experience of the transformational journey, using mindfulness meditation, healing guides (spiritual), and various other complementary/alternative medicine (CAM) self-care modalities.

Becoming a Healer

The initiation of a healer in ancient cultures was a rigorous process that included a personal journey of inner development and transformation. For centuries, various cultures have treated inner transformation as a necessary and desired component of life. The universal aspects of shamanism work with the inner aspects of healing through the use of altered states of consciousness (Grof & Grof, 1990). Like the Greek mythological figure Chiron, shamans, as wounded healers, have the gift for healing others while remaining unable to heal themselves. A nurse's transformational healing journey is a living-out of both the woundedness of Chiron and current knowledge about one's ability and need to connect with the inner healer (Santorelli, 2000).

Barriers, Stressors, and Needs

At the end of the first decade of the 21st century, the rapid transformation of our health care systems and health profession education has placed great demands on the time, energy, spirit, and health of professionals and students. Nurses and other health care employees are often caught in the crossfire of mergers, downsizing, redesign, and other changes that create uncertainty and anxiety in the work environment (Disch & Towey, 1998). The current national economic crisis in health care has created challenges for all health professionals and is making work environments more stressful. Nursing professionals must rapidly acquire new information to accomplish their work. Limits of time and resources create challenges to health professionals and require new approaches in educating health science students.

Viewing time as the enemy creates stress that is not conducive to a healing environment in the workplace (Lofy, 2000). Bailey (1999) identifies the loss of quality relationships among workers as an unhealthy factor in many workplaces. However, healing requires interactions with others. Quiet times are also necessary, for a person to be able to listen to the voice of inner wisdom. Silence may help reduce stress (Rubin, 2000), and yet silent reflection is difficult to attain without intentionally setting aside time for quiet. This is a challenge for nurses working in busy health care settings. Taking a few minutes at the beginning of work may help the nurse to maintain calmness and focus during the shift. Uncertainty is another stressor in current health care settings. Finding ways to maintain hope and develop resiliency are needed in the face of uncertainty (Towey, 1995).

The Dalai Lama (1999) described the ethics he regarded as necessary in the 21st century. In addition to restraint, virtue, and compassion, he identified a need for discerning the truth in the unseen world; this requires a healthy level of spiritual development, discipline, and practice.

An accessible "practice" at work might be a brief (30- to 60-second) focus on breathing, a prayer or meditation. Pausing for a moment to set one's intention of being a healing presence for a patient may facilitate healing for both patient and nurse.

SPIRITUAL DIRECTION

Spiritual direction is a time-honored tradition of accompanying other persons as they seek to grow in their relationship with God or the sacred in their lives. Spiritual direction is not psychotherapy or pastoral counseling, even though it has similar professional boundaries, ethics, and listening skills in common with them. Spiritual direction does not try to fix problems, but instead helps the directee find meaning and purpose in their life circumstances. Spiritual directors have completed specialized graduate education and are undergoing continual direction and supervision themselves.

Some form of spiritual direction is found in many of the major religions of the world. Among traditional Native Americans a medicine man/woman will guide a "vision quest" and interpret the dreams and visions of the seeker. A Zen master gives spiritual guidance to a seeker in the Buddhist tradition. In Christianity, spiritual direction has existed since the 4th century A.D. Until recently, spiritual direction was exclusive to those in religious life; laypersons rarely sought direction (Moon, 2002). Today it is found in many Protestant denominations as well as in the Roman Catholic Church. Benner (2002) states that although large sectors within Christianity have never heard of spiritual direction until recently, seminaries and colleges of many denominations are now busy refashioning departments of Christian education into programs of spiritual formation. Clergy and laity alike are seeking opportunities to learn about spiritual direction. Susanka (2007) suggests it is often necessary to find a place of stillness within oneself and, through that stillness, an opening to the spiritual life.

The modern spiritual director has received education in the art and practice of spiritual direction and adheres to professional ethics such as those specified by Spiritual Directors International (SDI). SDI is a global organization of persons from many faiths who share a common concern and passion for the practice of spiritual direction. Opportunities are available for sharing of resources and ideas online at www.sdiworld .org. A person seeking direction should inquire about a director's educational preparation, supervision, and practice. A spiritual director, with permission of the directee, may collaborate with other professional persons working with a directee. When a directee is in crisis, working with both a counselor and a director may be very beneficial; for others, it may be best to work with a counselor first and then with a director.

Nurses who seek spiritual direction do so to reflect on how God or the sacred is present in their lived experience as a nurse and a person. The focus of spiritual direction is on the inward movement of the Spirit in the nurse's life. A nurse may seek direction during a life transition or crisis, or during ordinary times, to gain a deeper relationship with God or the sacred. All of life's experiences can be brought to bear, but always at the discretion of the person seeking direction (Munger, 2009). In the course of receiving direction, some of the circumstances of one's life may appear unchanged, yet the inner transformation may be evident in one's professional work and personal relationships, even in one's environment. Problems may resolve as a side benefit of direction. A nurse, for example, working with a group of women in transition from prison to society, said of herself, "I no longer *say* prayers; I *am* prayer." She went on to describe how she had become less judgmental and more accepting, more patient, more peaceful, more relaxed, and more joyful. The work was still the same, the women's problems just as serious, but she was different and, as a result, has become much more present to the women she works with.

Spiritual direction is especially useful to nurses whose working lives are spent in high-stress health care environments, dealing with life-and-death questions on a regular basis. Spiritual direction is about reflection on one's life in all of its complexity. At the heart of direction is one's unique relationship with the sacred. Direction can help nurses become more sensitive to God's presence in their work and God's desire to "partner" with them. Developing an awareness of this partnership with God provides a serenity that can prevent emotional and spiritual burnout so that relationships with patients, families, colleagues, and oneself become healthy and healing (Moore, 2008). Spiritual directors typically suggest ways of prayer and meditation. They may also recommend reading materials, as well as different ways of listening to the sacred in their lives, for instance, through journal writing, art, and music (Steinhauser, 1999).

Spiritual direction typically occurs monthly, more frequently if the individual desires it. Spiritual directors may meet with individuals over several years or months, depending upon the circumstances of the directee. Group spiritual direction is also available. The director and directee assess their work together periodically. For access to a spiritual director, individuals can contact their religious denomination or SDI. Directors are usually willing to see people from any religious tradition. Some directors will have expertise in areas such as addiction (Wood-bridge, 2000), different ways of praying, dream work, or particular life circumstances.

DREAMS

The ancients asserted the relationship of health and dreams. Greek temples served as places to receive a dream. The given dream would reveal the nature of a person's illness or need, enabling the physician to prescribe appropriate treatment. In the West, until the 5th century A.D., dreams were respected by all religions as revealing the divine. Subsequently, Christians were admonished to ignore dreams because their religious leaders considered them linked to the occult. This thinking prevailed until the 20th century, but changed with the discovery of a mistranslation of Scripture from the Greek to the Latin 15 centuries earlier. Fortunately, dreams are once again recognized for their importance to human health (Sanford, 1989). Jungian psychology has contributed greatly to the restoration of dreams as part of health and healing.

Dreams serve many functions for the psyche in healing and maintenance of health. They give emotional compensation, reveal truths about life situations that the ego resists, provide warnings, and uncommonly provide what Jung called archetypal understanding (Sanford, 1989). *Archetype* is a term used to denote an idea or image that is part of the collective unconscious of humanity across time. An example of emotional healing occurred through a dream a woman had following her husband's death. She was in deep grief until her husband appeared to her in a dream, reassuring her that he was happy and wanted her to be as well. She was freed to move on with her life. Similarly, after a recent tsunami disaster, a young physician had a dream in which an androgynous figure used hand signals to broadcast God's unconditional love for those who had died.

Experts claim that few dreams are prophetic. Nightmares occur when an issue needs to be brought into the person's consciousness. Dreams are specific to the individual and correct interpretations may be difficult. Friends, spiritual directors, or therapists may be helpful as the person tries to understand his or her dreams. For example, a dreamer with a new diagnosis of cancer saw herself riding a bicycle, hitting a bump in the road, falling off the bicycle, and then dusting herself off and riding on happily. Her trusted friend helped her see the relationship between the bump in the road and her cancer. The dream gave her hope that she would be able to continue her life journey and that her cancer was not the end.

All human beings and animals dream, but unless dreams are recorded, they are rarely remembered. A time-tested way to remember dreams is to jot them down even in the middle of the night (a pad and pencil at bedside aids in this process). When one awakens, the dream fades quickly and is not easily recalled unless it recurs. It is important to rewrite the dream in as much detail as possible, without interpreting it. Then, one notes the words, the feeling state, and the sequence of events in the dream. Once the dream is recorded without editing, interpretation can begin. Words may be looked up in the dictionary, and the dream can be meditated upon for further understanding. Dreams often have many levels of interpretation. If one keeps a journal and reviews it from time to time, the meaning of particular dreams may become clear as the person's life experience is seen in retrospect. For example, a woman dreamed about marine life displays in an aquarium. The next day, she made an unplanned visit to an aquarium and recognized the marine displays from her dream even though she had never seen them either live or in pictures before the dream. The journal serves as a record and, years later, new awareness of meaning may occur to the individual.

Dreams are gifts that help us find direction and resolve emotional and other life issues. They teach us about our lives and ourselves. Dreams do not lie. They are presented in images tailored exclusively for us. Recording one's dreams honors the gift that they are.

FUTURE RESEARCH

Research in the following areas will contribute to knowledge about self-care and the nurse as healer:

1. Qualitative studies on the transformational journeys of nurses
2. Studies about the health effects on nurses working with their dreams and/or the health effects on nurses receiving spiritual direction
3. Surveys of nurses to identify the therapies they use in self-care.

REFERENCES

American Holistic Nurses Association. (2009). *Code of ethics for holistic nurses.* Retrieved February 15, 2009, from www.ahna.org/Resourses/Publications/PositionStatements/tabid/1926/default.aspx/ p. 2

Bailey, J. (1999). *The speed trap: How to avoid the frenzy of the fast lane.* San Francisco: HarperCollins.

Benner, D. G. (2002). Nurturing spiritual growth. *Journal of Religion and Theology, 30,* 355–361.

Brennan, B. (1987). *Hands of light: A guide to healing through the human energy field.* New York: Bantam.

Dalai Lama. (1999). *Ethics for the new millennium.* New York: Riverhead.

Disch, J., & Towey, S. (1998). Unit III case study: The healthy work environment as core to an organization's success. In D. Mason & J. Leavitt (Eds.), *Policy and politics in nursing and health care* (pp. 332–346). Philadelphia: Saunders.

Dossey, B. M. (2000). *Florence Nightingale: Mystic, visionary, healer.* Springhouse PA: Springhouse Corporation.

Emmons, H. (2006). *The chemistry of joy: A three step program, for overcoming depression through Western science and Eastern wisdom.* New York: Fireside.

Gordon, J. (2008). *Unstuck: Your guide to the seven stage journey out of depression.* New York: Penguin Press.

Grof, S., & Grof, C. (1990). *The stormy search for the self.* New York: Tarcher-Putnam.

Gunnarsdottir, T., & Peden-McAlpine, C. (2004). The experience of using a combination of complementary therapies: A journey of balance through self-healing. *Journal of Holistic Nursing, 222,* 116–132.

Horrigan, B. (1999). Interview: Barbara Dossey, RN, MS, on holistic nursing, Florence Nightingale, and the healing rituals. *Alternative Therapies in Health and Medicine, 5*(1), 79–86.

Kabat-Zinn, J. (2005). *Coming to our senses: Healing ourselves and the world through mindfulness.* New York: Hyperion.

Lewis, C. (1996). *Green nature/human nature: The meaning of plants in our lives.* Urbana & Chicago: University of Illinois Press.

Lofy, M. (2000). *A matter of time: Power, control, and meaning in people's everyday experience of time.* Unpublished doctoral dissertation, The Fielding Institute, Santa Barbara, CA.

Moon, G. W. (2002). Spiritual direction: Meaning, purpose, and implications for mental health professionals. *Journal of Religion and Theology, 30,* 264–275.

Moore, M. S. (2008). Listening the other into free speech. *Presence: The Journal of Spiritual Directors International, 14*(1), 29–33.

Munger, C., 2009. Field notes: Spiritual direction. *Listen: A Seeker's Resource for Spiritual Direction, 3*(1), 1.

Palmer, P. (2004). *A hidden wholeness: The journey toward an undivided life.* San Francisco: Jossey-Bass.

Rubin, A. (2000). *The power of silence: Using technology to create free structure in organizations.* Unpublished master's thesis, The Fielding Institute, Santa Barbara, CA.

Sanford, J. (1989). *Dreams: God's forgotten language.* San Francisco: Harper & Row.

Santorelli, S. (2000). *Heal thyself: Lessons on mindfulness in medicine.* NewYork: Bell Tower.

Steinhauser, J. (1999). Art prayer: A dance with the holy. *Presence. The Journal of Spiritual Directors International, 5*(3).

Susanka, S. (2007). *The not so big life: Making room for what really matters.* New York: Random House.

Towey, S. (1995). Personal and professional skills for living with uncertainty. *Creative Nursing, 1*(1), 9–11.

Woodbridge, B. (2000). Spiritual direction with an addicted person (pp. 37–47). In N. Vest (Ed.), *Still listening: New horizons in spiritual direction.* Harrisburg, PA: Moorehouse.

Presence

SUE PENQUE
MARIAH SNYDER

Presence is an intervention that is integral to the administration of all complementary therapies, though it can be used independently of them, or other therapies. It is closely related to the therapy of active listening, and the two share many similar characteristics. Although presence has been recognized for centuries within nursing, research on the subject has been initiated only recently. This research has largely been conducted in conjunction with the concept of caring.

DEFINITION

Philosophical views of existentialism assisted with the development of the concept of presence for nursing. Sartre (1943/1984) described awareness as a means toward knowing a person and a way of presence. Sartre coined the term *authentic self* as bringing self to "being with" a person. Heidegger (1962), in his philosophical teachings, introduced the term *Dasein* or "being there" for another. "Being" is the unique quality of a person and is experienced through sharing one's authentic self (Heidegger). According to nursing author T. P. Nelms (1996), "being" is presence and the heart of nursing practice.

The connection between philosophy and nursing regarding the use of the concept of presence began to emerge in the 1960s. Vaillot (1962) used the phenomenon of presence to describe therapeutic relationships as crucial to patient care. Two other pioneers in this field, Paterson and Zderad (1976), described presence as the process of being available with the whole of oneself and open to the experience of another through a reciprocal interpersonal encounter. According to Paterson and Zderad, presence is an intervention the nurse uses to establish a relationship with the patient.

Benner (1984) coined the verb *presencing* to denote the existential practice of being with a patient. *Presencing* is one of the eight competencies Benner identifies as constituting the helping role of the nurse. This view of presence in nursing is supported by Parse (1998), who characterized presence as "the primary mode of nursing practice" (p. 40). Parse (1998) identified three dimensions of presence: (a) illuminating meaning, which is clarifying what is happening through language; (b) synchronizing rhythms through connection and separation; and (c) mobilizing transcendence. Gardner (1992) expanded on the definition of presence by adding specifics related to physical and psychological presence. Presence is defined as "the physical being there and the psychological being with a patient for the purpose of meeting the patient's health care needs" (p. 191).

Presence is reciprocal. The interaction is meaningful to both the patient and the nurse. According to Liehr (1989), the nurse needs to genuinely engage with the patient for true presence to occur and add to a spiritual experience for the patient. The interaction must be deemed meaningful by the patient for presence to produce positive patient outcomes (Pettigrew, 1990). This transactional characteristic of presence was emphasized by McKivergin and Day (1998): In presence, the nurse is available to the patient with the wholeness of his or her unique individual being. Presence can be characterized as an exchange in which meaningful awareness on the part of the nurse helps to bring integration and balance to the life of the patient (Snyder, Brandt, & Tseng, 2000). The reciprocal nature of presence may add more satisfaction and meaning to the life of the nurse.

Two classifications of presence have been developed (McKivergin & Daubenmire, 1994; Osterman & Schwartz-Barcott, 1996). The continuum in both classifications extends from merely being physically present with the patient to being available with the wholeness of self. Exhibit

Exhibit 3.1

Types of Presence

Types of Presence	Example
Physical presence	Nurse is competent in carrying out patient care; has minimal interaction with patient and is seemingly unaware of non-verbal communication; exits room without noting future plan of care.
Full presence	Nurse enters room and greets patient by name; nurse carries out cares while communicating with patient; senses patient's nonverbal communication; plans care in collaboration with patient.
Transcendent presence	Before entering patient's room, nurse centers self so entire focus will be on patient; greets patient by name and uses touch. During the time with the patient the nurse conveys complete interest and is responsive to patient's holistic needs. This is done while providing competent care.

3.1 describes the categories of presence and provides an example of each type of presence. It is only the transcendent (Osterman & Schwartz-Barcott) or therapeutic presence (McKivergin & Daubenmire) that constitutes the complementary therapy designated as presence.

The universality of presence and caring has been documented (Endo, 1998; Jonsdóttir, Litchfield, & Pharris, 2004). Presence transcends cultures and modes of communication. The Buddhist way of life through mindfulness implies one is attentive, aware, and fully present in the moment (Kabat-Zinn, 1990). Even if the nurse and patient are unable to communicate verbally, the patient perceives the presence of a caring nurse. The psychological evidence of presence is apparent. According to Paulson (2004), presence requires an emotional, subjective interaction in which the nurse conveys genuine concern for patients, not just as patients but as human beings.

SCIENTIFIC BASIS

Paterson and Zderad (1976) recognized presence as an integral component of their theory of humanistic nursing. Presence implies openness, receptivity, readiness, and availability on the part of the nurse. Many nursing situations require close proximity to another person, but that in itself does not constitute presence. To experience the lived dialogue of nursing, the nurse responds with an openness to a "person-with-needs" and with an "availability-in-a-helping way" (Paterson & Zderad). Reciprocity often emerges through the dialogue.

Many nurse scientists have described presence as a subconstruct of the broad concept of caring (Watson, 1985; Nelms, 1996; Sherwood, 1997). Presence involves the nurse as "co-participant" in the caring process (Watson, 1985). Caring requires the nurse to be keenly attentive to the needs of the patient, the meaning the patient attaches to the illness or problem, and how the patient wishes to proceed. According to Watson, "a truly caring nurse/artist is able to destroy in the consciousness of the recipient the separation between him- or herself and the nurse" (p. 68). The use of presence helps lead the patient to healing, discovery of others, and the finding of meaning in life.

The body of knowledge documenting patients' perceptions of the value of presence is evolving. Much of the research on presence is found within studies on caring. Nurse researchers have sought to elicit patients' views of the caring behaviors of nurses. In a qualitative study by Riemen (1986) of patients' perceptions of nurses' behaviors, noncaring actions were described as having minimal contact with the patient and/or being physically present but emotionally distant. Availability, kindness, and consideration were desired characteristics identified by patients in a study by Cronin and Harrison (1988). Engaging in a reciprocal process with the nurse was one of the caring behaviors identified by patients who had been discharged from a critical care unit (Burfitt, Greiner, Miers, Kinney, & Branyon, 1993). In a study of hospitalized patients, presence was validated as a caring behavior by Hegedus (1999). The therapeutic benefits of presence are noticed and experienced by patients and families and add meaning to the health care experience.

Research on the expert practice of critical care nurses has demonstrated the importance of presence. Minick (1995) found that connectedness with the patient was important not only as a caring behavior but also because it assisted the nurse in the early identification of postoperative problems. Therapeutic presence may help nurses to be more attentive and to detect subtle changes that may not be evident without it. Nurses who lacked this connectedness were perceived by their patients as detached. Hanneman (1996) explored the effects of expert nurses on care outcomes and found that these nurses displayed two characteristics: presence with the patient and focused assessment of a patient's situation. Wilkin and Slevin (2004) further validated the fact that the importance of the critical care nurse being present to the patient was as essential a part of nursing care as were the skills needed to reach unresponsive and intubated patients.

Mohnkern (1992) asked 15 nurses to identify the antecedents, defining attributes, and consequences of presence. Antecedents included a patient who trusts the nurse and has a need to have her or his life processes facilitated, and a nurse who possesses a sense of mission, has an altruistic desire to help the patient, and is willing and strong enough to be open to the experience of the patient. Attributes of presence were physical closeness between the nurse and the patient, a metaphysical connection between nurse and patient in which energy is exchanged, and the nurse's use of a range of skills to facilitate the patient's experience. Other antecedents found in research include connection through personal stories, informal interactions, and empathic interactions (Evans, Coon, & Crogan, 2007). These factors are important to establishing presence with a patient.

When presence is used as a complementary therapy, consequences or effects occur for the patient, family, and nurse. Easter (2000) reported a decrease in pain for the patient, increase in satisfaction for the nurse, and improved mental well-being for the nurse through presence. According to Drick (2003), presence creates healing and changes the atmosphere in the nurse–patient relationship. Jonas and Crawford (2004) reported calcium flux at the cellular level and lower, more stable heart rates as a result of healing presence within minutes to hours of the intervention. Taverneir (2006) identified three consequences of presence: (1) relationship; (2) healing; and (3) reward. The importance of presence in care has been recognized and valued as a key nursing intervention. Further research on why and how presence plays a positive and vital role in health outcomes needs to be encouraged.

INTERVENTION

The description of presence related by Mitch Albom (1997) in *Tuesdays with Morrie* succinctly captures its essential elements. Albom is reporting how Morrie, a man with advanced amyotrophic lateral sclerosis, viewed presence:

> I believe in being fully present. That means you should be with the person you're with. When I'm talking with you now, Mitch, I try to keep focused only on what is going on between us. I am not thinking about something we said last week. I am not thinking about what's coming up this Friday. I am not thinking about doing another Koppel show, or about medications I'm talking. I am talking to you, I am thinking about you. (pp. 135–136)

Centering

Presence entails conscious attention to the upcoming interaction with the patient. The nurse must be available with the whole self and be open to the personal and care needs of the patient. This process is called centering, a meditative state. The nurse takes a short time, sometimes only 10 or 20 seconds, to eliminate distractions, so that the focus can be on the patient. Some people find that taking a deep breath and closing the eyes helps in freeing them of distractions and becoming centered. This may be done outside the room (or other setting) in which the encounter will occur. Centering may also be as simple as the nurse's pausing before contact with the patient and repeating the patient's name to help focus attention on that person.

Technique

Exhibit 3.2 lists the key components of presence and the skills necessary for practicing it. Sensitivity to others requires the nurse to be an excellent listener and observer. (Active listening is addressed in chapter 4.) Good observation skills assist nurses in identifying nuances in expression and communication that may reveal the real concerns of the patient. Presence often means periods of silence in which subtle interchanges occur. Continuing attentiveness on the part of the nurse is a critical aspect of this therapy. Both the nurse and the client experience a sense of union or joining for a moment in time. Focusing on the moment, not the past or future, is inherent in being present.

Little is known about the length of a therapy session or when therapeutic presence should be used. Often the nurse identifies it intuitively: "It just seems like this patient truly needs me now." Because

Exhibit 3.2

Skills for Implementing Presence

Key Component	Skills
Holistic attention to patient	Centering
	Active listening
	Openness to others
	Sensitivity
	Verbal communication that is at level of patient
	Use of touch
	Nonverbal demonstration of acceptance

of the intense nature of the interaction, the length of time the nurse is present to the patient may seem greater even though only a minute or two may have passed. Although presence is often used in conjunction with another therapy or treatment, identifying when a patient needs someone to just be present for a few minutes may be the most effective therapy.

Measurement of Effectiveness

Measuring outcomes of presence interventions involve both the patient and the nurse because of their reciprocal interaction. Comments from the patient about feeling cared for, being able to express concerns, and feeling understood are some outcome measures that can be derived from patient satisfaction tools. The consequences of presence identified by Mohnkern (1992) included improved psychosocial, spiritual, and emotional functioning; improved physical functioning; a peaceful death; and an appreciation of more interaction with the nurse. Some of these effects are routinely documented in patient satisfaction surveys. The correlation between high patient satisfaction and nursing care is well documented. Incorporating the effects of presence in patient surveys should be considered among the important outcomes indicating a positive health experience and healing. According to Mohnkern, one consequence noted by nurses was an affirmation of their role as nurses. Because of the intangibles that often occur with the use of presence, finding words or indices to measure presence may be challenging.

Precautions

The major precaution in the use of presence is to take one's cue from the patient and not force an encounter. A true presence encounter considers the wants and needs of the patient and is not for the nurse's primary benefit. If the nurse is "available with the whole of oneself and open to the experience" of the client, as the definition states, the nurse will act in accordance with the wishes and needs of the patient.

One negative consequence of presence identified by Mohnkern was nurses reporting that colleagues were critical of the time they spent with patients and families. Certainly this should not be a deterrent to the use of presence, but rather a concern that should be discussed and resolved by nursing staff.

USES

Presence can be used in any nursing situation. Persons struggling with a new diagnosis, an exacerbation of a condition, or a loss are especially in need of moments of presence. Moch (1995) included presence as part of a psychosocial intervention for women diagnosed with breast cancer and found the intervention to be helpful to these women. Presence is of particular value with hospice patients (Zerwekh, 1995).

Presence is also needed with patients in critical care settings (Wilkin & Slevin, 2004) and emergency departments (Wiman & Wikblad, 2004). Patients and their families often feel lost in high-tech critical care settings. The use of presence helps prevent critical care nurses from being viewed by their patients as emotionally distant and focusing only on the machines and technology (Marsden, 1990). Research suggests that incorporating the therapy of presence in critical care settings can reduce anxiety for patients and their families (Mohnkern, 1992).

CULTURAL APPLICATIONS

Culture is closely interlaced with nationality, race, ethnicity, social class, and even generations, and is important in considering the meaning of presence for the patient, family, and nurse. Presence may also hold a special interpretation for the individual based on past experience or family influence. The key is to identify and acknowledge its meaning for the patient and all family members in the relationship. Mitchell (2006) provides an exemplar of presence between the young, middle aged, and elderly. The themes of attentive presence and "being with" in the exemplar were apparent in each of the generations. As described by Mitchell, cultural connection is necessary to bringing meaning to life experience and was emotional and healing.

Each person has a preference for a communication style that may be influenced by their cultural background. In several cultures, gestures of respect and knowing the person hold high importance in establishing a relationship. In other cultures, too much eye contact may be seen as offensive. Communication and trust are shown to be the largest factors that create connection among Hispanic families (Evans, Coon, & Crogan, 2007). Conversational silence is important in some cultures as a mechanism to becoming present with another person or the environment. Buddhists use silence as a respectful technique to being present and are comfortable with long periods of silence, whereas other cultures may not be. Mindfulness, being in the "present" moment and aware of everything around you, is the Buddhist way of life (Cameron, 2002).

Nurses need to make an assessment of the cultural needs of patients before therapeutic presence can be attained. Presence has special meaning to the individual depending on their culture and according to their level of development. It is critical to understand how one connects with others and creates an intimate awareness.

FUTURE RESEARCH

Nurses document assessments made and treatments administered, but rarely do they document the use of presence and the outcomes of this therapy. Despite the challenges in identifying and documenting outcomes of presence, current interest in complementary therapies provides an opportunity for nurses to validate the positive outcomes of the use of presence. Areas in which research is needed include the following:

- Although every patient could benefit from presence, large caseloads often place restrictions on nurses' time. What are assessments that would alert nurses to patients who most need the therapy of presence?

- What are strategies that can be used to teach nursing students and other health professionals how to implement presence?
- With the advent of telemedicine, how can presence be introduced into these contacts with patients? Is physical presence essential or is presence a nonlocal phenomenon, like prayer?
- What are the barriers to becoming present?
- What needs to occur in the work environment for presence to have meaning for both the patient and the nurse?
- What are the cultural differences in the meaning of presence, and how can a nurse identify those differences?
- Is there a relationship between the quantity and/or quality of presence and patient outcomes?

REFERENCES

Albom, M. (1997). *Tuesdays with Morrie*. New York: Doubleday.

Benner, P. (1984). *From novice to expert: Excellence and power in clinical nursing practice*. Menlo Park, CA: Addison-Wesley.

Burfitt, S. N., Greiner, D. S., Miers, L. J., Kinney, M. R., & Branyon, M. E. (1993). Professional nurse caring as perceived by critically ill patients: A phenomenologic study. *American Journal of Critical Care, 2*, 489–499.

Cameron, M. E. (2002). *Karma and happiness: A Tibetan odyssey in ethics, spirituality and healing*. Minneapolis, MN: Fairview Press.

Cronin, S. N., & Harrison, B. (1988). Importance of nurse caring behaviors as perceived by patients after myocardial infarction. *Heart and Lung, 17*, 374–380.

Drick, C. A. (2003). Back to basics: The power of presence in nursing care. *Journal of Gynecologic Oncology Nursing, 13*(3), 13–18.

Easter, A. (2000). Construct analysis of four modes of being present. *Journal of Holistic Nursing, 18*, 362–377.

Endo, E. (1998). Pattern recognition as a nursing intervention with Japanese women with ovarian cancer. *Advances in Nursing Science, 20*(4), 49–51.

Evans, B. C., Coon, D., Crogan, N. L. (2007). Personalismo and breaking barriers: Accessing hispanic populations for clinical services and research. *Geriatric Nursing, 28*(5), 289–296.

Gardner, D. L. (1992). Presence. In G. M. Bulechek & J. C. McCloskey (Eds.), *Nursing interventions: Essential nursing treatments* (2nd ed., pp. 191–200). Philadelphia: Saunders.

Hanneman, S. K. (1996). Advancing nursing practice with a unit-based clinical expert. *Image: Journal of Nursing Scholarship, 28*, 331–337.

Hegedus, K. S. (1999). Providers' and consumers' perspective of nurses' caring behaviors. *Journal of Advanced Nursing, 30*, 1090–1096.

Heidegger, M. (1962). *Being and time* (J. Macquarrie, E. Robinson, Trans.). San Francisco: HarperCollins.

Jonas, W. B., & Crawford, C. C. (2004). The healing presence: Can it be reliably measured? *Journal of Alternative and Complementary Medicine, 10*(5), 751–756.

Jonsdóttir, H., Litchfield, M., & Pharris, M. D. (2004). The relational core of nursing practice in partnership. *Journal of Advanced Nursing, 47*, 241–248.

Kabat-Zinn, J. (1990). *Full Catastrophe Living.* New York: Delacorte Press.

Liehr, P. R. (1989). The core of true presence: A loving center. *Nursing Science Quarterly, 2*(1), 7–8.

Marsden, C. (1990). Ethical issues in critical care. *Heart and Lung, 19*, 540–541.

McKivergin, M., & Daubenmire, J. (1994). The essence of therapeutic presence. *Journal of Holistic Nursing, 12*(1), 65–81.

McKivergin, M., & Day, A. (1998). Presence: Creating order out of chaos. *Seminars in Perioperative Nursing, 7*, 96–100.

Minick, P. (1995). The power of human caring: Early recognition of patient problems. *Scholarly Inquiry for Nursing Practice: An International Journal, 9*, 303–317.

Mitchell, M. (2006). Understanding true presence with elders: A story of joy and sorrow. *Perspectives, 30*(3), 17–19.

Moch, S. D. (1995). *Breast cancer: Twenty women's stories.* New York: National League for Nursing Press.

Mohnkern, S. M. (1992). *Presence in nursing, its antecedents, defining attributes, and consequences.* Doctoral dissertation, University of Texas, Austin, TX.

Nelms, T. P. (1996). Living a caring presence in nursing: A Heideggerian hermeneutical analysis. *Journal of Advanced Nursing, 24*, 368–374.

Osterman, P., & Schwartz-Barcott, D. (1996). Presence: Four ways of being there. *Nursing Forum, 31*, 23–30.

Parse, R. R. (1992). Human becoming: Parse's theory of nursing. *Nursing Science Quarterly, 5*, 35–42.

Parse, R. (1998). *The human becoming school of thought: A perspective for nurses and other health professionals.* Thousand Oaks, California: Sage.

Paterson, J. G., & Zderad, L. T. (1976). *Humanistic nursing.* New York: Wiley.

Paulson, D. S. (2004). Taking care of patients and caring for patients are not the same. *AORN Online, 79*, 359–360, 362, 365–366.

Pettigrew, J. (1990). Intensive nursing care: The ministry of presence. *Critical Care Nursing Clinics of North America, 2*, 503–508.

Riemen, D. J. (1986). Noncaring and caring in the clinical setting: Patients' descriptions. *Topics in Clinical Nursing, 8*, 30–36.

Sartre, J. P. (1943/1984). *Being and nothingness.* New York: Washington Square Press.

Sherwood, G. (1997). Meta-synthesis of qualitative analyses of caring: defining a therapeutic model of nursing. *Advance Practice Nursing Quarterly, 3*, 32–42.

Snyder, M., Brandt, C. L., & Tseng, Y. (2000). Use of presence in the critical care unit. *AACN Clinical Issues, 11*, 27–33.

Tavernier, S. (2006). An evidence-based conceptual analysis of presence. *Holistic Nursing Practice, 20*(3), 152–156.

Vaillot, S. M. C. (1962). *Commitment to nursing: A philosophic investigation.* Philadelphia: Lippincott.

Watson, J. (1985). *Nursing: Human science and human care: A theory of nursing.* Norwalk, CT: Appleton-Century-Crofts.

Wilkin, K., & Slevin, E. (2004). The meaning of caring to nurses: An investigation into the nature of caring work in an intensive care unit. *Journal of Clinical Nursing, 13,* 50–59.

Wiman, E., & Wikblad, K. (2004). Caring and uncaring encounters in nursing in an emergency department. *Journal of Clinical Nursing, 13,* 422–429.

Zerwekh, J. V. (1995). A family caregiving model for hospice nursing. *Hospice Journal, 10,* 27–44.

4 Therapeutic Listening

SHIGEAKI WATANUKI
MARY FRAN TRACY
RUTH LINDQUIST

The most basic of all human needs is the need to understand and be understood. The best way to understand people is to listen to them.

—Ralph Nichols

Listening is an active and dynamic process of interaction with a client, which requires intentional effort to attend to a client's verbal and nonverbal cues. Listening is an integral part of nurse–client relationships. In fact, it is one of the most effective therapeutic techniques available to nurses (Sundeen, Stuart, Rankin, & Cohen, 1998). The theoretical underpinnings of listening can be traced back to counseling psychology and psychotherapy. Rogers (1957) used counseling and listening to foster independence and promote growth and development of clients and emphasized that empathy, warmth, and genuineness with clients were necessary and sufficient for therapeutic changes to occur. Listening has been identified as a significant component of therapeutic communication with patients and therefore fundamental to a therapeutic relationship between the nurse and her or his patient (Foy & Timmins, 2004).

DEFINITION

A variety of modifiers is used with the word *listening*, including *active*, *therapeutic*, *empathic*, and *holistic*. The choice of modifier seems to

47

depend more on an author's paradigm than on differences in the descriptions of listening (Fredriksson, 1999). Unless active listening was explicitly used by researchers in the articles reviewed, the term therapeutic listening is used in this chapter to focus on the formal, deliberate actions of listening for therapeutic purposes (Lekander, Lehmann, & Lindquist, 1993). Therapeutic listening is defined as "an interpersonal, confirmation process involving all the senses in which the therapist attends with empathy to the client's verbal and nonverbal messages to facilitate the understanding, synthesis, and interpretation of the client's situation" (Kemper, 1992, p.22).

SCIENTIFIC BASIS

Therapeutic listening is a topic of interest and concern to a variety of disciplines. A number of qualitative and quantitative studies provide a scientific basis of intervention effects in relation to process (e.g., behavioral changes of providers that foster communication) and outcomes (e.g., client satisfaction, improved clinical indicators).

A systematic review of 20 intervention studies that aimed at improving patient–doctor communication revealed the effectiveness of interventions that typically increased patient participation and clarification (Harrington, Noble, & Newman, 2004). Although few improvements in patient satisfaction were found, significant improvements in perceptions of control over health, preferences for an active role in health care, adherence to recommendations, and clinical outcomes were achieved. Likewise, preferable client outcomes were found in another study in nursing. A survey of 195 parents of hospitalized pediatric patients showed that health care providers' use of immediacy and perceived listening were positively associated with satisfaction, care, and communication (Wanzer, Booth-Butterfield, & Gruber, 2004).

Qualitative studies provide rich understanding of the nature of therapeutic listening and explore the meaning and experience of being listened to in the context of real-world settings. Self-expression opportunities that enable clients to be listened to and understood can promote clients' self-discovery, meaning reconstruction, and healing (Sandelowski, 1994). A discourse analysis of 20 nurse–patient pairs at community hospitals, however, indicated insufficient active listening skills on the part of nurses (Barrere, 2007). The study results showed that nurses often missed cues that patients needed nurses to listen to their concerns, or overlooked potential opportunity for health teaching, especially in "asymmetrical" communication patterns (i.e., dominance of nurse or patient) as compared to "symmetrical" patterns (i.e., nurse–patient communication involving active listening).

Studies evaluating training of health care providers in therapeutic communication skills have shown that training can be effective in improving therapeutic communication skills. A randomized controlled study tested the efficacy of 25-hour training sessions in self-control techniques and communication skills with 61 nurse volunteers. The participating nurses were presented with simulated encounters with relatives of seriously ill patients and their role-plays were evaluated by blinded raters. The results showed significant improvements in the skills of listening, empathizing, not interrupting, and coping with emotions after controlling for baseline performance scores (Garcia de Lucio, Garcia Lopez, Marin Lopez, Mas Hesse, & Caamano Vaz, 2000).

A combination of learning sessions (cognitive interventions) and administrative support and coaching activities (affective and behavioral interventions) enables long-term improvement in communication styles of nurses. A quasiexperimental study tested the effectiveness of an integrated communication skills training program for 129 nurses at a hospital in China. Continued significant improvements in overall basic communication skills, self-efficacy, outcome expectancy beliefs, and perceived support in the training group were observed after 1 and 6 months of training intervention. No significant improvement was found in the control group (Liu, Mok, Wong, Xue, & Xu, 2007).

These studies attempted to identify complex relationships among multiple phenomena and variables, including the immediate and long-term efficacy of training interventions, clinical supervision and support, and cognitive and behavioral changes on the part of nurses. Further systematic studies are needed to enhance knowledge related to intervention effectiveness, especially the link between client characteristics, client satisfaction, and type of interventions.

INTERVENTION

Therapeutic listening enables clients to better understand their feelings and to experience being understood by another caring person. Effective engagement in therapeutic listening requires nurses to be aware of verbal and nonverbal communication that conveys explicit and implicit messages. When verbalized words contradict nonverbal messages, communicators rely more often on nonverbal cues; facial expression, tone of voice, and silence become as important as words in determining the meaning of a message (Kacperek, 1997). Nonverbal communication is inextricably linked to verbal communication and can change, emphasize, or distract from the words that are spoken (Bush, 2001).

Guidelines

Listening is an active process, incorporating explicit behaviors as well as attention to choice of words, quality of voice (pitch, timing, and volume), and full engagement in the process (Burnard, 1997). Therapeutic listening requires a listener to tune in to the client and to use all the senses in analyzing, inferring, and evaluating the stated and underlying meaning of the client's message. Therapeutic listening requires concentration and an ability to differentiate between what is actually being said and what one wants or expects to hear. Listeners are cautioned to avoid making assumptions that might lead them to hear what they think the client ought to say (Schlesinger, 1994). It may be difficult to listen accurately and interpret messages that one finds difficult to relate to, or to listen to information that one may not want to hear. Therapeutic listening is both a cognitive and an emotional process (Arnold & Underman Boggs, 2007). When not fully engaged, it can be easy to become distracted or to start formulating a response rather than to stay focused on the message. Three components have been identified as being foundational to therapeutic listening:

1. Rephrasing the patient's words and thoughts to ensure clarity and accuracy
2. Conveying an understanding of the speaker's perceptions
3. Asking questions and prompting to clarify (De Vito, 2006).

These and other techniques for therapeutic listening intervention are presented in Exhibit 4.1.

Therapeutic listening with pediatric patients can be even more complex, as it frequently becomes triangular between the nurse, the child, and the child's caregiver(s) (Whaley & Wong, 1996). This may

Exhibit 4.1

Therapeutic Listening Techniques

Active Presence: Active presence involves focus on the client to interpret the message that he/she is trying to convey, recognition of themes, and hearing what is left unsaid. Short responses such as "yes" or "uh-huh" with appropriate timing and frequency may promote clients' willingness to talk.

Accepting Attitude: Conveying an accepting attitude is assuring, and can help clients to feel more comfortable about expressing themselves. This can be demonstrated by short affirmative responses or gestures.

Clarifying Statements: Clarifying statements and summarizing can help the listener verify message interpretation and create clarity. Encourage specificity rather than vague statements to facilitate communication. Rephrasing and reflection can assist the client in self-understanding. Using phrases such as "tell me more about that" or "what was that like?" may be helpful, rather than asking "why," which may elicit a defensive response from the client.

Use of Silence: Use of silence can encourage the client to talk, facilitate the nurse's focus on listening rather than the formulation of responses, and reduce the use of leading questions. Sensitivity toward cultural and individual variations in the seconds of silence may be developed by paying detailed attention to the patterns of client communication.

Tone: Tone of voice can express more than the actual words through empathy, judgment, or acceptance. Match the intensity of the tone to the message received to avoid minimizing or overemphasizing.

Nonverbal Behaviors: Clients relaying sensitive information may be very aware of the listener's body language and will be viewed as either accepting of the message or closed to it, judgmental, and/or disinterested. Eye contact, or a nodding head, is essential to convey the listener's true interest and attention. Maintaining a conversational distance and judicious use of touch may increase the client's comfort. Cultural and social awareness is important to avoid undesired touch.

Environment: Distractions should be eliminated to encourage the therapeutic interchange. Therapeutic listening may require careful planning to provide time for undivided attention or may occur spontaneously. Some clients may feel very comfortable having family present; others may feel inhibited when others are present.

take particular skill on the part of the nurse as he or she attends to both the spoken messages as well as the nonverbal communication/reactions of two or three persons simultaneously. In addition, the nurse must be sensitive to the clarification of information and cues in front of either the child or the caregiver, depending on the child's age and developmental stage.

Adolescents may especially appreciate talking with an adult who is not a member of their family (Whaley & Wong, 1996). They may, however, respond quickly and abruptly to any perceived indications of judgment, indifference, or disrespect on the part of the listener. It is especially important with adolescents to be fully attentive, allow for complete expression of thoughts, and avoid statements or facial expressions that imply disapproval or that can be misinterpreted.

Because therapeutic listening involves both cognitive and emotional processes, it is important that nurses recognize the role of emotional intelligence in their therapeutic interactions. Emotional intelligence is defined as an ability to recognize emotions in self and other, and understand and utilize these emotions in thinking processes and interactions with others (Vitello-Cicciu, 2002). Nursing requires a significant amount of emotional labor, resulting in expectations of expressions of caring, understanding, and empathy with patients and families. Strategies such as reflection, empathizing, and skilled therapeutic listening can promote a healing environment for patients and families (Molter, 2003).

A relatively new type of listening intervention targeting behavioral change of health care providers has been described and tested, a technique referred to as *change-oriented reflective listening* (Strang, McCambridge, Platts, & Groves, 2004). This technique has been adapted from the core principles of motivational interviewing (Rollnick et al., 2002). Change-oriented reflective listening is a brief motivational enhancement intervention that has a strong potential for incorporation into the repertoire of nursing interventions. Change-oriented reflective listening is a method to encourage providers' consideration of the quality of primary care, and then stimulate their intent to change. This method takes the form of a brief telephone conversation (15–20 min), where reflective listening statements are interspersed with open questions about the issue at hand. A menu of questions with the range of possible areas for discussion is constructed in advance. The technique has been successfully piloted with general practitioners to motivate them to intervene with opiate users and as part of alcohol intervention (McCambridge, Platts, Whooley, & Strang, 2004; Strang et al., 2004).

Measurement of Outcomes

Inclusion of multiple measurements, such as self-report, behavioral observation, physiological indicators, and qualitative accounts, provides rich data for the study of therapeutic listening. Challenges to outcome measurement include (a) the isolation of an independent variable (therapeutic listening as an intervention) from other confounding variables, and (b) the complexity of the multifaceted phenomenon of therapeutic listening, which may necessitate multivariate study design (Bennett, 1995). Antecedents to interventions (e.g., clients' characteristics) have to be taken into consideration; likewise, the process-related components of interventions (e.g., short- and long-term improvements in nurses' knowledge, skills, attitudes, and behavior after training) and client outcomes need to be evaluated (Harrington et al., 2004; Kruijver et al., 2000).

Positive changes in psychological variables such as anxiety, depression, hostility, or nursing care satisfaction are potential client outcomes of therapeutic listening. It may also be useful to examine physiological measures (e.g., heart rate, blood pressure, respiratory rate, temperature, oxygen saturation, electroencephalography results) as outcomes of therapeutic interchange. Outcomes may also include clinical variables such as length of stay, response to illness, mood, adherence, disease control, morbidity, and health care cost.

Precautions

Therapeutic listening has at its heart the intent to be helpful; however, a few precautions are warranted. Questions that start with the word "why" may take clients out of the context of their experience or feelings and direct them into an intellectual thinking mode or cause defensive responses. Rather, phrases such as *"Tell me more about that"* or *"What was that like?"* (Shattell & Hogan, 2005, p.31) may be helpful.

Maintaining professional boundaries during therapeutic listening is important; empathy is to be demonstrated, but within the professional and therapeutic relationship with clients. Referrals for professional counseling may be indicated in such cases as psychiatric crises. Ethical dilemmas may result if the principle of respecting clients' autonomy and confidentiality conflicts with the principle of maintaining professional responsibility and integrity (e.g., taking action based on sensitive information shared in the therapeutic exchange).

USES

Therapeutic listening is an intervention that is applicable to a virtually unlimited number of care situations. It is a vital technique that may

Exhibit 4.2

Selected Uses of Listening With Patient Populations or in Care Settings

Adolescent mental health (Street & Svanberg, 2003; Claveirole, 2004)

Cancer (Reid-Ponte, 1992; Liu et al., 2007)

Culturally diverse populations (Davidhizar, 2004)

Day surgery (Foy & Timmins, 2004)

Emergency care (O'Gara & Fairhurst, 2004; O'Hagan, Webb, & Moore, 2004)

Heart failure: To improve self-care (Riegel et al., 2006)

Older adults (Williams, Kemper, & Hummert, 2004)

Perinatal care (Battersby & Deery, 2001)

Post-traumatic stress (Gidron et al., 2001)

Relatives of critically ill patients: Use of training simulation for providers (Garcia de Lucio et al., 2000)

Terminal care (Cherin, Enguidanos, & Brumley, 2001)

Traumatic stress/disasters (Liehr, Mehl, Summers, & Pennebaker, 2004)

Women with breast cancer (Harris & Templeton, 2001)

be used to elicit the patient's perspective on their illness (Simpson et al., 1991). It is beneficial for practitioners to continue listening to a patient throughout the entire visit; patients have been known to disclose vital information in the closing moments of an appointment (White, Levinson, & Roter, 1994). Selected patient population–based examples in which the use of listening is described are included in Exhibit 4.2. Managers in the health care field may also reap benefits from active listening (Boyd, 1998; Kubota, Mishima, & Nagata, 2004). Exhibit 4.3 presents Web sites of national and international professional organizations where online resources for therapeutic listening can be found.

Technology is becoming increasingly important in assuring that patients have effective means to communicate and a way to be fully heard and understood. Devices such as Passy-Muir tracheal valves that can allow mechanically ventilated patients to speak, computer programs that can "speak" the patient's electronic input, and laryngeal devices

Exhibit 4.3

> **Professional Organizations and Online Resources for Therapeutic Listening**
>
> **National:**
>
> The National Communication Association http://www.natcom.org
> The Focusing Institute http://www.focusing.org
>
> **International:**
>
> The International Communication Association http://www.icahdq.org/
> The International Listening Association http://www.listen.org/
> Communication Institute for Online Scholarship http://www.cios.org/

are now more frequently available and expected to promote communication. Nonverbal communication when alternative methods are being used is even more important to observe and monitor.

CULTURAL APLICATIONS

Sensitivity and awareness toward cultural variations in communication styles are vital to intervention effectiveness. Cultural differences in meanings of certain words, styles, and approaches, or in certain nonverbal behaviors such as silence, touch, eye contact, or smile may adversely affect the effectiveness of therapeutic communication. For example, there may be tendencies for clients from certain cultures to talk loudly, to be direct in conversation, and to come to the point quickly. Clients from other cultures may tend to talk softly, be indirect in their communication, or "talk around" points while emphasizing attitudes and feelings. In some cultures, it is believed that open expression of emotions is unacceptable. Whether in the dominant culture or in nondominant cultures, however, persons may simply smile when they do not comprehend. The skills of therapeutic listening are particularly useful in ensuring that communication in such cases is effective. It is important that nurses explore and understand clients' cultural values and assumptions, as well as their patterns of behaviors related to communication, while avoiding stereotyping (Seidel, Ball, Dains, & Benedict, 2006).

Interpreter-mediated health care encounters can be a challenge for therapeutic interchange. The issue of translation and interpretation in health care includes more than the differences in language use. Interpretation should be founded on a word-for-word translation while incorporating nuances and maintaining semantic equivalency of communication. Difficulties in translation and interpretation in health care encounters is illustrated, for example, in a study by Flores et al. (2003) of Spanish–English interpretations in pediatric encounters. The study found that there were, on average, 31 errors in medical interpretation per clinical encounter. Most errors were typed as "omissions" of important information, and had potential clinical consequences. Those serious errors were more likely to be committed by "ad hoc" interpreters (e.g., nonprofessional interpreters including nurses, social workers, siblings) as compared with those committed by hospital interpreters. Use of appropriately trained and experienced interpreters is a necessity for clients who have language barriers.

FUTURE RESEARCH

Many research questions have potential for exploration in the area of therapeutic listening. Systematic studies are needed to develop a body of knowledge. The study designs will require new paradigms other than traditional randomized controlled trials, for ethical and feasibility reasons among other things. Qualitative studies, case reports, or mixed method designs may be better options for understanding the nature and effects of therapeutic listening. Some potential questions for future research are:

- Can therapeutic listening via phone or other interactive technology (synchronous or asynchronous) be effective at a distance?
- What are the effects of the use of listening by health care providers on patient satisfaction and other outcomes of care?
- Are interventions to enhance listening on the part of health care providers cost-effective and legitimate areas on which to focus continuous quality improvement to increase patient safety and quality of care?
- How do multicultural differences manifest themselves in the processes and effectiveness of therapeutic listening?

REFERENCES

Arnold, E. C., & Underman Boggs, K. (2007). *Interpersonal relationships: Professional communication skills for nurses* (5th ed.). London: W.B. Saunders.

Barrere, C. C. (2007). Discourse analysis of nurse-patient communication in a hospital setting: Implications for staff development. *Journal of Nurses in Staff Development, 23,* 114–122.

Battersby, S., & Deery, R. (2001). Midwifery and research: Comparable skills in listening and the use of language. *Practising Midwife, 4*(9), 24–25.

Bennett, J. A. (1995). Methodological notes on empathy: Further considerations. *Advances in Nursing Science, 18*(1), 36–50.

Boyd, S. D. (1998). Using active listening. *Nursing Management, 29*(7), 55.

Burnard, P. (1997). *Effective communication skills for health professionals* (2nd ed.). Cheltenham, UK: Nelson Thornes.

Bush, K. (2001). Do you really listen to patients? *RN, 64*(3), 35–37.

Cherin, D., Enguidanos, S., & Brumley, R. (2001). Reflection in action in caring for the dying: Applying organizational learning theory to improve communications in terminal care. *Home Health Care Services Quarterly, 19*(4), 65–78.

Claveirole, A. (2004). Listening to young voices: Challenges of research with adolescent mental health service users. *Journal of Psychiatric & Mental Health Nursing, 11*(3), 253–260.

Davidhizar, R. (2004). Listening—a nursing strategy to transcend culture. *Journal of Practical Nursing, 54*(2), 22–24.

De Vito, J. A. (2006). *The interpersonal communication book* (11th ed.). Needham Heights, MA: Allyn & Bacon.

Flores, G., Laws, M. B., Mayo, S. J., Zuckerman, B., Abreu, M., Medina, L., et al. (2003). Errors in medical interpretation and their potential clinical consequences in pediatric encounters. *Pediatrics, 111*(1), 6–14.

Foy, C. R., & Timmins, F. (2004). Improving communication in day surgery settings. *Nursing Standard, 19*(7), 37–42.

Fredriksson, L. (1999). Modes of relating in a caring conversation: A research synthesis on presence, touch and listening. *Journal of Advanced Nursing, 30,* 1167–1176.

Garcia de Lucio, L., Garcia Lopez, F. J., Marin Lopez, M. T., Mas Hesse, B., & Caamano Vaz, M. D. (2000). Training programme in techniques of self-control and communication skills to improve nurses' relationships with relatives of critically ill patients: A randomized controlled study. *Journal of Advanced Nursing, 32,* 425–431.

Gidron, Y., Gal, R., Freedman, S., Twiser, I., Lauden, A., Snir, Y., et al. (2001). Translating research findings to PTSD prevention: Results of a randomized-controlled pilot study. *Journal of Traumatic Stress, 14,* 773–780.

Harrington, J., Noble, L. M., & Newman, S. P. (2004). Improving patients' communication with doctors: A systematic review of intervention studies. *Patient Education and Counseling, 52*(1), 7–16.

Harris, S. R., & Templeton, E. (2001). Who's listening? Experiences of women with breast cancer in communicating with physicians. *Breast Journal, 7,* 444–449.

Kacperek, L. (1997). Non-verbal communication: The importance of listening. *British Journal of Nursing, 6,* 275–279.

Kemper, B. J. (1992). Therapeutic listening: Developing the concept. *Journal of Psychosocial Nursing and Mental Health Services, 30*(7), 21–23.

Kubota, S., Mishima, N., & Nagata, S. (2004). A study of the effects of active listening on listening attitudes of middle managers. *Journal of Occupational Health, 46*(1), 66–67.

Kruijver, I. P., Kerkstra, A., Francke, A. L., Bensing, J. M., & van de Wiel, H. B. (2000). Evaluation of communication training programs in nursing care: A review of the literature. *Patient Education and Counseling, 39,* 129–145.

Lekander, B. J., Lehmann, S., & Lindquist, R. (1993). Therapeutic listening: Key nursing interventions for several nursing diagnoses. *Dimensions of Critical Care Nursing, 12,* 24–30.

Liehr, P., Mehl, M. R., Summers, L. C., & Pennebaker, J. W. (2004). Connecting with others in the midst of stressful upheaval on September 11, 2001. *Applied Nursing Research, 17*(1), 2–9.

Liu, J. E, Mok, E., Wong, T., Xue, L., & Xu, B. (2007). Evaluation of an integrated communication skills training program for nurses in cancer care in Beijing, China. *Nursing Research, 56,* 202–209.

McCambridge, J., Platts, S., Whooley, D., & Strang, J. (2004). Encouraging GP alcohol intervention: Pilot study of change-oriented reflective listening (CORL). *Alcohol & Alcoholism, 39*(2), 149–149.

Molter, N. C. (2003). Creating a healing environment for critical care. *Critical Care Nursing Clinics of North America, 15,* 295–304.

O'Gara, P. E., & Fairhurst, W. (2004). Therapeutic communication: Part 2. Strategies that can enhance the quality of the emergency care consultation. *Accident and Emergency Nursing, 12,* 201–207.

O'Hagan, B., Webb, L., & Moore, K. (2004). Listening and learning from patients. *Emergency Nurse, 12*(7), 12–14.

Reid-Ponte, P. (1992). Distress in cancer patients and primary nurses' empathy skills. *Cancer Nursing, 15,* 283–292.

Riegel, B., Dickson, V. V., Hoke, L., McMahon, J. P., Reis, B. F., & Sayers, S. (2006). A motivational counseling approach to improving heart failure self-care: Mechanisms of effectiveness. *Journal of Cardiovascular Nursing, 21,* 232–241.

Rogers, C. R. (1957). The necessary and sufficient conditions of therapeutic personality change. *Journal of Consulting Psychology, 21,* 95–103.

Rollnick, S., Allison, J., Ballasiotes, S., Barth, T., Butler, C. C., Rose, G. S., & Rosengren, D. B. (2002). Variations on a theme: Motivational interviewing and its adaptations. In W. R. Miller & S. Rollnick (Eds.), *Motivational interviewing: Preparing people for change* (2nd ed., pp. 270–283). New York: Guilford.

Sandelowski, M. (1994). We are the stories we tell: Narrative knowing in nursing practice. *Journal of Holistic Nursing, 12,* 23–33.

Schlesinger, H. J. (1994). How the analyst listens: The pre-stages of interpretation. *International Journal of Psycho-Analysis, 75,* 31–37.

Seidel, H. E., Ball, J. W., Dains, J. E., & Benedict, G. W. (Eds.). (2006). Cultural awareness. In H. E. Seidel, J. W. Ball, J. E. Dains, & G. W. Benedict (Eds.), *Mosby's guide to physical examination* (6th ed., pp.38–50). St Louis, Missouri: Mosby.

Shattell, M., & Hogan, B. (2005). Facilitating communication: How to truly understand what patients mean. *Journal of Psychosocial Nursing and Mental Health Service. 43*(10), 29–32.

Simpson, M., Buckman, R., Stewart, M., Maguire, P., Lipkin, M., Novack, D., & Till, J. (1991). Doctor–patient communication: The Toronto Consensus Statement. Consensus Development Conference. *British Medical Journal, 303*(6814), 1385–1387.

Strang, J., McCambridge, J., Platts, S., & Groves, P. (2004). Engaging the reluctant GP in care of the opiate users. *Family Practice, 21*(2), 150–154.

Street, C., & Svanberg, J. (2003, July–August). Listening to young people. *Mental Health Today,* 28–30.

Sundeen, S. J., Stuart, G. W., Rankin, E. A. D., & Cohen, S. A. (1998). *Nurse–client interaction: Implementing the nursing process* (6th ed.). St. Louis, MO: Mosby.

Vitello-Cicciu, J. M. (2002). Exploring emotional intelligence: Implications for nursing leaders. *Journal of Nursing Administration, 32*(4), 203–210.

Wanzer, M. B., Booth-Butterfield, M., & Gruber, K. (2004). Perceptions of health care providers' communication: Relationships between patient-centered communication and satisfaction. *Health Communication, 16,* 363–384.

Whaley, L., & Wong, D. (1996). *Essential of pediatric nursing* (5th ed). St Louis: C. V. Mosby.

White, J., Levinson, W., & Roter, D. (1994). "Oh by the way": the closing moments of the medical visit. *Journal of General Internal Medicine, 9,* 24–28.

Williams, K., Kemper, S., & Hummert, M. L. (2004). Enhancing communication with older adults: Overcoming elderspeak. *Journal of Gerontological Nursing, 30*(10), 17–25.

Mind–Body–Spirit Therapies

PART II

OVERVIEW

The National Center for Complementary/Alternative Medicine (NCCAM) uses the designator *mind–body therapies* for this category. However, from a holistic perspective, *spirit* is included, as this aspect of human beings is an integral part of a number of the therapies discussed in this section, such as prayer, meditation, and yoga. NCCAM defines this category as encompassing therapies that promote the mind's capacity to have an impact on the functioning of the body. In keeping with the perspective of the inclusion of the spirit, this would also encompass the impact that the spirit can have on physical parameters. The NCCAM definition continues to emphasize the Western focus on the body in health and the impact that the mind and spirit may have on the body; it does not convey that the converse may be true—that the functioning of the body may have an impact on the mind and spirit. One only has to think about the impact that a headache has on one's mind and spirit and the consequent difficulties in reading or praying.

Mind–body–spirit therapies stand in opposition to the beliefs that underlie Western biomedicine. The philosophy of Rene Descartes, in which the body and mind are separated, has predominated in that discipline. During the past few decades, nursing curricula have begun to emphasize a holistic basis for nursing practice. Course content on mind–body–spirit therapies are now included in nursing curricula. Thus, nursing practice is moving away from the dichotomy between mind and body and beginning to see persons from a holistic perspective.

There is now a substantial body of research supporting the use of mind–body–spirit therapies. Since Herbert Benson's research in the 1960s on transcendental meditation, research on mind–body–spirit therapies such as prayer, music, and imagery continues. New developments in measurement indices to determine the outcome of these therapies continue to emerge.

Many of the therapies in this category—imagery, music, prayer, meditation, humor—continue to be a part of the armamentarium used by nurses. Nurses need to be aware of mind–body–spirit therapies used by persons from other cultures. Therapies that are spirit-focused are prominent in many cultures. *Time* magazine (Walsh, 2009) highlighted a number of healing practices found in cultures around the world that differ significantly from those that nurses encounter and use on a daily basis. Basic knowledge about therapies of other cultures will assist nurses in understanding their patients and giving consideration to how these therapies may have an impact on health outcomes.

REFERENCES

Walsh, B. (2009). How the world heals. *Time, 173*(7), 81–83.

Imagery

MAURA FITZGERALD
MARY LANGEVIN

Imagery is a mind–body intervention that uses the power of the imagination to bring about change in physical, emotional, or spiritual dimensions. Throughout our daily lives we constantly see images, feel sensations, and register impressions. A picture of lemonade makes our mouths water, a song makes us happy or sad, a smell takes us back to a past moment. Images evoke physical and emotional responses and help us understand the meaning of events.

Imagery is commonly used in health care, most often in the form of guided imagery, clinical hypnosis, or self-hypnosis. In the mid-1950s, the American Medical Association and the American Psychiatric Association recognized hypnosis as a therapeutic tool (Lee, 1999). Nurses, physicians, psychologists, and others use it in their practice with adults and children for treatment of acute and chronic illness, relief of symptoms, and enhancement of wellness. Imagery is a hallmark of stress-management programs and has become a standard therapy to alleviate anxiety, promote relaxation, improve coping and functional status, gain psychological insight, even to make progress on a chosen spiritual path.

DEFINITION

Imagery is the formation of a mental representation of an object, place, event, or situation that is perceived through the senses. It is a cognitive–

behavioral strategy that uses the individual's own imagination and mental processing and can be practiced as an independent activity or guided by a professional. Imagery employs all the senses—visual, aural, tactile, olfactory, proprioceptive, and kinesthetic. Although imagery is often referred to as "visualization," it includes imagining through any sense and not just being able to "see something" in the mind's eye.

Van Kuiken (2004) describes four types of guided imagery: pleasant, physiologically focused, mental rehearsal or reframing, and receptive imagery. While inducing imagery, the individual often imagines seeing, hearing, smelling, tasting, and/or touching something in the image. The image used can be active or passive (playing volley ball versus lying on the beach). Although for many participants physical and mental relaxation tends to facilitate imagery, this is not necessary, particularly for children, who often do not need to be in a relaxed state. Imagery may be receptive, with the individual perceiving messages from the body, or it may be active, with the individual evoking thoughts or ideas. Active imagery can be outcome- or end-state–oriented, in which the individual envisions a goal, such as being healthy and well; or it can be process-oriented, in which the mechanism of the desired effect is imagined, such as envisioning a strong immune system fighting a viral infection or tumor.

Imagery and clinical hypnosis are closely related. Clinical hypnosis is a strategy in which a professional guides the participant into an altered state of deep relaxation and suggestions for changes in subjective experience and alterations in perception are made. Both hypnosis and guided imagery incorporate the use of relaxation techniques, such as diaphragmatic breathing or progressive muscle relaxation to assist the participant to focus the attention. In hypnosis, this is referred to as an induction. Guided imagery is often used within the context of hypnosis to further deepen the state of relaxation and in both techniques suggestions for positive growth, change, or improvement are often made. Because of the close association between these two processes selected studies on hypnosis will be discussed in this chapter.

SCIENTIFIC BASIS

Imagery can be understood as an activity that generates physiologic and somatic responses. It is based on the cognitive process known as mental imagery. Mental imagery is a central element of cognition that operates when mental representations are created in the absence of sensory input. Functional magnetic resonance imaging (fMRI) has demonstrated that the mental construction of an image activates the same neural pathways and central nervous system structures as are engaged when an individual is actually utilizing one or more of the senses (Djordjevic, Zatorre, Petrides, Boyle, & Jones-Gotaman, 2005; Formisano et al., 2002; Gulyas, 2001; Kosslyn, Ganis, & Thompson, 2001; Kraemer, Macrae, Green, & Kelley, 2005). For example, if an individual is imagining hearing a sound, the brain structures associated with hearing will become activated. Mental rehearsal of movements will activate motor areas and can be incorporated into stroke rehabilitation and sports improvement programs (Braun, Beurskens, Borm, Schack, & Wade, 2006; Lacourse, Turner, Randolph-Orr, Schandler, & Cohen, 2004).

Andrasik and Rime (2007) postulate that cognitive tasks, such as mental imagery, can be conceptualized as neuromodulators. Neuromodulation is generally defined as the interaction between the nervous system and electrical or pharmacological agents that block or disrupt the perception of pain. By distraction, imagery alters processing in the central, peripheral, and autonomic nervous systems. The perception of a symptom such as pain or nausea is reduced or eliminated.

A key mechanism by which imagery modifies disease and reduces symptoms is thought to be by reducing the stress response. The stress response is triggered when a situation or event (perceived or real) threatens physical or emotional well-being or when the demands of the situation exceed available resources. It activates complex interactions between the neuroendocrine system and the immune system. Emotional responses to situations trigger the limbic system and signal physiologic changes in the peripheral and autonomic nervous systems, resulting in the characteristic fight-or-flight stress response. Over time, chronic stress results in adrenal and immune suppression and may be most harmful to cellular immune function, impairing the ability to ward off viruses and tumor cells (Pert, Dreher, & Ruff, 1998).

The complexity of the human response to stress is best understood through psychoneuroimmunology (PNI), an interdisciplinary field of study that explains the mechanisms by which the brain and body communicate through cellular interactions. Early work was based on extensive rat model research by Robert Ader and Nicholas Cohen, which confirmed that the immune system could be conditioned by expectations and beliefs (Ader & Cohen, 1981; Ader, Felten, & Cohen, 1991; Fleshner & Laudenslager, 2004). Subsequent research focused on the mechanisms of brain and body communication through cellular interactions and identified receptors for neuropeptides, neurohormones, and cytokines that reside on neural and immune cells and induce biochemical changes when activated by neurotransmitters.

A cascade of signaling events in response to perceived or actual stress results in the release of hormones from the hypothalamus, pituitary gland, adrenal medulla, adrenal cortex, and peripheral sympathetic nerve terminals. Psychosocial and physical stressors have the potential to upregulate this hypothalamic-pituitary-adrenal (HPA) axis. Chronic hyperactivation of the HPA axis and sympathetic nervous system with the associated increased levels of cortisol and catecholemines can deregulate immune function, whereas moderate levels of circulating cortisol may enhance immune function (Langley, Fonseca, & Iphofen, 2006). Cytokines are secreted by cells participating in the immune response and act as messengers between the immune system and the brain (McCance & Huenther, 2002). They also function as neurotransmitters crossing the blood–brain barrier or affecting sensory neurons. Through these channels, cytokines induce symptoms of fever, increased sensitivity to pain, anorexia, and fatigue, which are adaptive responses that may facilitate recovery and healing (Langley et al., 2006). These interactions between the brain and the immune system are bidirectional and changes in one system will influence the others. The stress response can therefore become a double-edged sword that can either enhance or suppress optimal immunity (Flescher & Laudenslager, 2004).

Although immune responses to emotional states are extremely complex, in general, acute stress activates cardiac sympathetic activity and increases plasma catecholamines and natural killer (NK) cell activity, whereas chronic stress (or inescapable or unpredictable stress) is associated with suppression of NK cells and interleukin-1-beta and other proinflammatory cytokines (Cacioppo et al., 1998; Glaser et al., 2001). These effects appear to be mediated by the influence of stress hormones on T helper components (Th1 and Th2) (Maes et al., 1998). Imagery, by inducing deep relaxation and reprocessing of stressful triggers, interrupts or alters the stress response and supports the immune system. In a recent review of guided imagery studies examining immune system function, Traktenberg (2008) concluded that there is evidence to support a relationship between the immune system and stress or relaxation.

The degree of response to stress varies among individuals. Cacioppo and colleagues (1998) hypothesized that persons who have large physiologic responses to everyday stressors have "high stress reactivity" and are at greater risk for disease susceptibility, even when coping, performance, and perceived stress are comparable. One of the goals of imagery is to reduce stress reactivity by reframing stressful situations from negative responses of fear and anxiety to positive images of healing and well-being (Dossey, 1995; Kosslyn, Ganis, & Thompson, 2001). Donaldson (2000) proposed that thoughts produce physiological responses and activate appropriate neurons. Using imagery to increase emotional awareness and restructure the meaning of a remembered situation by changing negative responses to positive images and meaning alters the physiological response and improves outcomes.

INTERVENTION

Techniques and Guidelines

Imagery has been used extensively in children, adolescents, and adults. Children as young as age 4 who have language skills adequate to understand the suggestions can benefit from imagery (Olness & Kohen, 1996). Young children often are better at imagery because of their natural, active use of their imaginations. Imagery may be practiced independently, or with a coach or teacher, or with a videotape or audiotape. The most effective imagery intervention is one that is specific to individuals' personalities, their preferences for relaxation and specific settings, their age or developmental stage, and the desired outcomes. The steps of a general imagery session are outlined in Exhibit 5.1.

Imagery sessions for adults and adolescents are usually 10 to 30 minutes in length, whereas most children tolerate 5 to 15 minutes. The session typically begins with a relaxation exercise, which enables the participant to focus or "center." A technique that works well both for children and for adults is to engage in slow and expansive breathing, which facilitates relaxation as the breath moves lower into the chest and the diaphragm while the abdominal muscles begin to be used more than the upper chest muscles. Other techniques include progressive

Exhibit 5.1

General Guided Imagery Technique

1. Achieving a relaxed state
   A. Find a comfortable sitting or reclining position (not lying down).
   B. Uncross any extremities.
   C. Close your eyes or focus on one spot or object in the room.
   D. Focus on breathing with abdominal muscles—being aware of the breath as it enters through your nose and leaves through your mouth. With your next breath let the exhalation be just a little longer and notice how the inhalation that follows is deeper. And as you notice that, let your body become even more relaxed. Continue to breathe deeply, gradually letting the exhalation become twice as long as the inhalation.
   E. Feel your body becoming heavy and warm—from the top of your head to the tips of your fingers and toes.
   F. If your thoughts roam, bring your mind back to thinking of your breathing and your relaxed body.

2. Specific suggestions for imagery
   A. In your mind, go to a place you enjoy and where you feel good.
   B. What do you see—hear—taste—smell—and feel?
   C. Let yourself enjoy being in this place.
   D. Now imagine yourself the way you want to be—(describe the desired goal specifically).
   E. Imagine what steps you will need to take to be the way you want to be.
   F. Practice these steps now—in this place where you feel good.
   G. What is the first thing you are doing to help you be the way you want to be?
   H. What will you do next?
   I. When you reach your goal of the way you want to be—feel yourself, touch yourself, embrace yourself, listen to the sounds surrounding you.

3. Summarize process and reinforce practice
   A. Remember that you can return to this place, this feeling, and this way of being anytime you want.
   B. You can feel this way again by focusing on your breathing, relaxing, and imagining yourself in your special place.
   C. Come back to this place and envision yourself the way you want to be every day.

4. Return to present
   A. Be aware again of the favorite place.
   B. Bring your focus back to your breathing.
   C. Become aware of the room you are in (drawing attention to the temperature, sounds, or lights).
   D. You will feel relaxed and refreshed and be ready to resume your activities.
   E. When you are ready you may open your eyes.

muscle relaxation or focusing on a word or object. Some children may use their bodies to demonstrate or respond to their image. Although most participants close their eyes, some, especially young children, will prefer to have eyes open.

Once the participant is in a relaxed or in an "altered" state, the practitioner suggests an image of a relaxing, peaceful, or comforting place or introduces an image suggested by the client. Scenes commonly used to induce relaxation include watching a sunset or clouds, sitting on a warm beach or by a fire, or floating through water or space. Some participants, particularly young children, may prefer active images that involve motion, such as flying or playing a sport. The scene used is one that the client finds relaxing or engaging. It is often introduced as a "favorite" place. Huth, VanKuiken, and Broome (2006) interviewed children who were participants in a guided imagery research study, to determine the content of their imagery. The children reported their favorite images as the park, swimming at a beach, amusement parks, and vacationing. They also visualized a variety of familiar places, such as sports events and places that included pets and other animals.

Although mental relaxation is often accompanied by muscle relaxation, this is not always a goal. Participants of any age, but particularly preschool and school-age children, may imagine in an active state. For example, a group of 9- to 12-year-old boys with sickle cell disease were being taught guided imagery as a pain-control technique. When asked what special place they would like to go to, they requested a trip to a local amusement park and a ride on the roller coaster. During the imagery many of them were physically and vocally active, swaying from side to side and moving their arms up and down. At the end of the visualization they all reported feeling like they had been in the park (absorption) and gave examples of things they felt, saw, heard, or smelled.

For directed imagery, the practitioner guides the imagery, using positive suggestions to alleviate specific symptoms or conditions (outcome or end-state imagery) or to rehearse or "walk through" an event (process imagery). Images do not need to be anatomically correct or vivid. Symbolic images may be the most powerful healing images because they are drawn from individual beliefs, culture, and meaning. A cancer patient might imagine sweeping cancer cells away or an asthma patient might picture the lungs as an expanding tree.

The ability to use guided imagery is related to the individual's hypnotic ability or the ability to enter an altered state of consciousness and to become involved or absorbed in the imagery (Kwekkeboom, Huseby-Moore, & Ward, 1998; Kwekkeboom, Wanta, & Bumpus, 2008). Hypnotizability increases through early childhood, peaking somewhere between ages 7 and 14 and then leveling off into adolescence and adulthood (Olness & Kohen, 1996). Some individuals have naturally high hypnotic abilities: they recall pictures more accurately, generate more complex images, have higher dream-recall frequency in the waking state, and make fewer eye movements in imagery than poor visualizers. However, most individuals can utilize imagery if the experience is adjusted to their needs and preferences (Carli, Cavallaro, & Santarcangelo, 2007; Olness, 2008). Recognizing individual, cultural, and developmental preferences for settings, situations, and preference for either relaxation or stimulation can improve the effectiveness of the imagery and reduce time and frustration with learning it. Practicing imagery oneself is extremely helpful in guiding others.

Measurement of Outcomes

Evaluating and measuring outcomes are important in determining the effectiveness and value of imagery in clinical practice. The clinical outcomes of imagery are related to the context in which it is used and include: physical signs of relaxation; lower levels of anxiety and depression; alteration in symptoms; improved functional performance or quality of life; a sense of meaning, purpose, and/or competency; and positive changes in attitude or behavior. Health services benefits may include reduced costs, morbidity, and reduced length of stay.

The outcomes measured should reflect the client's situation and the conceptual framework providing the rationale for the use of imagery. If imagery is used to facilitate rehabilitation or performance, outcomes would include functional measures such as improved gait or ability to perform a specific task. If imagery is used to control symptoms in clients undergoing chemotherapy for cancer, expected outcomes might include reduced nausea, vomiting, and fatigue, enhanced body image, positive mood states, and improved quality of life. When imagery is used to reduce the stress response and promote relaxation, outcomes may include increased oxygen saturation levels, lower blood pressure and heart rate, warmer extremities, reduced muscle tension, greater alpha waves on electroencephalography, and lower anxiety.

Factors that may influence imagery's success include dose, client characteristics, and condition being treated. Great variability exists in how frequently imagery is recommended. In an attempt to quantify this effect, Van Kuiken (2004) conducted a meta-analysis of 16 published studies going back to 1996. Although the final sample of 10 studies was too small for statistical analysis, Van Kuiken concluded that imagery practice up to 18 weeks increases the effectiveness of the intervention. A minimum dose was not determined and further study is needed to explore a dose relationship with outcomes. To help with standardization of imagery interventions and generalizability, other documentation should include a detailed description of the specific interventions used, outcomes affected by the imagery, and factors influencing effectiveness.

Individual differences such as imaging ability, outcome expectancy, preferred coping style, relationship with the imagery practitioner, and disease state may all affect the outcome of an imagery experience. In a crossover-design pilot study comparing progressive muscle relaxation therapy (PMRT) and imagery to control the combined intervention groups demonstrated improved pain control (Kweekeboom, Wanta, & Bumpus, 2008). However, the individual responder analysis revealed that subjects did not respond equally to each therapy and only half of the participants had reduced pain from each intervention. Imagery sessions were more likely to have positive results when participants had greater imaging ability, positive outcome expectancy, and fewer symptoms. A study of 323 adult medical patients who received six interactive guided imagery sessions with a focus on gaining insight and self-awareness demonstrated that participants' ability to engage in the guided imagery process and the relationship with the practitioner were strong influences on outcome (Scherwitz, McHenry, & Herrero, 2005).

One of the most difficult determinations to make is whether the outcomes are the result solely of imagery or of a combination of factors. Learning and practicing imagery often changes other health-related behaviors, such as getting more sleep, eating a healthier diet, smoking cessation, or exercising regularly. The therapist's presence, attention, and compassion also may constitute an intervention independent of the imagery process.

Precautions

Imagery is generally a safe intervention, as noted in a systematic review of guided imagery for cancer, in which there were no reports of adverse events or side effects (Roffe, Schmidt, & Ernst, 2005). However, occasionally a participant will react negatively to relaxation or to the imagery. Kwekkeboom and colleagues (1998) reported increased anxiety in 3 of 15 subjects using imagery specifically to reduce anxiety associated with a stressful task although the subjects perceived the imagery as pleasant. Huth, Broome, and Good (2004) reported that two children became distressed during guided imagery practice sessions; hence, the authors encourage pre-screening. Some individuals have anecdotally reported increased discomfort or airway constriction or difficulty breathing when they focus on diaphragmatic breathing. This is most likely to occur if the participant is experiencing a symptom such as abdominal pain or dyspnea. Using another centering method, such as focusing on an object in the room or repeating a mantra, can reduce this distressing response and still induce relaxation. Some participants may report feeling out of control or "spacey" when deeply relaxed. The guide can help participants to become more grounded by focusing on an image such as a tree with strong roots or do more alert relaxation such as having eyes open and focusing on an object. Participants may report dizziness which is often related to mild hyperventilation and can be relieved by encouraging them to breathe slower and less deeply.

The expertise and training of the nurse should guide judgment in using imagery to achieve outcomes in practice. Imagery techniques can be easily applied to managing symptoms (pain, nausea, vomiting) and facilitating relaxation, sleep, or anxiety reduction. Advanced techniques often associated with hypnosis, such as age regression and management of depression or posttraumatic stress disorder, require further training.

USES

Imagery has been used therapeutically in a variety of conditions and populations (Exhibit 5.2). Pain and cancer are two conditions in which imagery has been helpful both in adults and in children.

Pain

Pain is a uniquely subjective experience, and proper management depends on individualizing interventions that recognize determinants af-

Exhibit 5.2

Conditions for Which Imagery Has Been Tested

Clinical Condition	Selected Sources
In children and adolescents	
Abdominal pain	Anbar (2001a); Ball, Sharpiro, Monheim, Weydert (2003); Youssef et al. (2004); Weydert et al. (2006); Vlieger, Blink, Tromp, & Benninga (2008)
Asthma	Hackman, Stern, & Gershwin (2000)
Cancer	Richardson, Smith, McCall, & Pilkington (2006)
Chronic dyspnea	Anbar (2001b)
Habit cough	Anbar & Hall (2004)
Headache	Fichtel & Larsson (2004); Olness et al. (1999)
Hospice care	Russell, Smart, & House (2007)
Procedural pain	Butler et al. (2005); Cyna, Tomkins, Moddock, & Barker (2007); Uman, Chambers, McGrath, & Kisely (2008)
Post traumatic stress disorder	Gordon, Staples, Blyta, Bytyqi, & Wilson (2008)
Pain	Baumann (2002); Culbert, Friedrichsdorf, & Kuttner (2008); Wood & Bioy (2008)
Periopertive symptom management (pain, nausea, anxiety, behavioral disorders)	Huth, Broome, & Good (2004); Calipel, Lucas-Polomeni, Wodey, & Ecoffey (2005); Mackenzie & Frawley (2007); Polkki, Pietila, Vehvilainen-Julkunen, Laukkala, & Kiviluoma (2008)
Psychiatry	Anbar (2008)
Sickle cell anemia	Gil et al. (2001)
In adults	
Asthma	Epstein et al. (2004)
Autoimmune disorders	Collins & Dunn (2005); Torem (2007)
Cancer treatment—physical and emotional side effects	Roffe, Schmidt, & Ernest (2005); Yoo, Ahn, Kim, Kim, & Han (2005); Leon-Pizarro et al. (2007); Sloman (2002)
Chronic obstructive pulmonary disease	Louie (2004)

(continued)

Exhibit 5.2 *(continued)*

Clinical Condition	Selected Sources
Counseling	Heinschel (2002); Elliott (2003)
Depression	Chou & Lin (2006)
Fibromyalgia	Creamer, Singh, Hochberg, & Berman (2000); Menzies et al. (2006); Menzies & Kim (2008)
Health and well-being	Watanabe, Fukuda, & Shirakawa (2005); Watanabe et al. (2006)
Immune response in breast cancer	Nunes et al. (2007); Lengacher et al. (2008)
Medical conditions (general)	Scherwitz, McHenry, & Herrero (2005); Toth et al. (2007)
Osteoarthritis	Baird & Sands (2004); Baird & Sands (2006)
Pain–cancer	Kwekkeboom et al. (2008); Kwekkeboom, Wanta & Bumpus (2008); Kwekkeboom, Kneip, & Pearson (2003)
Pain–chronic	Lewandowski, Good, & Draucker (2005); Carrico, Peters, & Diokno (2008); Proctor, Murphy, Pattison, Suckling, & Farquhar (2008); Turk, Swanson, & Tunks (2008)
Pain–postoperative	Antall & Kresevic (2004); Haase et al. (2005)
Pain–phantom limb	Oakley, Whitman, & Halligan (2002); MacIver, Lloyd, Kelly, Roberts, & Nurmikko (2008)
Pain–procedural	Flory, Salazar, & Lang (2007)
Pregnancy	DiPietro, Costigan, Nelson, Gurewitsch, & Laudenslager (2007)
Rehabilitation	Braun et al. (2006), Dunsky, Dickstein, Marcovitz, Levy, & Deutsch (2008)
Sleep	Richardson (2003); Krakow & Zadra (2006)
Smoking cessation	Wynd (2005)
Sports medicine	Newmark & Bogacki (2005); Driediger, Hall, & Callow (2006)

fecting the pain response. Age, temperament, sex, ethnicity, and stage of development are all considerations when developing a pain management plan (Gerik, 2005; Young, 2005). Whether pain is from illness, side effects of treatment, injury, or physical stress on the body, emotional factors contribute to pain perception, and mind–body interventions such as imagery can help make pain more manageable (Reed, 2007). Stress, anxiety, and fatigue decrease the threshold for pain, making the perceived pain more intense. Imagery can break this cycle of pain–tension–anxiety–pain. Relaxation with imagery decreases pain directly by reducing muscle tension and related spasms and indirectly by lowering anxiety and improving sleep. Imagery also is a distraction strategy; vivid, detailed images using all senses tend to work best for pain control. In addition, cognitive reappraisal/restructuring used with imagery can increase a sense of control over the ability to reframe the meaning of pain.

There is a considerable body of research examining the efficacy of guided imagery as a therapy to treat adult pain. Studies have explored the effectiveness of guided imagery in treating cancer pain (Kwekkeboom, Hau, Wanta, & Bumpus, 2008; Kwekkeboom, Wanta, & Bumpus, 2008), dysmenorrhea (Proctor, Murphy, Pattison, Suckling, & Farquhar, 2008), orthopedic pain (Antall & Kresevic, 2004), interstitial cystitis (Carrico, Peters, & Diokno, 2008), and fibromyalgia (Menzies & Kim, 2008; Menzies, Taylor, & Bourguignon, 2006), among others. Results have been variable, but favorable enough to indicate guided imagery may help relieve some forms of pain, especially when used as an adjunct to standard care measures. Although Haase, Schwenk, Hermann, and Muller (2005) found no change in report of pain or analgesic use in a population of colorectal surgery patients, they note that patients responded positively to guided imagery, 79% perceiving a benefit from listening to tapes of either guided imagery or relaxation.

There are many causes of chronic pain, but, whatever the underlying etiology, it is generally challenging and costly to treat and has an impact on many aspects of an individual's life. Analgesic therapy often falls short of achieving adequate pain relief, and successful management frequently depends on the use of cognitive–behavioral techniques, such as imagery (Turk, Swanson, & Tunks, 2008). Two conditions leading to chronic pain in adults are osteoarthritis and fibromyalgia. In a randomized trial of 28 women with osteoarthritis, participants received either standard care or a 12-week program of guided imagery with relaxation (Baird & Sands, 2006). Participants in the intervention group improved in scores of health-related quality of life (HRQOL). Analysis noted that improvement in scores was not completely explained by improved mobility and pain reduction and that the guided imagery and relaxation intervention may have had a positive effect on social and emotional functioning.

Fibromyalgia is a condition of chronic wide-spread pain accompanied by fatigue, disturbed sleep, stiffness, and depression (Menzies & Kim, 2008). In a feasibility study, 20 subjects were enrolled in an 8-week group intervention (Creamer, Singh, Hochberg, & Berman, 2000). Each session included education (30 minutes), relaxation and meditation (1 hour), and Chinese movement therapy–Qi Gong (1 hour). Significant improvement was seen in a number of indicators, including difficulty sleeping, fatigue, social functioning and pain. However, given the small sample, lack of control, and multimodal approach, it is difficult to determine the specific effect of the imagery. Menzies and colleagues investigated the effect of guided imagery on fibromyalgia in a randomized, control trial of 48 subjects (Menzies et al., 2006). Subjects in the intervention group received guided imagery audio tapes and were instructed to use them daily. The control group received usual care. There was improvement in functional status and self-efficacy, but no change in report of pain. Subsequently a small (10-subject) pilot study of Hispanic adults was conducted to assess a 10-week course of imagery with relaxation (Menzies & Kim, 2008). Improvement was seen in daily pain, functional status, and self-efficacy measures, but no improvement was seen in psychological distress and other pain measures. This study has limited generalizability due to its small sample size, lack of control, and use of self-report measures.

In spite of the many advances made in the treatment of pediatric pain, the American Academy of Pediatrics and American Pain Society (2001) report that children's pain continues to be inadequately assessed and managed. They recommend a multimodal approach to pain management to include both pharmacological and nonpharmacological interventions. There are adverse short-term and long-term effects of inadequate pain management in children, including hypoxemia, immobility, altered pulmonary function, posttraumatic stress, and adverse psychological and behavioral patterns (Grunau, Oberlander, & Whitfield, 2001; Lux, Algren, & Algren, 1999; Taddio, Katz, & Ilersich, 1997).

Distraction imagery is particularly helpful in getting a child through a medical procedure with a safe and effective level of sedation/analgesia and as little movement as possible (Butler, Symons, Henderson, Shortliffe, & Spiegel, 2005). Suggestions to breathe deeply and to relax or be comfortable are combined with vivid images of a favorite place or pleasant experience that draw the attention away from the pain. It is best to introduce the child to breathing techniques and explore favorite images prior to the procedure. However, in critical or emergency situations imagery has been successfully employed without pre-work (Kohen, 2000). In a randomized study of 44 children from 4 to 15 years of age undergoing voiding cystourethrography, children who were taught self-hypnotic visual imagery before the procedure were compared with controls that received routine care. Results indicated benefits for the intervention group in the form of parental perception of decreased trauma, decreased observational ratings of distress, increased ease of procedure by physician report, and decreased time to complete the procedure (Butler et al., 2005). In a systemic review of controlled trials of interventions for needle-related procedural pain and distress distraction, combined cognitive–behavioral interventions and hypnosis showed the most promise (Uman, Chambers, McGrath, & Kisely, 2008).

Chronic abdominal pain in childhood can be challenging to treat and has significant impact on the child's quality of life and engagement in school and social activities. The efficacy of imagery and relaxation on abdominal pain was assessed in two studies. Youssef et al. (2004) reported significant improvement over baseline, with overall improvement of pain, fewer pain episodes, decreased intensity, fewer missed school day per month, and improved quality-of-life scores; however, sample size was small and there was no control group. Weydert et al. (2006), in a randomized trial, compared guided imagery to a control group that was taught breathing exercises. The imagery group had significantly fewer days with pain at one and two months. In addition, children in the imagery group had less than four pain episodes a month and did not miss any activities on account of pain. Both of these studies reported no adverse effects.

Huth, Broome, and Good (2004) examined the use of guided imagery as an adjunct to routine analgesics for postoperative tonsillectomy and/or adenoidectomy pain. Significantly less pain was found in the treatment group 1 to 4 hours after surgery, but not at 22 to 24 hours after surgery. Children in the imagery group had 28% less sensory pain,

10% less anxiety, and 8% less affective pain than the children in the control group. A correlation between state of anxiety and sensory pain was high at both points and there were no differences in analgesic use between groups. The researchers reported two adverse events in which children became distressed during the practice sessions.

Cancer Treatment

Imagery interventions in oncology have focused on physiological and psychological responses to cancer treatment. Areas that have been researched are: efficacy in management of symptoms (pain, nausea); influence on surgical outcomes; improvement in quality of life; psychological states (depression, anxiety); and changes in immunity (Lee, 1999; Roffe et al., 2005). Roffe and colleagues, in a systemic literature search that spanned three decades, uncovered 103 articles investigating guided imagery in cancer care. Of these, 27 were case studies, 56 combined imagery with another treatment (PMRT, music therapy, hypnosis, etc.), 12 were uncontrolled trials, and 2 were non-randomized. The authors reviewed in detail 6 randomized control trials. The collective data suggests that guided imagery is most beneficial on psychosocial and quality-of-life indicators. No effects were found on physical symptoms, which may be partially explained by a paucity of distressing symptoms in the subjects. When guided imagery was compared with other relaxation strategies, all study arms did better than the control, indicating that other relaxation strategies are also beneficial or that there is significant overlap between strategies.

In clinical cancer care, relaxation strategies such as PMRT are often paired with imagery. This combination was investigated in a randomized controlled trial of 60 women undergoing chemotherapy treatment for breast cancer (Yoo, Ahn, Kim, Kim, & Han, 2005). Guided imagery was paired with PMRT to determine their effect on nausea and vomiting and quality of life. Thirty patients received PMRT and guided imagery one hour before treatment for six chemotherapy cycles, and were given a tape to use at home. The 30 patients in the control group received standard therapy. Both groups received an antiemetic one-half hour before chemotherapy administration. Patients in the intervention group demonstrated improvement in anticipatory nausea, postchemotherapy nausea, and quality of life. Positive treatment effects on quality of life were present at 3 months and 6 months posttherapy. Similarly, Leon-Pizarro, et al. (2007) conducted a randomized controlled trial of 66 gynecologic and breast cancer patients who were undergoing brachy-therapy (placement of a radioactive source near or within the tumor source). The intervention group had a ten-minute training in relaxation and guided imagery and an individualized cassette for home use while the control group received standard care. The treatment group had statistically significant reductions in anxiety, depression, and body discomfort.

In pediatric oncology, the focus of research has largely been on procedural pain and on the use of hypnosis. A review of seven randomized controlled trials and one nonrandomized controlled clinical trial (Richardson, Smith, McCall, & Pilkington, 2006) reported reductions in pain and anxiety for hypnosis in pediatric oncology patients undergoing procedures (bone marrow aspiration, lumbar puncture, venipuncture). Both this review and a previous one (Wild & Espie, 2004) cite methodological limitations, including: small, underpowered samples; lack of reporting on the method of randomization; concealment of allocation and/or blinding; lack of information on standard care; and wide variation in procedures used.

The role of imagery in improving cancer outcomes has been studied for over two decades. It continues to be difficult to identify the significance of imagery in long-term survival when so many related factors must be considered in cancer survival. Most recently, Sahler, Hunter, and Liesveld (2003) showed reduced time to engraftment in 23 patients undergoing bone marrow transplant. A common explanation for how imagery may improve cancer outcomes is postulated through increasing cellular immune function. Some studies have demonstrated increases in natural killer (NK) cytotoxicity (Fawzy et al., 1990, 1993; Gruber, Hall, Hersh, & Dubois, 1988; Gruber et al., 1993; Gruzelier, 2002; Lengacher et al., 2008; Walker et al., 1996), NK cell numbers (Bakke, Purtzer, & Newton, 2002), and T cell responses (Gruber et al., 1988; Gruber et al., 1993), whereas others have found no differences (Nunes et al., 2007; Post-White et al., 1996; Richardson et al., 1997) or decreases (Zachariae & Bjerring, 1994) in NK numbers and cytotoxicity. Despite inconclusive effects on cancer outcome, imagery interventions have consistently improved coping responses and psychological states in patients with cancer, suggesting that imagery may mediate psychoneuroimmune outcomes in breast and other cancers (Walker, 2004). Further study is needed to determine the clinical significance of immunological effects.

Guided imagery has been identified as one of the 10 most frequently recommended integrative therapies for cancer on the Internet (Schmidt & Ernst, 2004). The low methodological quality of the studies suggests that rigorous research in imagery for cancer is not as prevalent as actual use in clinical practice.

CULTURAL APPLICATIONS

Modern day imagery owes it roots to the use of imagery in traditional healing. Acterberg (1985) describes the image as "the world's oldest and greatest healing resource" (p. 3), and notes that use of imagery is foundational to the shamanic healing found in many healing traditions. Shamanic healing is a centuries-old practice in which imagery is used within an ecstatic or altered state to access the patient's subconscious mind and belief system (Reed, 2007). This opens communication between mind, body, and spirit so as to cure, alleviate suffering, and facilitate spiritual transformation. Epstein (2004) notes that in spiritual life, experiences are images reflecting us back to ourselves.

The interest in imagery as part of a therapeutic treatment plan is found globally. In addition to the many studies from the United States, research on the use and effectiveness of imagery is prevalent in many other countries, including Spain (Leon-Pizarro et al., 2007), Brazil (Nunes, et al., 2007), Korea (Yoo et al., 2005), and Japan (Watanabe, Fukuda, Hara, Maeda, & Ohira, 2006; Watanabe, Fukuda, & Shirakawa, 2005).

It is important to always consider individual preferences and use images that are understandable and acceptable to the participant. As a rule, the most powerful and meaningful image is one that the participant creates rather than one that is supplied by the "guide." Participants will be more likely to choose images that are congruent with their cultural, spiritual, and personal beliefs. The guide or therapist is there to help them utilize that image.

FUTURE RESEARCH

Despite documented relationships between the mind and the body, there continues to be a lack of high-quality intervention trials testing the effectiveness of guided imagery and other mind–body interventions. Although the body of evidence is growing, with many reports of clinical efficacy, more scientifically rigorous research testing outcomes are needed. For example, Richardson et al. (2006) concluded that there is sufficient evidence for the efficacy of hypnosis to manage procedural pain in pediatric oncology, but they note a number of methodological limitations. Small sample sizes, lack of standardized control groups, and inadequate reporting of research methods limit the generalizability of the findings of many imagery studies.

Key questions remain to be answered regarding specific physiologic responses to imagery, the influence of imagery on clinical outcomes and quality of life, and the effect of individual factors. As a low-cost, noninvasive intervention, imagery has the potential to be effective in reducing symptoms and distress across several conditions. Questions to be pursued include:

1. What is the role of imagery in maintaining health and wellness? Should imagery be a component of preventive medicine? Over time, can imagery reduce stress, improve coping, enhance well-being, create healthier lifestyles, and reduce illness in individuals?
2. What is the effect of imagery on clinical outcomes relevant to quality-of-life and health/ illness states and does it have an impact on cost-effectiveness and quality of care?
3. What is the relationship between imagery and other relaxation strategies? Are they more effective when paired or should they be used alone?
4. Does the type of imagery (outcome or process) produce different outcomes? What imagery protocols or processes are most appropriate in specific conditions (use of tape recorder or session with a practitioner; duration and number of sessions)?
5. Is it possible to predict the usefulness of an imagery intervention in specific individuals? Are there certain characteristics of individuals that determine their ability to respond to imagery and produce desired outcomes? Are there certain individuals or conditions for which imagery should not be recommended?
6. What are the long-term effects of imagery?
7. What is the role of practitioner characteristics (type of training, practitioner style, number of different practitioners) in outcomes?

WEB SITES FOR IMAGERY

The following Web sites contain additional information on guided imagery:

Academy for Guided Imagery (2008). Workshops and resources: http://www.academyforguidedimagery.com

American Holistic Nurses Association (2008). Web site: http://www.ahna.org/home/

American Society of Clinical Hypnosis (2008). Certification, workshops, and resources: http://www.asch.net

Association for Music and Imagery (2008). Bonny method of guided imagery and music therapy: http://www.ami-bonnymethod.org

Beyond Ordinary Nursing (2008). Integrative Imagery Training for Health Professionals. Certificate program and continuing education credits for health care professionals: http://www.sdbp.org

Imagination, Mental Imagery, Consciousness, and Cognition: Scientific, Philosophical, and Historical Approaches by Nigel Thomas (November 12, 2008): http://www.imagery-imagination.com

National Center for Complementary and Alternative Medicine (2008). Overview of mind-body medicine: http://nccam.nih.gov/health/backgrounds/mindbody.htm

Society for Developmental and Behavioral Pediatrics (2008). Training in pediatric hypnosis: http://www.sdbp.org

ACKNOWLEDGMENT

The authors would like to acknowledge Janice Post-White, PhD, RN, for her past work on this chapter.

REFERENCES

Achterberg, J. (1985). *Imagery in healing: Shamanism and modern medicine.* Boston: Shambhala.

Ader, R., & Cohen, N. (1981). Conditioned immunopharmacologic responses. In R. Ader (Ed.), *Psychoneuroimmunology* (pp. 281–319). New York: Academic Press.

Ader, R., Felten, D. L., & Cohen, N. (1991). *Psychoneuroimmunology* (2nd ed.). San Diego: Academic Press.

American Academy of Pediatrics Committee on Psychosocial Aspects of Children and Family Health and American Pain Society Task Force on Pain in Infants, Children and Adolescents. (2001). The assessment and management of acute pain in infants, children and adolescents. *Pediatrics, 10*(8), 793–797.

Anbar, R. D. (2001a). Self-hypnosis for the treatment of functional abdominal pain in childhood. *Clinical Pediatrics, 40*(8), 447–451.

Anbar, R. D. (2001b). Self-hypnosis for management of chronic dyspnea in pediatric patients. *Pediatrics, 107*(2):e21 [electronic version].

Anbar, R. D. (2008). Subconscious guided therapy with hypnosis. *American Journal of Clinical Hypnosis, 50*(4), 323–334.

Anbar, R. D., & Hall, H. R. (2004). Childhood habit cough treated with self-hypnosis. *Journal of Pediatrics, 144*, 213–217.

Andrasik, F., & Rime, C. (2007). Can behavioural therapy influence neuromodulation? *Neurological Sciences, 28* (Suppl. 2), S124–S129.

Antall, G. F., & Kresevic, D. (2004). The use of guided imagery to manage pain in an elderly orthopaedic population. *Orthopedic Nursing, 23*(5), 335–340.

Baird, C. L., & Sands, L. (2004). A pilot study of the effectiveness of guided imagery with progressive muscle relaxation to reduce chronic pain and mobility difficulties of osteoarthritis. *Pain Management Nursing, 5*(3), 97–104.

Baird, C. L., & Sands, L. (2006). Effect of guided imagery with relaxation on health-related quality of life in older women with osteoarthritis. *Research in Nursing and Health, 29*, 442–451.

Bakke, A. C., Purtzer, M. Z., & Newton, P. (2002). The effect of hypnotic-guided imagery on psychological well-being and immune function in patients with prior breast cancer. *Journal of Psychosomatic Research, 53*(6), 1131–1137.

Ball, T. M., Shapiro, D. E., Monheim, C. J., & Wydert, J. A. (2003). A pilot study of the use of guided imagery for the treatment of recurrent abdominal pain in children. *Clinical Pediatrics, 42*(6), 527–532.

Baumann, R. J. (2002). Behavioral treatment of migraine in children and adolescents. *Pediatric Drugs, 4*(9), 555–561.

Braun, S. M., Beurskens, A. J., Borm, P. J., Schack, T., & Wade, D. T. (2006). The effects of mental practice in stroke rehabilitation: A systematic review. *Archives of Physical Medicine and Rehabilitation, 87*, 842–852.

Butler, L. D., Symons, B. K., Henderson, S. L., Shortliffe, L. D., & Spiegel, D. (2005). Hypnosis reduces distress and duration of an invasive medical procedure for children. *Pediatrics, 115*(1), e77–e85.

Cacioppo, J. T., Berntson, G. G., Malarkey, W. B., Kiecolt-Glaser, J. K., Sheridan, J. F., Poehlmann, K., et al. (1998). Autonomic, neuroendocrine, and immune responses to psychological stress: The reactivity hypothesis. *Annals of the New York Academy of Sciences, 1*(840), 664–673.

Calipel, S., Lucas-Polomeni, M. M., Wodey, E., &, Ecoffey, C. (2005). Premedication in children: Hypnosis versus midazolam. *Pediatric Anesthesia, 15*, 275–281.

Carli, G., Cavallaro, F. I., & Santarcangelo, E. L. (2007). Hypnotizability and imagery modality preference: Do highs and lows live in the same world? *Contemporary Hypnosis, 24*(2), 64–75.

Carrico, D. J., Peters, K. M., & Diokno, A. C. (2008). Guided imagery for women with interstitial cystitis: Results of a prospective, randomized controlled pilot study. *Journal of Alternative and Complementary Medicine, 14*(1), 53–60.

Chou, M. H., & Lin, M. F. (2006). Exploring the listening experiences during guided imagery and music therapy of outpatients with depression. *Journal of Nursing Research, 14*(2), 93–102.

Collins, M. P., & Dunn, L. F. (2005). The effects of meditation and visual imagery on an immune system disorder: Dermatomyositis. *Journal of Alternative and Comlementary Medicine, 11*(2), 275–284.

Creamer, P., Singh, B. B., Hochberg, M. C., & Berman, B. M. (2000). Sustained improvement produced by nonpharmacologic intervention in fibromyalgia: Results of a pilot study. *Arthritis Care and Research, 13*(4), 198–204.

Culbert, T., Friedrichsdorf, S., & Kuttner, L. (2008). Mind-body skills for children in pain. In H. Breivik, W. I. Campbell, & M. K. Nicholas (Eds.), *Clinical pain management: Practice and procedures* (2nd ed., pp. 478–495). London: Hodder Arnold.

Cyna, A. M., Tomkins, D., Maddock, T., & Bardker, D. (2007). Brief hypnosis of severe needle phobia using switch-wire imagery in a 5-year-old. *Pediatric Anesthesia, 17,* 800–804.

DiPietro, J. A., Costigan, K. A., Nelson, P., Gurewitsch, E. D., & Laudenslager, M. L. (2008). Fetal responses to induced maternal relaxation during pregnancy. *Biological Psychology, 77,* 11–19.

Djordjevic J., Zatorre, R. J., Petrides, M., Boyle, J. A., & Jones-Gotaman, M. (2005). Functional neuroimaging of odor imagery. *Neuroimage, 24*(3), 791–801.

Donaldson, V. W. (2000). A clinical study of visualization on depressed white blood cells in medical patients. *Applied Psychophysiology and Biofeedback, 25*(2), 230–235.

Dossey, B. (1995). Complementary modalities. Part 3: Using imagery to help your patient heal. *American Journal of Nursing, 96*(6), 41–47.

Driediger, M., Hall, C., & Callow, N. (2006). Imagery use by injured athletes: A qualitative analysis. *Journal of Sports Sciences, 24*(3), 261–271.

Dunsky, A., Dickstein, R., Marcovitz, E., Levy, S., & Deutsch, J. (2008). Home-based motor imagery training for gait rehabilitation of people with chronic poststroke hemiparesis. *Archives in Physical Medicine and Rehabilitation, 89,* 1580–1588.

Elliot, H. (2003). Imagework as a means for healing and personal transformation. *Complementary Therapies in Nursing and Midwifery, 9,* 118–124.

Epstein, G. (2004). Mental imagery: The language of spirit. *Advances, 20*(3), 4–10.

Epstein, G. N., Halper, J. P., Barrett, E. A., Birdsal, C., McGee, M., Baron, K. P., et al. (2004). A pilot study of mind–body changes in adults with asthma who practice mental imagery. *Alternative Therapies, 10*(4), 66–71.

Fawzy, F. I., Fawzy, N. W., Hyun, C. S., Elashoff, R., Guthrie, D., Fahey, J. L., et al. (1993). Malignant melanoma: Effects of an early structured psychiatric intervention, coping and affective state on recurrence and survival 6 years later. *Archives of General Psychiatry, 50,* 681–689.

Fawzy, F. I., Kemeny, M. E., Fawzy, N. W., Elashoff, R., Morton, D., Cousins, N., & Fahey, J. L. (1990). A structured psychiatric intervention for cancer patients II. Changes over time in immunological measures. *Archives of General Psychiatry, 47,* 729–735.

Fichtel, A., & Larsson, B. (2004). Relaxation treatment administered by school nurses to adolescents with recurrent headaches. *Headache, 44,* 545–554.

Fleshner, M., & Laudenslager, M. L. (2004). Psychoneuroimmunology: Then and now. *Behavioral and Cognitive Neuroscience Reviews, 3* (2), 114–130.

Flory, N., Salazar, G. M. M., & Lang, E. V. (2007). Hypnosis for acute distress management during medical procedures. *International Journal of Clinical and Experimental Hypnosis, 55*(3), 303–317.

Formisano, E., Linden, D. E. J., DiSalle, F., Trojano, L., Esposito, F., Sack, A.T., et al. (2002). Tracking the mind's image in the brain: Time-resolved fMRI during visuospatial mental imagery. *Neuron, 35,* 185–194.

Gerik, S. M. (2005). Pain Management in children: Developmental considerations and mind–body therapies. *Southern Medical Journal, 98*(3), 295–301.

Gil, K. M., Anthony, K. K., Carson, J. W., Redding-Lallinger, R., Daescher, C. W., & Ware, R. E. (2001). Daily coping practice predicts treatment effects in children with sickle cell disease. *Journal of Pediatric Psychology, 26*(3), 163–173.

Glaser, R., MacCallum, R. C., Laskowski, B. F., Malarkey, W. B., Sheridan, J. F., & Kiecolt-Glaser, J. K. (2001). Evidence for a shift in the Th-1 to Th-2 cytokine response associated with chronic stress and aging. *Journal of Gerontology. A: Biological Science and Medical Science, 56*(8), M477–M482.

Gordon, J. S., Staples, J. K., Blyta, A., Bytyqi, M., & Wilson, A. (2008). Treatment of posttraumatic stress disorder in postwar Kosovar adolescents using mind–body skills groups: A randomized controlled trial. *Journal of Clinical Pyschiatry, 69*(9), 1469–1476.

Gruber, B. L., Hall, N. R., Hersh, S. P., & Dubois, P. (1988). Immune system and psychologic changes in metastatic cancer patients while using ritualized relaxation and guided imagery: A pilot study. *Scandinavian Journal of Behavioral Therapy, 17,* 25–46.

Gruber, B. L., Hersh, S. P., Hall, N. R., Waletzky, L. R., Kunz, J. F., Carpenter, J. K., et al. (1993). Immunological responses of breast cancer patients to behavioral interventions. *Biofeedback and Self Regulation, 18*(1), 1–22.

Grunau, R. E., Oberlander, T. F., & Whitfield, M. F. (2001). Demographic and therapeutic determinants of pain reactivity in very low birth weight neonates at 32 weeks postconception age. *Pediatrics, 107,* 105–117.

Gruzelier, J. H. (2002). A review of the impact of hypnosis, relaxation, guided imagery and individual differences on aspects of immunity and health. *Stress, 5*(2), 147–163.

Gulyas, B. (2001). Neural networks for internal reading and visual imagery of reading: A PET study. *Brain Research Bulletin, 54*(3), 319–328.

Haase, O., Schwenk, W., Hermann, C., & Muller, J. M. (2005). Guided imagery and relaxation in conventional colorectal resections: A randomized, controlled, partially blinded trial. *Diseases of the Colon and Rectum, 48*(10), 1955–1963.

Hackman, R. M., Stern, J. S., & Gershwin, M. E. (2000). Hypnosis and asthma: A critical review. *Journal of Asthma, 37*(1), 1–15.

Heinschel, J. A. (2002). A descriptive study of the interactive guided imagery experience. *Journal of Holistic Nursing, 20*, 325–346.

Huth, M. M., Broome, M. E., & Good, M. (2004). Imagery reduces children's postoperative pain. *Pain, 110*(1–2), 439–448.

Huth, M. M., VanKuiken, D. M., & Broome, M. E. (2006). Playing in the park: What school age children tell us about imagery. *Journal of Pediatric Nursing, 21*(2), 115–125.

Kohen, D. (2000, June). *Integrating hypnosis into practice.* Presented at the Introductory Workshop in Clinical Hypnosis. St. Paul, MN: University of Minnesota and the Minnesota Society of Clinical Hypnosis.

Kosslyn, S. M., Ganis, G., & Thompson, W. (2001). Neural foundations of imagery. *Nature Reviews, 2*, 635–642.

Kraemer, D. J., Macrae, C. N., Green, A. E., & Kelley, W. M. (2005). Musical imagery: Sound of silence activates auditory cortex. *Nature, 434*(7030), 158.

Krakow, B., & Zadra, A. (2006). Clinical management of chronic nightmares: Imagery rehearsal therapy. *Behavioral Sleep Medicine, 4*(1), 45–70.

Kwekkeboom, K., Huseby-Moore, K., & Ward, S. (1998). Imaging ability and effective use of guided imagery. *Research in Nursing and Health, 21*, 189–198.

Kwekkeboom, K., Kneip, J., & Pearson, L. (2003). A pilot study to predict success with guided imagery for cancer pain. *Pain Management Nursing, 4*(3), 112–123.

Kwekkeboom, K. L., Hau, H., Wanta, B., & Bumpus, M. (2008). Patients' perceptions of the effectiveness of guided imagery and progressive muscle relaxation interventions used for cancer pain. *Complementary Therapies in Clinical Practice, 14*, 185–194.

Kwekkeboom, K. L., Wanta, B., & Bumpus, M. (2008). Individual difference variables and the effects of progressive muscle relaxation and analgesic imagery interventions on cancer pain. *Journal of Pain and Symptom Management, 36*(6), 604–615.

Lacourse, M. G., Turner, J. A., Randolph-Orr, E., Schandler, S. L., & Cohen, M. J. (2004). Cerebral and cerebellar sensorimotor placticity following motor imagery-based mental practice of a sequential movement. *Journal of Rehabilitation Research and Development, 41*(4), 505–524.

Langley, P., Fonseca, J., & Iphofen, R. (2006). Psychoneuroimmunology and health from a nursing perspective. *British Journal of Nursing, 15*(29), 1126–1129.

Lee, R. (1999). Guided imagery as supportive therapy in cancer treatment. *Alternative Medicine Alert, 2*(6), 61–64.

Lengacher, C. A., Bennett, M. P., Gonzalez, L., Gilvary, D., Cox, C. E., Cantor, A., et al. (2008). Immune responses to guided imagery during breast cancer treatment. *Biological Research in Nursing, 9*(3), 205–214.

Leon-Pizarro, C., Gich, I., Barthe, E., Rovirosa, A., Farrus, B., Casa, F., et al. (2007). A randomized trial of the effect of training in relaxation and guided imagery techniques in improving psychological and quality-of-life indices for gynecologic and breast brachytherapy patients. *Psycho-Oncology, 16*, 971–979.

Lewandowski, W., Good, M., & Draucker, C. B. (2005). Changes in the meaning of pain with the use of guided imagery. *Pain Management Nursing, 6*(2), 58–67.

Louie, S. W. (2004). The effects of guided imagery relaxation in people with COPD. *Occupational Therapy International, 11*(3), 145–159.

Lux, M., Algren, C. L., & Algren, J. T. (1999). Management strategies for ensuring adequate analgesia in children. *Disease Management Health Outcomes, 6*(1), 37–44.

McCance, K. L., & Huether, S. E. (2002). *Pathophysiology: The biologic basis for disease in adults and children* (4th ed.). St. Louis, MO: Mosby.

MacIver, K., Lloyd, D. M., Kelly, S., Roberts, N., & Nurmikko, T. (2008). Phantom limb pain, cortical reorganization and the therapeutic effect of mental imagery. *Brain, 131,* 2181–2191.

Mackenzie, A., & Frawley, G. P. (2007). Preoperative hypnotherapy in the management of a child with anticipatory nausea and vomiting. *Anesthesia and Intensive Care, 35,* 784–787.

Maes, M., Song, C., Lin, A., De Jongh, R., Van Gastel, A., Kenis, G., et al. (1998). The effects of psychological stress on humans: Increased production of pro-inflammatory cytokines and a Th1-like response in stress-induced anxiety. *Cytokine, 10*(4), 313–318.

Menzies, V., & Kim, S. (2008). Relaxation and guided imagery in Hispanic persons diagnosed with fibromyalgia: A pilot study. *Family and Community Health, 31*(3), 204–212.

Menzies, V., Taylor, A. G., & Bourguignon, C. (2006). Effects of guided imagery on outcomes of pain, functional status, and self-efficacy in persons diagnosed with fibromyalgia. *Journal of Alternative and Complementary Medicine, 12*(1), 12–30.

Newmark, T. S., & Bogacki, D. F. (2005). The use of relaxation, hypnosis, and imagery in sport psychiatry. *Clinics in Sports Medicine, 21,* 973–977.

Nunes, D. F. T., Rodriguez, A. L., Hoffman, F. S., Luz, C., Filho, A. P. F. B., Muller, M. C., & Bauer, M. E. (2007). Relaxation and guided imagery program in patients with breast cancer undergoing radiotherapy is not associated with neuroimmunomodulatory effects. *Journal of Psychosomatic Research, 63,* 647–655.

Oakley, D. A., Whitman, L. G., & Halligan, P. W. (2002). Hypnotic imagery as a treatment for phantom limb pain: Two case reports and a review. *Clinical Rehabilitation, 16,* 368–377.

Olness, K. (2008). Helping children and adults with hypnosis and biofeedback. *Cleveland Clinic Journal of Medicine, 75*(2), S39–S43.

Olness, K., Hall, H., Rozniecki, J. J., Schmidt, W., & Theoharides, T. C. (1999). Mast cell activation in children with migraine before and after training in self-regulation. *Headache, 39,* 101–107.

Olness, K., & Kohen, D. (1996). *Hypnosis and hypnotherapy with children* (3rd ed.). New York: Guilford.

Pert, C. B., Dreher, H. E., & Ruff, M. R. (1998). The psychosomatic network: Foundations of mind–body medicine. *Alternative Therapies, 4*(4), 30–41.

Polkki, T., Pietila, A. M., Vehvilainen-Julkunen, K., Laukkala, H., & Kiviluoma, K. (2008). Imagery-induced relaxation in children's postoperative pain relief: A randomized pilot study. *Journal of Pediatric Nursing, 23*(3), 217–224.

Post-White, J., Schroeder, L., Hannahan, A., Johnston, M. K., Salscheider, N., & Grandt, N. (1996). Response to imagery/support in breast cancer survivors. *Oncology Nursing Forum, 23*(2), 355.

Proctor, M. L., Murphy, P. A., Pattison, H. M., Suckling, J., & Farquhar, C. M. (2008). Behavioural interventions for primary and secondary dysmenorrhoea (review). *Cochrane Library, 4,* 1–24.

Reed, T. (2007). Imagery in the clinical setting: A tool for healing. *Nursing Clinics of North America, 42,* 261–277.

Richardson, J., Smith, J. E., McCall, G., & Pilkington, K. (2006). Hypnosis for procedure-related pain and distress in pediatric cancer patients: A systematic review of effectiveness and methodology related to hypnosis interventions. *Journal of Pain and Symptom Management, 31*(1), 70–84.

Richardson, M. A., Post-White, J., Grimm, E. A., Moye, L. A., Singletary, S. E., & Justice, B. (1997). Coping, life attitudes, and immune responses to imagery and group support after breast cancer. *Alternative Therapies in Health and Medicine, 3*(5), 62–70.

Richardson, S. (2003). Effects of relaxation and imagery on the sleep of critically ill adults. *Dimensions of Critical Care Nursing, 22*(4), 182–190.

Roffe, L., Schmidt, K., & Ernst, E. (2005). A systematic review of guided imagery as an adjuvant cancer therapy. *Psycho-oncology, 14,* 607–617.

Russell, C., Smart, S., House, D. (2007). Guided imagery and distraction therapy in paediatric hospice care. *Paediatric Nursing, 19*(2) 24–25.

Sahler, O. L., Hunter, B. C., & Liesveld, J. L. (2003). The effect of using music therapy with relaxation imagery in the management of patients undergoing bone marrow transplantation: A pilot feasibility study. *Alternative Therapies in Health & Medicine, 9*(6), 70–74.

Scherwitz, L. W., McHenry, P., & Herrero, R. (2005). Interactive guided imagery therapy with medical patients: Predictors of health outcomes. *Journal of Alternative and Complementary Medicine, 11*(1), 69–83.

Schmidt, K., & Ernst, E. (2004). Assessing websites on complementary and alternative medicine for cancer. *Annals of Oncology, 15,* 733–742 [electronic version].

Sloman, R. (2002). Relaxation and imagery for anxiety and depression control in community patients with advanced cancer. *Cancer Nursing, 25*(6), 432–435.

Taddio, A., Katz, J., & Ilersich, A. L. (1997). The effects of neonatal circumcision on pain response during subsequent routine vaccination. *Lancet, 349,* 599–603.

Torem, M. S. (2007). Mind-body hypotic imagery in the treatment of auto-immune disorders. *American Journal of Clincal Hypnosis, 50*(2), 157–170.

Toth, M., Wolsko, P. M, Foreman, J., Davis, R. B., Delbance, T., & Phillips, R. S. (2007). A pilot study for a randomized, controlled trail on the effect of guided imagery in hospitalized medical patients. *Journal of Alternative and Complementary Medicine, 13*(2), 194–197.

Trakhtenberg, E. C. (2008). The effects of guided imagery on the immune system: A critical review. *International Journal of Neuroscience, 118,* 839–855.

Turk, D. C., Swanson, K. S., & Tunks, E. R. (2008). Psychological approaches in the treatment of chronic pain patients—when pills, scalpels and needles are not enough. *Canadian Journal of Psychiatry, 53*(4), 213–223.

Uman, L. S., Chambers, C. T., McGrath, P. J., & Kisely, S. (2008). A systematic review of randomized controlled trials examining psychological interventions for needle-related procedural pain and distress in children and adolescents: An abbreviated Cochrane review. *Journal of Pediatric Psychology, 33*(8), 842–854.

Van Kuiken, D. (2004). A meta-analysis of the effect of guided imagery practice on outcomes. *Journal of Holistic Nursing, 22*(2), 164–179.

Vlieger, A. M., Blink, M., Tromp, E., & Benninga, M. (2008). Use of complementary and alternative medicine by pediatric patients with functional and organic gastrointestinal diseases: Results from a multicenter survey. *Pediatrics, 122*, e446–e451. Online version; retrieved November 2008, from http://www.pediatrics.org/cgi/content/full/122/2/e446

Walker, L. G. (2004). Hypnotherapeutic insights and interventions: A cancer odyssey. *Contemporary Hypnosis, 21*(1), 35–45.

Walker, L. G., Miller, I., Walker, M. B., Simpson, E., Ogston, K., Segar, A., et al. (1996). Immunological effects of relaxation training and guided imagery in women with locally advanced breast cancer. *Psycho-Oncology, 5*(3), (Suppl. 16), 16.

Watanabe, E., Fukuda, S., Hara, H., Maeda, Y., & Ohira, H. (2006). Differences in relaxation by means of guided imagery in a healthy community sample. *Alternative Therapies, 12*(2), 60–66.

Watanabe, E., Fukuda, S., & Shirakawa, T. (2005). Effects amoung healthy subjects of the duration of regularly practicing a guided imagery program. *BMC Complementary and Alternative Medicine, 5*(21), 1–8. [doi:10.1186/1472-6882-5-21].
Accessible online at http://www.biomedcentral.com/1472-6882/5/21

Weydert, J. A., Shapiro D. E., Acra, S. A., Monheim, C. J., Chambers, A. S., & Ball, T. M. (2006). Evaluation of guided imagery as treatment for recurrent abdominal pain in children: A randomized controlled trial. *BMC Pediatrics, 6*(29), 1–10. Accessible online at http://www.biomedcentral.com/1471-2431/6/29

Wild, M. R., & Espie, C. A. (2004). The efficacy of hypnosis in the reduction of procedural pain and distress in pediatric oncology: A systematic review. *Developmental and Behavioral Pediatrics, 25*(3), 207–213.

Wood, C., & Bioy, A. (2008). Hypnosis and pain in children. *Journal of Pain and Symptom Management, 35*(4), 437–446.

Wynd, C. A. (2005). Guided health imagery for smoking cessation and long-term abstinence. *Journal of Nursing Scholarship, 37*(3), 245–250.

Yoo, H. J, Ahn, S. H, Kim, S. B., Kim, W. K., & Han, O. S.. (2005). Efficacy of progressive muscle relaxation training and guided imagery in reducing chemotherapy side effects in patients with breast cancer and in improving their quality of life. *Supportive Care in Cancer, 13*, 826–833.

Young, K. D. (2005). Pediatric procedural pain. *Annals of Emergency Medicine, 45*(2), 160–171.

Youssef, N. N., Rosh, J. R., Loughran, M., Schuckalo, S. G., Cotter, A. N., Verga, B. G., et al. (2004). Treatment of functional abdominal pain in childhood with cognitive behavioral strategies. *Journal of Pediatric and Gastroenterological Nutrition, 39*(2), 192–196.

Zachariae, R., & Bjerring, P. (1994). Laser-induced pain-related brain potentials and sensory pain ratings in high and low hypnotizable subjects during hypnotic suggestions of relaxation, dissociated imagery, focused analgesia, and placebo. *International Journal of Clinical and Experimental Hypnosis, XLII* (1), 56–80.

6 Music Intervention

LINDA L. CHLAN

Music has been used throughout history as a treatment modality. From the time of the ancient Egyptians, the power of music to affect health has been noted. Nursing pioneer Florence Nightingale recognized the healing power of music (1860/1969). Today, nurses can use music in a variety of settings to benefit patients and clients.

DEFINITIONS

The *American Heritage Dictionary*® *of the English Language* (2000) defines music as "the art of arranging sounds in time so as to provide a continuous, unified and evocative composition, as through melody, harmony, rhythm, and timbre." Alvin (1975) delineated five main elements of music. The character of a piece of music and its effects depend on the qualities of these elements and their relationships to one another:

- **Frequency** or **pitch** is produced by the number of vibrations of a sound—the highness or lowness of a musical tone, noted by the letters A, B, C, D, E, F, G. Rapid vibrations tend to act as a stimulant, whereas slow vibrations bring about relaxation.

- **Intensity** creates the volume of the sound, related to the amplitude of the vibrations. A person's like or dislike of certain music partially depends on intensity, which can be used to produce intimacy (soft music) or power (loud music).
- **Tone color** or **timbre** is a nonrhythmical, subjective property that results from harmony. Psychological significance results from the timbre of music because of associations with past events or feelings.
- **Interval** is the distance between two notes related to pitch, which creates melody and harmony. Melody results from how musical pitches are sequenced and the interval between them. Harmony results from the way pitches are sounded together, described by the listener as consonant (conveying the feeling of restfulness) or dissonant (conveying the feeling of tension). Cultural norms determine what a listener deems enjoyable and pleasant.
- **Duration** creates rhythm and tempo. Duration refers to the length of sounds, and rhythm is a time pattern fitted into a certain speed. Rhythm is what influences one to move with music in a certain manner and can convey peace and security, whereas repetitive rhythms can elicit feelings of depression. Continuous sounds that are repeated at a slow pace and become gradually slower produce decreased levels of responsiveness. Strong rhythms can awaken feelings of power and control.

From a nursing perspective, music intervention is the use of music for therapeutic purposes to promote patient/client health and well-being. Music therapists are employed in many health care facilities, and countless situations arise in which nurses can implement music intervention in a patient's plan of care. So as not to confuse the practice of music therapy with the use of music from a nursing perspective, the term *music intervention* will be used in this chapter.

SCIENTIFIC BASIS

Music is complex and affects the physiological, psychological, and spiritual dimensions of human beings. Individual responses to music can be influenced by personal preferences, the environment, education, and cultural factors.

Entrainment, a physics principle, is a process whereby two objects vibrating at similar frequencies will tend to cause mutual sympathetic resonance, resulting in their vibrating at the same frequency (Maranto, 1993). Music and physiological processes (heartbeat, blood pressure, body temperature, adrenal hormones, etc.) involve vibrations that occur in a regular, periodic manner and consist of oscillations (Saperstein, 1995). Rhythm and tempo of music can be used to synchronize or entrain body rhythms (e.g., heart rate, respiratory pattern) with resultant changes in physiological states. Certain properties of music (less than 80 beats per minute with fluid, regular rhythm) can be used to promote relaxation by causing body rhythms to slow down or "entrain" with the slower beat and regular, repetitive rhythm (Robb, Nichols, Rutan, Bishop, & Parker, 1995).

Likewise, music can decrease anxiety by occupying attention channels in the brain with meaningful, distractive auditory stimuli (Bauldoff, Hoffman, Zullo, & Sciurba, 2002). Music intervention provides a patient/client with a familiar, comforting stimulus that can evoke pleasurable sensations while refocusing the individual's attention onto the music instead of on stressful thoughts or other environmental stimuli.

INTERVENTION

Determining a patient's music preferences through assessment is essential; among the tools developed for this purpose is an assessment instrument by Chlan and Tracy (1999), which elicits information on how frequently music is listened to, the type of musical selections preferred, and the person's reasons for listening to music. For some people the purpose of listening to music may be to relax, whereas others may prefer music that stimulates and invigorates. After assessment data have been gathered, appropriate techniques with specific music can then be devised and implemented.

Techniques

The use of music can take many forms, such as (passively) listening to selected compact discs (CDs) or individual music downloads from the Internet, or actively singing or drumming. A number of factors should be kept in mind when considering the specific technique: the type of music and personal preferences, active versus passive and/or individual versus group involvement, length of time involved, and desired outcomes. Two of the more commonly used music intervention techniques will be discussed here: individual listening and group work.

Individual Music Listening

Providing the means for patients to listen to music is the intervention technique most frequently implemented by nurses. CDs or MP3 downloads from a reputable Internet source (such as www.MyMusicInc.com or iTunes) make it easy to provide music intervention for patients/ clients in a wide range of settings. CD players are relatively inexpensive; they are small and can be used in even the most crowded confines, such as critical care units. CD players have superior sound clarity and track-seeking that allows immediate selection of a desired piece. Comfortable headphones allow patients private listening that does not disturb others. Equipment selected for music intervention should be easy for patients to use with minimal effort. Small, MP3 players, like the Apple iPod®, are more expensive than CD players and should be reserved for patients with intact dexterity and sufficient visual acuity to operate the small unit.

With only a very modest outlay of money, a nursing unit can establish a library containing a wide variety of selections to suit various musical preferences. The Public Radio Music Source (www.prms.org) offers a great variety of music for purchase. It is also easy to individualize CDs/MP3 files to accommodate the preferences of each patient. Attention to copyright laws is necessary when reproducing CDs or downloading music from Internet sites (go to www.copyright.gov for guidance).

Although various musical genres are available on the radio, commercial messages and talking are deterrents to using them for music intervention. Likewise, one cannot control the quality of the radio signal reception or the specific music selections.

Group Music Making

Music can be used for patient groups as a powerful integrating force. Music creates interrelationships among the members as well as between the listener and the music. One method of group music making is drumming, a form of rhythmic auditory stimulation. Drumming has been found to reduce posttraumatic stress disorder (PTSD) symptoms in a small group of soldiers, both by serving as an outlet for rage and for regaining a sense of control (Bensimon, Amir, & Wolf, 2008). Drumming circles induce relaxation by entraining theta and alpha brain waves, leading to altered states of consciousness by activation of the limbic brain region with the lower brain (Winkelman, 2003). Drumming circles have been used effectively to reduce burnout and improve mood in nursing students (Bittman et al., 2004) and to enhance recovery from a variety of chemical addictions (Winkelman, 2003).

Before implementing this type of group music making, nurses should consult with experts in drumming. The American Music Therapy Association Web site (www.musictherapy.org) can provide assistance in locating a music therapist. Further, diversity in the preferences, interests, and abilities of individuals in a group or the difficulties of securing an appropriate site for a group session may necessitate implementing music on an individual basis; group sessions also require more planning than do individual sessions.

Types of Music for Intervention

Careful attention to the selection of the music contributes to its therapeutic effect. For example, music to induce relaxation has a regular rhythm (less than 80 beats per minute), no extreme pitch or dynamics, and a melodic sound that is smooth and flowing (Robb et al., 1995). Past experiences can influence one's response to music as well.

Older persons may prefer patriotic and popular songs from an earlier era or hymns with slower tempos played with familiar instruments (Moore, Staum, & Brotons, 1992). Religious music may be welcomed by persons who are unable to attend religious services.

Classical music is thought to evoke greater enjoyment and interest with repeated listening, whereas popular music declines in effectiveness with repetition (Bonny, 1986). Bonny believes that patients in a weakened state respond less to popular music and more to the stimulus of classical music that has endured over time. In any event, providing a choice and considering a person's musical preferences are imperative.

New Age, synthesized, or nontraditional music has become very popular. This type of music differs from traditional music, which is characterized by tension and release (Guzzetta, 1995). However, some experts think that this type of synthesized music is not appropriate for relaxation because of the novelty of the stimulus and the absence of the usual forms found in more traditional music (Bonny, 1986; Hanser, 1988). Music perceived as unfamiliar will cause an orienting response that may undermine goals for intervention (Maranto, 1993).

Guidelines

Music intervention for the purpose of relaxation uses music as a pleasant stimulus to block out sensations of anxiety, fear, and tension and to divert attention from unpleasant thoughts (Thaut, 1990). A minimum of 20 minutes of music is necessary to induce relaxation, along with some form of relaxation exercise, such as deep breathing, prior to initiating music intervention (Guzzetta, 1995).

Although the definition of relaxing music may vary by individual, factors affecting response include musical preferences, familiarity of selections, and cultural background. Relaxing music should have a tempo at or below a resting heart rate (less than 80 beats per minute); predictable dynamics; fluid melodic movement; pleasing harmonies; regular rhythm without sudden changes; and tonal qualities that include strings, flute, piano, or specially synthesized music (Robb et al., 1995). One of the most widely used classical music selections for relaxation is Pachelbel's Canon in D Major, which is frequently included in commercially available relaxation CDs. Exhibit 6.1 outlines the basic steps for implementing music intervention for promoting relaxation.

Measurement of Outcomes

The outcome indices for evaluating the effectiveness of music vary, depending on the purpose for which the music is implemented. Outcomes may be physiological or psychological alterations and include a decrease in anxiety or stress arousal, promotion of relaxation, increase in social interaction, reduction in the need for medications, and increase in overall well-being. The nurse should carefully consider the goals of intervention and select outcome measurements accordingly.

Precautions

Adaptation occurs if the auditory system is continually exposed to the same type of stimulus (Farber, 1982). Neural adaptation can occur after 3 minutes of continuous exposure, with the result that music is no

Exhibit 6.1

Guidelines for Music Intervention for Relaxation

1. Ascertain that patient has adequate hearing.
2. Ascertain patient's like/dislike for music.
3. Assess music preferences and previous experience with music for relaxation.
4. Provide a choice of relaxing selections; assist with CD/MP3 selections as needed.
5. Determine agreed-upon goals for music intervention with patient.
6. Complete all nursing care prior to intervention; allow for a minimum of 20 minutes of uninterrupted listening time.
7. Gather equipment (CD or MP3 player, CDs, headphones, fresh batteries) and ensure all are in good working order.
8. Assist patient to a comfortable position as needed; ensure call-light is within easy reach and assist patient with equipment as needed.
9. Enhance environment as needed (draw blinds, close door, turn off lights, etc.).
10. Post a "Do Not Disturb" sign to minimize unnecessary interruptions.
11. Encourage and provide patient with opportunities to "practice" relaxation with music.
12. Document patient responses to music intervention.
13. Revise intervention plan and goal(s) as needed.

longer a stimulant and may not have the intended calming influence. Use of stimulation such as music in the first phase following head injury may increase intracranial pressure. Music of a stimulating quality should be delayed until the autonomic nervous system has stabilized. Quiet music may be used to induce relaxation and block irritating sounds from the environment; however, the patient's individual response to music should be monitored.

Careful control of volume is essential. Permanent ear damage results from exposure to high frequencies and volumes. Decibels higher than 90 dBSL cause discomfort (Idzoriek, 1982), and fatigue occurs more frequently when stimulation is at higher frequencies (Farber, 1982).

Initiating music intervention without first assessing a person's likes and dislikes may produce deleterious effects. Because of music's effect on the limbic system, it can bring about intense emotional responses. Use of portable players with headphones may be inappropriate for patients in psychiatric settings, who may use the equipment cords for self-harm.

USES

Music has been tested as a therapeutic intervention with many different patient populations, with a majority of the nursing literature focusing

on individualized music listening. Exhibit 6.2 shows those patient populations and the numerous therapeutic purposes which music has served.
Two frequent uses will be highlighted here.

Decreasing Anxiety and Stress

One of the strongest effects of music is anxiety reduction (Standley,
1986). Music can enhance the immediate environment, provide a diver-
sion, and lessen the impact of potentially disturbing sounds for pediatric
patients (Barrera, Rykov, & Doyle, 2002; Klein & Winkelstein, 1996),
for patients experiencing a variety of surgical procedures (Augustin &
Hains, 1996; Yung, Chui-Kam, French, & Chan, 2002), for coronary
care unit patients (Hamel, 2001; White, 1992, 1999), and for ventilator-
dependent intensive care unit (ICU) patients (Chlan, 1998; Wong,
Lopez-Nahas, & Molassiotis, 2001). Specially designed music can be
effective in enhancing relaxation in an out-patient oncology setting for
children (Kemper, Hamilton, McClean, & Lovato, 2008). Music can be
an effective intervention for enhancing the neonatal ICU environment
and reducing stress (Kemper, Martin, Block, Shoaf, & Woods, 2004)
with such improvements as enhanced oxygenation during suctioning
(Chou, Wang, Chen, & Pai, 2003) and increased feeding rates
(Standley, 2003).

Distraction

Music is an effective intervention for creating distraction, particularly
for procedures that induce untoward symptoms and distress, such as
pain and anxiety with hemodialysis (Pothoulaki et al., 2008). It can
reduce noise annoyance in the ICU for cardiac surgery patients (Byers &
Smyth, 1997). It has been found to be an effective diversional adjunct
in the care of persons with burns (Fratianne et al., 2001; Prensner,
Yowler, Smith, Steele, & Fratianne, 2001), in management of nausea
and vomiting induced by chemotherapy (Ezzone, Baker, Rosselet, &
Terepka, 1998), in nausea and pain intensity after bone marrow transplantation (Sahler, Hunter, & Liesveld, 2003), for distress in children
undergoing immunizations (Megel, Houser, & Gleaves, 1998), in persons undergoing regular hemodialysis (Pothoulaki et al., 2008), and
for reduction in the amount of sedation required for adults during
colonoscopy (Lee et al., 2002; Smolen, Topp, & Singer, 2002).

Exhibit 6.2

Uses of Music Intervention

Orientation/minimizing disruptive behaviors

Elders (Clark, Lipe, & Bilbrey, 1998; Gerdner, 1997; Janelli, Kanski, Jones, & Kennedy, 1995; Sambandham & Schism, 1995)

Decreasing anxiety

Restrained patients (Janelli & Kanski, 1998)

Pediatrics (Barrera et al., 2002; Kemper et al., 2008; Klein & Winkelstein, 1996)

Surgical patients (Augustin & Hains, 1996; Yung et al., 2002)

Cardiac patients (Hamel, 2001; White, 1992, 1999)

Flexible sigmoidoscopy (Chlan, Evans, Greenleaf, & Walker, 2000)

Ventilator-dependent ICU patients (Chlan, 1998; Wong et al., 2001)

Pain management

Acute pain (Good, 1995; Good et al., 1999; Good et al., 2001; Laurion & Fetzer, 2003; Shertzer & Keck, 2001)

Chronic pain (Schorr, 1993)

Nursing care procedures/pediatrics (Whitehead-Pleaux, Zebrowski, Baryza, & Sheridan, 2007)

Invasive procedures/pediatrics (Berlin, 1998)

Stress reduction and relaxation

Elderly patients undergoing ophthalmic surgery (Golden & Izzo, 2001)

NICU patients (Burke, Walsh, Oehler, & Gingras, 1995; Kemper et al., 2004)

Nursing students (Bittman et al., 2004)

Stimulation

Depression in older adults (Hanser & Thompson, 1994)

Cognitive recovery and mood post-stroke (Sarkamo et al., 2008)

Sleep disturbances in older adults (Mornhinweg & Voignier, 1995) or college students (Harmat, Takacs, & Bodizs, 2008)

Increasing children's sociability (Aasgaard, 2001)

Head injury (Formisano et al., 2001; Jones, Hux, Morton-Anderson, & Knepper, 1994)

Distraction

Adjunct to spinal or general anesthesia (Lepage, Drolet, Girard, Grenier, & DeGagne, 2001; Nilsson, Rawal, Unesthahl, Zetterberg, & Unosson, 2001)

Burn care (Fratianne et al., 2001; Prensner et al., 2001)

Cardiac patients on bedrest (Cadigan et al., 2001)

Haemodialysis associated pain and anxiety (Pothoulaki et al., 2008)

High-dose chemotherapy (Ezzone et al., 1998)

Cardiac laboratory environmental enhancement (Thorgaard, Henriksen, Pedersbaek, & Thomsen, 2003)

CULTURAL APPLICATIONS

Although music may indeed be considered a universal phenomenon, there is no universal language to music. Various cultures structure music differently than what is usual to the average Western listener. For example, music from Eastern cultures contains very different tone structures and timbre, which can be foreign to the Western listener. Likewise, persons from a non-Western culture may find the classical music of Mozart or Beethoven as foreign sounding and irritating to the listener. These structural differences in what various cultures consider music are crucial to consider when implementing music-listening interventions.

Across five pain intervention studies, Caucasian persons preferred orchestral music, African American persons jazz, and Taiwanese persons harp music (Good et al., 2000). However, other investigators have found that minority elders tend to prefer music that is familiar to their own cultural background rather than Western music (Lai, 2004). These disparate findings highlight the need for careful music preference assessment prior to intervention.

FUTURE RESEARCH

Although the evidence base is increasing, the following are areas in which research is needed to further build the science of music intervention:

- Recent meta-analyses have been published on the strong, consistent effects of music intervention for premature infants (Standley, 2002) and for children and adolescents with autism (Whipple, 2004). A large body of work is available on music intervention for reducing anxiety and pain. An up-to-date meta-analysis articulating effect sizes for these symptoms that nurses typically manage would make a significant contribution to the scientific base of music intervention.
- Additional research into the management of symptom clusters would enhance the scientific base of music intervention. For example, persons with cancer typically experience nausea, vomiting, distress, and fatigue with treatments. Can the implementation of carefully selected music and its delivery improve a

constellation of symptoms? Can cancer patients be taught symptom management through the self-initiation of tailored music?

■ Cost and cost savings are significant issues in health care today. Little is known about the potential cost savings that could be realized with music intervention. Research is needed to determine whether music is a cost-effective or cost-neutral intervention and, if cost-effective, in which patient-care or symptom-management settings this is so.

■ Much of the nursing research focuses on immediate or short-term effects of music intervention. It is not known whether music can be effective for managing symptoms and distress in persons with chronic conditions or improving their quality of life.

■ There is a paucity of investigations as to the appropriate or optimal timing for delivery of music intervention to enhance effectiveness and for which specific patient populations or symptoms.

■ Many published studies have used convenience samples limited to single centers. Randomized, multisite clinical trials are needed to determine whether music indeed is effective in natural settings that are not as highly controlled by the investigator, under what conditions this may be so, and the importance of individual music preferences on the outcome of music-listening interventions.

Although intervention research itself is labor intensive, there is a need for additional research on music intervention. The knowledge base about music intervention for promotion of patient/client health and well-being can be expanded through high-quality research and by dissemination of those findings in a timely manner.

REFERENCES

Aasgaard, T. (2001). An ecology of love: Aspects of music therapy in the pediatric oncology environment. *Journal of Palliative Care, 17*(3), 177–181.

Alvin, J. (1975). *Music therapy*. New York: Basic Books.

American Heritage® dictionary of the English language (4th ed.). (2000). Boston, MA: Houghton Mifflin.

American Music Therapy Association. Retrieved September, 4, 2008, from www.musictherapy.org

Augustin, P., & Hains, A. (1996). Effect of music on ambulatory surgery patients' preoperative anxiety. *AORN Journal, 63*(4), 750–758.

Barrera, M., Rykov, M., & Doyle, S. (2002). The effects of interactive music therapy on hospitalized children with cancer: A pilot study. *Psycho-Oncology, 11*(5), 379–388.

Bauldoff, G., Hoffman, L., Zullo, T., & Sciurba, I. (2002). Exercise maintenance following pulmonary rehabilitation: Effect of distractive stimuli. *Chest, 122*(3), 948–954.

Bensimon, M., Amir, D., & Wolf, Y. (2008). Drumming through trauma: Music therapy with post-traumatic soldiers. *Arts in Psychotherapy, 35*(1), 34–48.

Berlin, B. (1998). Music therapy with children during invasive procedures: Our emergency department's experience. *Journal of Emergency Nursing, 24*(6), 607–608.

Bittman, B., Snyder, C., Liebfreid, F., Stevens, C., Westengard, J., & Umbach, P. (2004, July 9). Recreational music-making: An integrative group intervention for reducing burnout and improving mood states in first-year associate degree nursing students: Insights and economic impact. *International Journal of Nursing Education Scholarship, 1.* Retrieved September 4, 2008, from www.bepress.com/ijnes/vol1/iss1

Bonny, H. (1986). Music and healing. *Music Therapy, 6*(1), 3–12.

Burke, M., Walsh, J., Oehler, J., & Gingras, J. (1995). Music therapy following suctioning. *Neonatal Network, 14*(7), 41–49.

Byers, J., & Smyth, K. (1997). Effect of music intervention on noise annoyance, heart rate, and blood pressure in cardiac surgery patients. *American Journal of Critical Care, 6*(3), 183–191.

Cadigan, M., Caruso, N., Haldeman, S., McNamara, M., Noyes, D., Spadafora, M., et al. (2001). The effects of music on cardiac patients on bedrest. *Progress in Cardiovascular Nursing, 16*(1), 5–13.

Chlan, L. (1998). Effectiveness of a music therapy intervention on relaxation and anxiety for patients receiving ventilatory assistance. *Heart & Lung, 27*(3), 169–176.

Chlan, L., Evans, D., Greenleaf, M., & Walker, J. (2000). Effects of a single music therapy intervention on anxiety, discomfort, satisfaction, and compliance with screening guidelines in outpatients undergoing screening flexible sigmoidoscopy. *Gastroenterology Nursing, 23*(4), 148–156.

Chlan, L., & Tracy, M. (1999). Music therapy in critical care: Indications and guidelines for intervention. *Critical Care Nurse, 19*(3), 35–41.

Chou, L., Wang, R., Chen, S., & Pai, L. (2003). Effects of music therapy on oxygen saturation in premature infants receiving endotracheal suctioning. *Journal of Nursing Research, 11*(3), 209–215.

Clark, M., Lipe, A., & Bilbrey, M. (1998). Use of music to decrease aggressive behavior in people with dementia. *Journal of Gerontological Nursing, 24*(7), 10–17.

Ezzone, S., Baker, C., Rosselet, R., & Terepka, E. (1998). Music as an adjunct to antiemetic therapy. *Oncology Nursing Forum, 25*(9), 1551–1556.

Farber, S. (1982). *Neurorehabilitation.* Philadelphia: Saunders.

Formisano, R., Vinicola, V., Penta, F., Matteis, M., Brunelli, S., & Weckel, J. (2001). Active music therapy in the rehabilitation of severe brain injured patients during coma recovery. *Annali Dell Instituto Superiore di Sanità, 37*(4), 627–630.

Fratianne, R., Prensner, J., Huston, M., Super, D., Yowler, C., & Standley, J. (2001). The effect of music-based imagery and musical alternate engagement on the burn debridement process. *Journal of Burn Care & Rehabilitation, 22*(1), 47–53.

Gerdner, L. (1997). An individualized music intervention for agitation. *Journal of the American Psychiatric Nurses Association, 3*(6), 177–184.

Golden, A., & Izzo, J. (2001). Normalization of hypertensive responses during ambulatory surgical stress by perioperative music. *Psychosomatic Medicine, 63*(3), 487–492.

Good, M. (1995). A comparison of the effects of jaw relaxation and music on postoperative pain. *Nursing Research, 44*(1), 52–57.

Good, M., Picot, B., Salem, S., Chin, C., Picot, S., & Lane, D. (2000). Cultural differences in music chosen for pain relief. *Journal of Holistic Nursing, 18*(3), 245–260.

Good, M., Stanton-Hicks, M., Grass, J., Anderson, G., Choi, C., Schoolmeesters, L., et al. (1999). Relief of postoperative pain with jaw relaxation, music and their combination. *Pain, 81*(1, 2), 163–172.

Good, M., Stanton-Hicks, M., Grass, J., Anderson, G., Lai, H., Roykulcahroen, V., et al. (2001). Relaxation and music to reduce postsurgical pain. *Journal of Advanced Nursing, 33*(2), 208–215.

Guzzetta, C. (1995). Music therapy: Hearing the melody of the soul. In B. Dossey, L. Keegan, C. Guzzetta, & L. Kolkmeier (Eds.), *Holistic nursing* (pp. 670–698). Gaithersburg, MD: Aspen.

Hamel, W. (2001). The effects of music intervention on anxiety in the patient waiting for cardiac catheterization. *Intensive and Critical Care Nursing, 17*(2), 279–285.

Hanser, S. (1988). Controversy in music listening/stress reduction research. *Arts in Psychotherapy, 15*(2), 211–217.

Hanser, S., & Thompson, L. (1994). Effects of a music therapy strategy on depressed older adults. *Journal of Gerontology, 49*(6), 265–269.

Harmat, L., Takacs, J., & Bodizs, R. (2008). Music improves sleep quality in students. *Journal of Advanced Nursing, 62*(3), 327–335.

Idzoriek, P. (1982). *Comparison of auditory and strong tactile stimuli on responsiveness.* Unpublished Plan B Project. University of Minnesota, School of Nursing, Minneapolis, MN.

Janelli, L., & Kanski, G. (1998). Music for untying restrained patients. *Journal of the New York State Nurses Association, 29*(1), 13–15.

Janelli, L., Kanski, G., Jones, H., & Kennedy, M. (1995). Exploring music intervention with restrained patients. *Nursing Forum, 30*(4), 12–18.

Jones, R., Hux, C., Morton-Anderson, A., & Knepper, L. (1994). Auditory stimulation effect on a comatose survivor of traumatic brain injury. *Archives of Physical Medicine and Rehabilitation, 75*(1), 164–171.

Kemper, K., Hamilton, C., McClean, T., & Lovato, J. (2008). Impact of music on pediatric oncology patients. *Pediatric Research, 64*(1), 105–109.

Kemper, K., Martin, K., Block, S., Shoaf, R., & Woods, C. (2004). Attitudes and expectations about music therapy for premature infants among staff in the neonatal intensive care unit. *Alternative Therapies in Health & Medicine, 10*(2), 50–54.

Klein, S., & Winkelstein, M. (1996). Enhancing pediatric health care with music. *Pediatric Health Care, 10*(1), 74–81.

Lai, H. L. (2004). Music preference and relaxation in Taiwanese elderly people. *Geriatric Nursing, 25*(5), 286–291.

Laurion, S., & Fetzer, S. J. (2003). The effect of two nursing interventions on the postoperative outcomes of gynecologic laparoscopic patients. *Journal of Perianesthesia Nursing, 18*(4), 254–261.

Lee, D., Chan, K., Poon, C., Ko, C., Cha, K., Sin, K., et al. (2002). Relaxation music decreases the dose of patient-controlled sedation during colonoscopy: A prospective randomized controlled trial. *Gastrointestinal Endoscopy, 55*(1), 33–36.

Lepage, C., Drolet, P., Girard, M., Grenier, Y., & DeGagne, R. (2001). Music decreases sedative requirements during spinal anesthesia. *Anesthesia and Analgesia, 93,* 912–916.

Maranto, C. (1993). Applications of music in medicine. In M. Heal & T. Wigram (Eds.), *Music therapy in health and education* (pp. 153–174). London: Jessica Kingsley.

Megel, M., Houser, C., & Gleaves, L. (1998). Children's responses to immunization: Lullabies as a distraction. *Issues in Comprehensive Pediatric Nursing, 21*(3), 129–145.

Moore, R., Staum, M., & Brotons, M. (1992). Music preferences of the elderly: Repertoire, vocal ranges, tempos, and accompaniments for singing. *Journal of Music Therapy, 29*(4), 236–252.

Mornhinweg, G., & Voignier, R. (1995). Music for sleep disturbance in the elderly. *Journal of Holistic Nursing, 13*(3), 248–254.

Nightingale, F. (1860/1969). *Notes on nursing.* New York: Dover.

Nilsson, U., Rawal, N., Unesthahl, L., Zetterberg, C., & Unosson, M. (2001). Improved recovery after music and therapeutic suggestions during general anesthesia: A double-blind randomized controlled trial. *Acta Anesthesiologica Scandinavica, 45,* 812–817.

Pothoulaki, R., MacDonald, P., Flowers, E., Stamataki, V., Filiopoulos, D., Stamatiadis, D., & Stathakis, C. (2008). An investigation of the effects of music on anxiety and pain perception in patients undergoing haemodialysis treatment. *Journal of Health Psychology, 13*(7), 912–920.

Prensner, J., Yowler, C., Smith, L., Steele, A., & Fratianne, R. (2001). Music therapy for assistance with pain and anxiety management in burn treatment. *Journal of Burn Care & Rehabilitation, 22*(1), 83–88.

Public Radio Music Source. Available at: www.prms.org

Robb, S., Nichols, R., Rutan, R., Bishop, B., & Parker, J. (1995). The effects of music-assisted relaxation on preoperative anxiety. *Journal of Music Therapy, 32*(1), 3–12.

Sahler, O., Hunter, B., & Liesveld, J. (2003). The effect of using music therapy with relaxation imagery in the management of patients undergoing bone marrow transplantation: A pilot feasibility study. *Alternative Therapies in Health & Medicine, 9*(6), 70–74.

Sambandham, M., & Schism, V. (1995). Music as a nursing intervention for residents with Alzheimer's disease in long-term care. *Geriatric Nursing, 16*(2), 79–83.

Saperstein, B. (1995). The effects of consistent tempi and physiologically interactive tempi on heart rate and EMG responses. In T. Wigram, B. Saperstein, & M. West (Eds.), *The art and science of music therapy: A handbook* (pp. 58–79). Newark, NJ: Harwood Academic Publishers.

Sarkamo, T., Tervaniemi, M., Laitinen, S., Forsblom, A., Soinila, S., Mikkonene, M., et al. (2008). Music listening enhances cognitive recovery and mood after middle cerebral artery stroke. *Brain, 131,* 866–876.

Schorr, J. (1993). Music and pattern change in chronic pain. *Advances in Nursing Science, 15*(4), 27–36.

Shertzer, K., & Keck, J. (2001). Music and the PACU environment. *Journal of PeriAnesthesia Nursing, 16*(2), 90–102.

Smolen, D., Topp, R., & Singer, L. (2002). The effect of self-selected music during colonoscopy on anxiety, heart rate and blood pressure. *Applied Nursing Research, 16*(2), 126–130.

Standley, J. (1986). Music research in medical/dental treatment: Meta-analysis and clinical applications. *Journal of Music Therapy, 23*(2), 56–122.

Standley, J. (2002). A meta-analysis of music therapy for premature infants. *Journal of Pediatric Nursing, 17*(2), 107–113.

Standley, J. (2003). The effect of music-reinforced sucking on feeding rate of premature infants. *Journal of Pediatric Nursing, 18*(3), 169–173.

Thaut, M. (1990). Physiological and motor responses to music stimuli. In R. Unkefer (Ed.), *Music therapy in the treatment of adults with mental disorders: Theoretical bases and clinical interventions* (pp. 33–49). New York: Schirmer Books.

Thorgaard, B., Henriksen, B., Pedersbaek, G., & Thomsen, I. (2003). Specially selected music in the cardiac laboratory—an important tool for improvement of the well-being of patients. *European Journal of Cardiovascular Nursing, 3*(1), 21–26.

Whipple, J. (2004). Music in intervention for children and adolescents with autism: A meta-analysis. *Journal of Music Therapy, 41*(2), 90–106.

White, J. (1992). Music therapy: An intervention to reduce anxiety in the myocardial infarction patient. *Clinical Nurse Specialist, 6*(2), 58–63.

White, J. (1999). Effects of relaxing music on cardiac autonomic balance and anxiety after acute myocardial infarction. *American Journal of Critical Care, 8*(4), 220–230.

Whitehead-Pleaux, A., Zebrowski, N., Baryza, M., & Sheridan, R. (2007). Exploring the effects of music therapy on pediatric pain: Phase 1. *Journal of Music Therapy, 34*(3), 217–241.

Winkelman, M. (2003). Complementary therapy for addiction: "Drumming out drugs." *American Journal of Public Health, 93*(4), 647–651.

Wong, H., Lopez-Nahas, V., & Molassiotis, A. (2001). Effects of music therapy on anxiety in ventilator-dependent patients. *Heart & Lung, 30*(5), 376–387.

Yung, P., Chui-Kam, S., French, P., & Chan, T. (2002). A controlled trial of music and pre-operative anxiety in Chinese men undergoing transurethral resection of the prostate. *Journal of Advanced Nursing, 39*(4), 352–359.

7 Humor

KEVIN L. SMITH

A merry heart doeth good like a medicine, but a broken spirit
drieth the bones.
                                                    —*Proverbs 17:22*

Throughout history, human beings have accorded a beneficial effect to
joy and mirth. Greek philosophers including Plato and Aristotle wrote
treatises on humor (McGhee, 1979). The German philosopher Imman-
uel Kant, in 1790, set forth similar physical effects of humor and characterized it as a talent that enabled one to look at things from a different
perspective (Haig, 1988). In medieval physiology, humor referred to
the four principal fluids of the body: blood, phlegm, choler (yellow
bile), and melancholy (black bile). A proper balance of the four was
called good humor, and a preponderance of any one constituted ill
humor (Robinson, 1991).

That humor and laughter can improve our ability to cope with
difficulties and to stay healthy is a popular notion. Interest in this area
has increased since Norman Cousins's account of the role of laughter
in his recovery from a painful collagen disorder (1979). The belief
that humor and laughter positively influence health persists, and the
scientific evidence supporting this belief will be reviewed to provide a
basis for the use of humor by nurses and others providing health care.

Nursing journal articles continue to address many facets of humor, such as laughter and stress management (Paquet, 1993; Smith, 2003; Woodhouse, 1993), humor as a nursing intervention (Hunt, 1993; Mornhinweg & Voignier, 1995), humor and the older adult (Herth, 1993), humor and healing (Macaluso, 1993), and the positive physiologic effects of humor (Lambert & Lambert, 1995). Humor organizations and publications are proliferating, humor workshops are being offered to nurses and other health care providers, and many continuing education offerings are incorporating humorous presentations or activities.

Humor can be used as a specific therapy or with other therapies as a concurrent intervention. The goals in using humor as an intervention are to enhance the well-being of the client, to enhance the therapeutic relationship between the nurse and the client, and to bring hope and joy to the situation. Humor creates an outlet for stress for both client and nurse. It can be used to foster trust and a comfortable environment for the client. In addition to incorporating humor into the health care setting with patients, the use of humor in daily and work life is a significant self-care practice for health care professionals. Virtually anyone can develop the requisite skills needed to use humor as an intervention.

DEFINITIONS

Humor is the good-natured side of truth.
                                    —*Mark Twain*

The Association for Applied and Therapeutic Humor (2000) defines therapeutic humor as follows:

> Any intervention that promotes health and wellness by stimulating a playful discovery, expression, or appreciation of the absurdity or incongruity of life's situations. This intervention may enhance work performance, support learning, improve health, or be used as a complementary treatment of illness to facilitate healing or coping, whether physical, emotional, cognitive, social, or spiritual. (www.aath.org)

Nurse and humor expert, Vera Robinson (1978), described the phenomenon of humor as "any communication which is perceived by any of the interacting parties as humorous and leads to laughing, smiling or a feeling of amusement" (p. 193). *Webster's* dictionary defines it as "the quality of being funny," and "the trait of appreciating (and being able to express) the humorous" (*Webster's online dictionary*, n.d.). Humor can be the process of either producing or perceiving the comical. What is personally defined or perceived as funny and its physical manifestations vary among individuals. However, there are predictable stimuli for laughter and usual responses.

WHY DO WE LAUGH?

We laugh for many different reasons. Sometimes the response is simply for the fun of it; sometimes it is for more important reasons. Here we will discuss four basic theories for the laughter response: surprise, superiority, incongruity, and release.

1. **Surprise:** Good humor or a good joke may catch one off guard. The surprise in itself causes a person to laugh. Another type of surprise humor is shock humor. This could be a startling or loud punch line or something taboo or vulgar. Shock humor is not recommended in clinical or therapeutic settings.
2. **Superiority:** The theory of superiority laughter (Robinson, 1991) involves situations in which laughter occurs when one feels superior to another individual or group. One's laughter is in response to the inferiority, stupidity, or misfortunes of others. In its most simple form, this is slapstick humor; a more sophisticated form is political satire. It has been suggested that the essential effect of humor is derived from a sense of mastery or ego strength (Lefcourt & Martin, 1986).
3. **Incongruity:** Schaefner (1981) concisely describes this theory as laughter occurring because of "a perception of an incongruity in a ludicrous context." For example, a man walks into a psychiatrist's office with a duck on his head. The duck says, "Doc, you got to help me get this guy off my tail." Two ideas are juxtaposed in an impossible or absurd situation. The incongruity theory advanced by Kant and other philosophers such as Schopenhauer and Spencer emphasized the importance of a sudden surprise, shock, conflict of ideas, or incongruity as a trigger for laughter

(Liechty, 1987). Asimov (1992) argues that incongruities put the listener, for a brief moment, in a fantasy world. This suspension of reality readies the listener for the crowning bit of fantasy or the punch line that results in laughter.

4. **Release**: The basic premise of the release theory, as a laughter stimulus, is that humor and laughter help to release tensions and anxieties. Freud (1905/1960) viewed humor as a coping tool that allows individuals to reduce tension by expressing hostile or obscene impulses in a socially acceptable manner. Morreal (1983) called this the relief theory and notes that humor that produces laughter is a method for venting nervous energy. This release type of laughter is often enhanced in group situations where many share the same anxiety.

HUMOR STYLES

Most of the humor employed on a daily basis with staff and patients is of the spontaneous type: situational humor that arises out of the normal absurdities of the day's activities. This type of humor is also a very effective communication tool when used to break the ice with patients or coworkers. An attempt is made to lighten the situation; this is a sign of caring and allows for a free exchange of thoughts and emotions. Formal humor, or premeditated acts of humor (Smith, 2008), include the sharing of jokes, cartoons, humorous articles or stories, novelty toys or gag gifts, and practical jokes. Formal humor, like most kinds of humor, is usually effective only when it is relevant to the situation in which it is presented. Other, more specific styles of humor include self-deprecating humor, puns and plays on words, ethnic humor, sarcastic humor, and gallows humor.

Self-deprecating humor may be the most effective and powerful humor tool that nurses can develop and use. To show that one is able to laugh at oneself demonstrates that one is a normal human being with weaknesses who at the same time displays confidence, self-awareness, and self-esteem. Ronald Reagan used this type of humor effectively when critics made derogatory comments about his age during his second run for the presidency. He quipped, "Andrew Jackson was seventy-five years old and still vigorous when he left the White House. I know because he told me" (Klein, 1989, p. 10). Paulsen (1989) stated that gently poking fun at oneself acts as a social lubricant. It shows that a person is at ease with the situation. People are often suspicious or afraid of those without a sense of humor.

Puns and plays on words are simple and straightforward humor styles. Some consider puns to be the lowest form of humor, but pun enthusiasts include Asimov and Freud. Puns (e.g., "With friends like you, who needs enemas?") typically produce groans rather than laughter.

Ethnic humor is often regional. Using one's own ethnicity or profession as the target of the joke is the most acceptable approach. Sarcastic humor is somewhat risky; overheard sarcasm can make patients or others think they are the target of the sarcastic comments.

Freud (1905) developed a theory about why people laugh at tragedy and death, which he called gallows humor. Such grim humor is typically seen when people are faced with considerable stress. He theorized that jokes allow people to express unconscious aggressive or sexual impulses. Obrldik (1942) asserted that the phenomenon of gallows humor has a definite social purpose. It provides a psychological escape and strengthens the morale of the group and in some situations undermines the morale of the oppressors. Gallows humor is frequently used in situations where individuals are under significant stress, such as emergency rooms, intensive care units, operating rooms, and morgues.

SCIENTIFIC BASIS

Many of the positive physiological effects of humor and laughter have been studied. Humor is the stimulus and laughter the response. Laughter creates a cascade of physiological changes in the body. Fry (1971) studied the effects of mirthful laughter on heart rate and on the oxygen saturation level of peripheral blood and respiratory phenomena. He found that both the arousal and cathartic effects are paralleled in the physiological. Laughter involves extensive physical activity. It increases respiratory activity and oxygen exchange, increases muscular activity and heart rate, and stimulates the cardiovascular system, the sympathetic nervous system, and the production of catecholamines. The arousal state is followed by the relaxation state, in which respiration rate, heart rate, and muscle tension return to normal. Although the oxygen saturation of peripheral blood is not affected during this relaxation state, blood pressure is reduced and a state exists similar to the impact of hearty exercise. Fry and Savin (1988) investigated the effects of humor on arterial blood pressure using direct arterial cannulization. Findings showed increases in systolic and diastolic blood pressure that were directly related to the intensity and duration of laughter. Blood pressure decreased immediately after the laugh to below the prelaughter baseline.

Many studies have found that humor and laughter increase levels of salivary immunoglobulin A (S-IgA), a vital immune system protein that is the body's first line of defense against respiratory illnesses. In a controlled study, Dillon, Minchoff, and Baker (1985) demonstrated increased levels of S-IgA in college students who viewed a humorous video. Martin and Dobbin (1988) measured subjects' sense of humor, stress levels, and S-IgA levels and demonstrated that subjects with low scores on the humor scales showed a greater negative relationship between stress and S-IgA than did subjects with high humor scores. Stone, Valdimarsdottir, Jandorf, Cox, and Neale (1987) found that the S-IgA response level was lower on days of negative mood and higher on days of positive mood. Lambert and Lambert (1995) produced similar findings with S-IgA levels in healthy fifth-grade students.

Berk, Tan, and Fry (1989) studied the effects of laughter on the neuroendocrine stress hormones and immune parameters (Berk, Tan, Napier, & Eby, 1989). They found a complex autonomic response with each catecholamine, suggesting that laughter may be an antagonist to the classical stress response. They demonstrated that laughter lowered serum cortisol levels, increased the amount of activated T-lymphocytes, and increased the number and activity of natural killer cells. Laughter stimulates the immune system, counteracting the immunosuppressive effects of stress. Berk, Felten, Tan, Bittman, and Westengard (2001) proposed that interventions of mirthful laughter may be capable of modulating neuroendocrine and neuroimmune parameters and may be an adjunct to other therapies.

Friedman and Ulmer (1984) assigned hundreds of heart attack survivors to one of two groups. The control group received standard advice regarding medications, diet, and exercise. The treatment group received additional counseling on relaxation, smiling, laughing at themselves and mistakes, taking time to enjoy life, and renewing their religious faith. Over 3 years, the treatment group experienced half as many repeat heart attacks as the control group.

In the pediatric oncology setting, Dowling, Hockenberry, and Gregory (2003) found a direct relationship between a well-developed sense of humor and psychological adjustment to cancer as well as a lower incidence of infection among children with high coping humor scores. Yet Schofield and colleagues (2004) found no evidence that a high level of optimism prior to treatment improved survival in patients with non–small-cell lung carcinoma.

Psychological Perspectives

Humor has been considered an adaptive coping mechanism. Freud (1905) regarded humor and laughter as two of the few socially acceptable means for releasing pent-up frustrations and anger, a cathartic mechanism for preserving psychic or emotional energy. Humor and laughter alter our perspective in various situations. Laughter can counteract negative emotions; it allows people to transcend predicaments, overcome painful circumstances, and cope with difficulties. By focusing energy elsewhere, humor can diffuse the stress of difficult events (Klein, 1989). The use of humor has been shown to reduce threat-induced anxiety (Yovetich, Dale, & Hudak, 1990).

INTERVENTION

There are many approaches, techniques, and tools that can be applied to using humor as an intervention. A first step in deciding how and when to use humor is to complete a humor assessment, first of yourself, then of your patient.

Assessment

A humor interview guide was developed to explore older adults' perceptions of humor (Herth, 1993; see Exhibit 7.1). This assessment could be adapted for use in clinical settings or used in research. The assessment is completed by the provider and then by the client.

When completing an assessment of one's own sense of humor, one should consider what type of humor seems most natural. Consider preferences for spontaneity versus formal humor. Like all skills, you can always work on improving your sense of humor. Strickland (1993)

Exhibit 7.1

Humor Assessment Interview Guide

1. When you think of humor, what kinds of images or thoughts come to mind?
2. Was humor a part of your life when you were younger?
3. Is humor still a part of your life?
4. How has humor been helpful or not helpful at this time in your life?
5. If humor is helpful, what do you do to maintain humor in your life?
6. Are there certain times when you appreciate humor more than other times?
7. When has humor been a negative experience?
8. What types of activities do you find amusing or enjoyable?

Note: From Herth (1993). Copyright 1993 by W. B. Saunders Company, Philadelphia, PA. Adapted with permission.

says that the first and biggest barrier to using humor is the fear of appearing foolish or of losing control over one's self-image.

Part of the humor assessment of a patient is determining what type of humor is appropriate to use for the patient and the particular situation. Humor that is divisive in any way should be avoided. Investigate the patient's and family's prior use of humor and whether they currently appreciate and value humor and laughter (Davidhizar & Bowen, 1992). Spontaneous humorous comments on a neutral topic such as the weather, equipment, or yourself can help you find out whether the individual is open to humor, though readiness for humor may not always be apparent.

Techniques

Exhibit 7.2 shows a variety of approaches to humor intervention. Ackerman, Henry, Graham, and Coffey (1994) developed a model for incorporating humor into the health care setting and described the steps to create a humor program. Humorous materials were made available to patients through a "chuckle wagon" cart that was taken to their rooms. A humor resource center was developed to assist nurses in incorporating humor into their patient care, and a patient satisfaction evaluation tool was developed to assess patients' response to the humor cart. Exhibit 7.3 provides several humor Web sites that contain material for humor interventions.

Exhibit 7.2

Selected Techniques and Activities to Provide and Support Humor Interventions

1. Assemble/collect humor resources (create humor rooms, humor carts, humor videos).
2. Invite guest performers (comedians, magicians, clowns).
3. Wear a humorous item, silly button, necktie, etc.
4. Display humorous photos of staff.
5. Have a cartoon bulletin board with favorites from staff and patients displayed each week.
6. Play music that encourages playful movement.
7. Support and applaud the efforts of staff and patients to use humor.

Exhibit 7.3

Selected Online Humor Resources

1. Association for Applied and Therapeutic Humor: http://www.aath.org
2. *The Joyful Noiseletter*: http://www.joyfulnoiseletter.com
3. The Humor Project: http://www.humorproject.com
4. International Society for Humor Studies (ISHS): http://www.hnu.edu/ishs/
5. World Laughter Tour: http://worldlaughtertour.com/
6. *Hospital Clown Newsletter*: http://hospitalclown.com/
7. Comedy Cures Foundation: http://www.comedycures.org
8. The Humor Collection: http://www.thehumorcollection.org/
9. Dr. Thorson's Humor Scale: http://www.spirituality-health.com/spirit/node/67
10. How Laughter Works: http://www.howstuffworks.com/laughter6.htm

Measurement of Effectiveness

Although physical laughter is not an essential outcome of humor, physical responses to a humor intervention are obvious indicators of effectiveness. According to Black (1984), the multiple physical manifestations of the laughter response cover a range from smiling to belly laughing. Other positive responses may be the relief of symptoms, facial expression, degree of involvement in activities, and strengthening of the relationship between caregiver and client.

Lefcourt and Martin (1986) developed the Situational Humor Response Questionnaire (SHRQ) for determining an individual's response to particular types of humor. It has been used in numerous studies and has been validated as effectively measuring humor. Diverse elements, such as developmental or cultural factors, may also influence an individual's response to humor. It is important to be alert to the variations and subtleties of a patient's response.

Precautions

There are a variety of factors that practitioners should consider when using humor. The timing of the use of humor in the clinical setting is crucial to its success. Leiber (1986) cautioned that one must assess the patient's receptiveness to humor. Crane (1987) states that there are times when humor is contraindicated. What may be funny to patients when they are feeling well may not seem funny during an illness episode. Humor and laughter have no place at the height of a crisis, although they can be useful to allay tension as the crisis subsides. Inside jokes among health care professionals can seem offensive or callous to outsiders who may overhear them. Laughing at others negates confidence and destroys team spirit, whereas laughing *with* others builds confidence, brings people together, and pokes fun at our common dilemmas (Goodman, 1992). Patients may use inappropriate or sexually aggressive remarks under the pretext of joking, in which case further assessment may be indicated to determine the underlying reason for the aggressive verbal behavior.

USES

Humor may be effectively used in highly stressful situations to overcome tensions and to facilitate patient catharsis or expression of fear and anxiety. Ziv (1984) described the use of humor as a defense mechanism for dealing with anxieties. As a provider of patient care, one must be sensitive to the fact that the patient's use of humor could be an attempt to avoid facing more serious issues or feelings. Humorous distraction may be used to reduce preoperative anxiety (Gaberson, 1991). Humor has also been used as an adjunct for enhancing postoperative recall of the exercise routines that were taught preoperatively (Parfitt, 1990). It may be used effectively for problems associated with communication, anxiety, grieving, powerlessness, or social isolation (Hunt, 1993).

The psychological impact of humor and laughter has been studied as an adjunct in the management of psychiatric patients (Saper, 1988, 1990) and may be an effective intervention as part of psychotherapy (Rosenheim & Golan, 1986). Moody (1978) studied and has incorporated the use of positive emotions and humor in dealing with the fear, anxiety, and pain that go along with cancer and other chronic conditions. In the oncology setting, humor provides benefits related to *psychological* aspects of patients, such as using humor as a defense mechanism; *communication,* by creating a more relaxed mood between patients and providers; and *social situations,* by using humor to establish relationships with the many individuals involved in their care (Joshua, Cotroneo, & Clarke, 2005). In a group of men with testicular cancer, humor was found to ease difficult interactions, but health care providers should take cues from their patients to determine whether the use of humor is appropriate (Chapple & Ziebland, 2004). In the palliative care setting, humor can help patients preserve their dignity, contend with challenging circumstances, and building relationships (Dean & Gregory, 2005). Humor has also been advocated as an intervention for elderly clients (Hulse, 1994).

CULTURAL APPLICATIONS

When using humor, cultural differences and perceptions should be considered. For example, Dean (2003) describes unique considerations in caring for Native American patients. Laughing and joking are considered to be signs of closeness that honor a relationship. Gentle teasing and the use of witticisms are common forms of relational humor among Native Americans.

Berger, Coulehan, and Belling (2004) describe potential risks and benefits of using humor in the clinical encounter. The recipient may find some aspect of the humor inappropriate and the health professional may risk embarrassment, which could harm the therapeutic relationship. The provider can start the encounter with low-risk humor, such as the self-deprecating kind, which can enhance communication without being offensive.

Humor may be used to increase comfort or raise the pain threshold. Cogan, Cogan, Waltz, and McCue (1987) studied the effects of laughter and relaxation on discomfort thresholds. In a group of volunteers, tolerance levels of physical discomfort were measured after members of the group listened to either a laughter-inducing narrative or an uninteresting narrative tape, or had no intervention. Patient discomfort thresholds increased (patients could handle more pain) in the laughter-inducing scenario.

The use of humor is particularly appropriate in situations involving short-term pain, such as some routine treatments (e.g., injections) as well as recovery from procedures or surgery.

FUTURE RESEARCH

The therapeutic use of humor by nurses has been and will continue to be an important aspect of providing patient care. Awareness of the importance of humor is increasing, as demonstrated by the plethora of articles published in support of humor as an intervention, numerous scientific studies regarding its use, and an increase in the number of educational offerings regarding humor intervention. A greater understanding is needed of how humor, laughter, and positive emotions benefit the physiology and potential healing capacity of individuals. Nurses can use this same information to incorporate humor into their own lives, to make their work and personal lives more enjoyable and become more effective providers of care. Research questions to be addressed include:

1. What are the physiological effects of humor on patients who are critically ill?
2. How can the use of humor be taught and the effectiveness of its use be measured?
3. Can the systematic use of humor speed healing or enhance outcomes of acute illness?
4. Can humor be utilized in care environments to reduce stress and enhance nurse satisfaction and retention?

REFERENCES

Ackerman, M., Henry, M., Graham, K., & Coffey, N. (1994). Humor won, humor too: A model to incorporate humor into the health care setting (revised). *Nursing Forum,* 29(2), 15–21.

Asimov, I. (1992). *Asimov laughs again.* New York: HarperCollins.

Association for Applied and Therapeutic Humor. (2000). Retrieved October 28, 2008, from www.aath.org

Berger J., Coulehan, J., & Belling, C. (2004). Humor in the physician–patient encounter. *Archives of Internal Medicine, 164*(8), 825–830.

Berk, L., Felten, D., Tan, S., Bittman, B., & Westengard, J. (2001). Modulation of neuroimmune parameters during the eustress of humor-associated mirthful laughter. *Alternative Therapies in Health and Medicine, 7*(2), 62–76.

Berk, L., Tan, S., & Fry, W. (1989). Neuroendocrine and stress hormone changes during mirthful laughter. *American Journal of Medical Sciences, 298*(6), 390–396.

Berk, L., Tan, S., Napier, B., & Eby, W. (1989). Eustress of mirthful laughter modifies natural killer cell activity. *Clinical Research, 37*(1), 115A.

Black, D. (1984). Laughter. *Journal of the American Medical Association, 25*(21), 2995–2998.

Chapple, A., & Ziebland, Z. (2004). The role of humor for men with testicular cancer. *Qualitative Health Research, 14*(8), 1123–1139.

Cogan, R., Cogan, D., Waltz, W., & McCue, M. (1987). Effects of laughter and relaxation on discomfort thresholds. *Journal of Behavioral Medicine, 10,* 139–144.

Cousins, N. (1979). *Anatomy of an illness.* New York: Norton.

Crane, A. L. (1987). Why sickness can be a laughing matter. *RN, 50,* 41–42.

Davidhizar R., & Bowen, M. (1992). The dynamics of laughter. *Archives of Psychiatric Nursing, 6*(2), 132–137.

Dean, R. A., (2003) Native American humor: Implications for transcultural care. *Journal of Transcultural Nursing, 14*(1), 62–65.

Dean, R. A. K., & Gregory, D. M. (2005) More than trivial: Strategies for using humor in palliative care. *Cancer Nursing, 28*(4), 292–300.

Dillon, K., Minchoff, B., & Baker, K. (1985). Positive emotional states and enhancement of the immune system. *International Journal of Psychiatry in Medicine, 15*(1), 3–17.

Dowling, J. S., Hockenberry, M., & Gregory, R. L. (2003). Sense of humor, childhood cancer stressors, and outcomes of psychosocial adjustment, immune function, and infection. *Journal of Pediatric Oncology Nursing, 20*(6), 271–292.

Freud, S. (1960). *Jokes and their relation to the unconscious.* New York: Norton. (Originally: *Der Witz und seine Beziehung zum Unbewussten.* Leipzig and Vienna: Durtricke, 1905.)

Friedman, M., & Ulmer, D. (1984). *Treating type A behavior–and your heart.* New York: Knopf.

Fry, W. (1971). Mirth and oxygen saturation of peripheral blood. *Psychotherapy and Psychosomatics, 19,* 76–84.

Fry, W. F., & Savin, M. (1988). Mirthful laughter and blood pressure. *Humor, 1,* 49–62.

Gaberson, K. (1991). The effect of humorous distraction on preoperative anxiety. *AORN Journal, 54*(6), 1258–1264.

Goodman, J. (1992). Laughing matters: Taking your job seriously and yourself lightly. *Journal of the American Medical Association, 267*(13), 1858.

Haig, R. A. (1988). *The anatomy of humor: Biopsychosocial and therapeutic perspectives.* Springfield, IL: Charles C Thomas.

Herth, K. A. (1993). Humor and the older adult. *Applied Nursing Research, 6*(4), 146–153.

Hulse, J. (1994). Humor: A nursing intervention for the elderly. *Geriatric Nursing, 15*(2), 88–90.

Hunt, A. H. (1993). Humor as a nursing intervention. *Cancer Nursing, 16*(1), 34–39.

Joshua, A., Cotroneo, A., & Clarke, S. (2005). Humor and oncology. *Journal of Clinical Oncology, 23*(3), 645–648.

Klein, A. (1989). *The healing power of humor.* Los Angeles: Jeremy P. Tarcher.

Lambert, R., & Lambert, N. K. (1995). The effects of humor on secretory immunoglobulin-A levels in school-aged children. *Pediatric Nursing, 21*(1), 16–19.

Lefcourt, H. M., & Martin, R. A. (1986). *Humor and life stress: Antidote to adversity.* New York: Springer Verlag.

Leiber, D. B. (1986). Laughter and humor in critical care. *Dimensions in Critical Care Nursing, 5*(3), 162–170.

Liechty, R. D. (1987). Humor and the surgeon. *Archives of Surgery, 122,* 519–522.

Macaluso, M. C. (1993). Humor, health and healing. *American Nephrology Nurses Association Journal, 20*(1), 14–16.

Martin, R., & Dobbin, J. (1988). Sense of humor, hassles, and immunoglobulin evidence for a stress-moderating effect of humor. *International Journal of Psychiatry in Medicine, 18*(2), 93–105.

McGhee, P. (1979). *Humor: Its origin and development.* San Francisco: Freeman.

Moody, R. A. (1978). *Laugh after laugh.* Jacksonville, FL: Headwaters.

Mornhinweg, G., & Voignier, R. (1995). Holistic nursing interventions. *Orthopaedic Nursing, 14*(4), 20–24.

Morreal, J. (1983). *Taking laughter seriously.* Albany: State University of New York Press.

Obrldik, A. (1942). Gallows humor: A sociological phenomenon. *American Journal of Sociology, 47,* 709–716.

Paquet, J. (1993, November/December). Laughter and stress management. *Today's OR Nurse,* 13–17.

Parfitt, J. M. (1990). Humorous preoperative teaching: Effect of recall of postoperative exercise routines. *AORN Journal, 52*(1), 114–120.

Paulsen, T. (1989). *Making humor work: Take your job seriously and yourself lightly.* Los Altos, CA: Crisp.

Robinson, V. (1978). Humor in nursing. In C. Carlson & B. Blackwell (Eds.), *Behavioral concepts and nursing interventions* (pp. 129–152). Philadelphia: Lippincott.

Robinson, V. M. (1991). *Humor and the health professions* (2nd ed.). Thorofare, NJ: Slack.

Rosenheim, E., & Golan, G. (1986). Patients' reactions to humorous interventions in psychotherapy. *American Journal of Psychotherapy, 40*(1), 110–124.

Saper, B. (1988). Humor in psychiatric healing. *Psychiatric Quarterly, 59*(4), 306–319.

Saper, B. (1990). The therapeutic use of humor for psychiatric disturbances in adolescents and adults. *Psychiatric Quarterly, 61*(4), 261–272.

Schaefner, N. (1981). *The art of laughter.* New York: Columbia University Press.

Schofield, P., Ball, D., Smith, J., Borland, R., O'Brien, P., Davis, S., et al. (2004). Optimism and survival. *Cancer, 100*(6), 1276–1282.

Smith, K. (2003). Clinical wit and wisdom. *Advances for Nurse Practitioners, 11*(12), 83.

Smith, K. L. (2008, April). *Humor as a clinical skill: Are you joking?* Paper presented to National Association of Pediatric Nurse Practitioners (NAPNP) Annual Conference, Nashville, TN.

Stone, A., Valdimarsdottir, H., Jandorf, L., Cox, D., & Neale, J. (1987). Evidence that IgA antibody is associated with daily mood. *Journal of Personality and Social Psychology, 52,* 988–993.

Strickland, D. (1993, November/December). Seriously, laughter matters. *Today's OR Nurse,* 19–24.

Webster's Online Dictionary. Retrieved July 28, 2009, from http://www.websters-online-dictionary.org/definition/humor

Woodhouse, D. K. (1993). The aspects of humor in dealing with stress. *Nursing Administration Quarterly, 18*(1), 80–89.

Yovetich, N. A., Dale, A., & Hudak, M. (1990). Benefits of humor in reduction of threat induced anxiety. *Psychological Reports, 66,* 51–58.

Ziv, A. (1984). *Personality and sense of humor.* New York: Springer Verlag.

8 Yoga

MIRIAM E. CAMERON

Anyone can benefit from yoga, regardless of health, beliefs, age, or culture (Danhauer et al., 2008). The systematic practice of yoga heals the body and the mind (Agte & Chiplonkar, 2008). Yoga's do-it-yourself prescription for stress management and well-being has no side effects and does not require medications or expensive equipment and treatments (Duncan, Leis, & Taylor-Brown, 2008). Nurses practice yoga themselves and use yoga as a complementary, alternative, and primary therapy. Millions of people around the world practice yoga, primarily for physical fitness and relaxation (Birdee et al., 2008); however, yoga has a much deeper dimension (Cameron, 2008).

Yoga consists of a systematic ethical and spiritual path of transformation of consciousness, as yogis in India and Tibet have advocated for centuries and Western researchers now are discovering (DiStasio, 2008). As practitioners let go of ego, which is thought to underlie suffering and most illnesses, they realize that they are linked to every being, the environment, and the larger forces of the universe. Grateful for this vast interconnectedness, they reach out to relieve suffering in other living beings. They sift out the unreal from the real and allow their true natures to shine forth. Then their inner wisdom flows spontaneously through all the cells of the body, promoting optimal health, inner

123

freedom, creativity, peace, and joy (Cameron & Parker, 2004; Kabat-Zinn, 2005).

DEFINITION

Yoga, an ancient art and science developed in India, and later in Tibet, means "integration" or "joining together" of body and mind with each other and the universe. Two millennia ago, the Indian sage Patanjali systematized yoga into the *Yoga Sutra*, a treatise consisting of 196 compact observations. This unique blend of theoretical knowledge and practical application is the primary text for all schools of yoga. In the *Yoga Sutra*, Patanjali analyzed how we know what we know and why we suffer. He described a meditative program through which to fulfill the primary purpose of consciousness: to see things as they really are and achieve freedom from suffering. Through yoga, he explained, we can rein in our tendency to gravitate toward external things, identify with them, and try and find happiness through them. Only by turning inward and becoming aware of our true nature, he wrote, can we understand how to develop happiness and wisdom. By becoming still, we can abide in this deep, absorptive knowing (Hartranft, 2003).

In the *Yoga Sutra*, Patanjali described yoga as consisting of eight interconnected limbs, or aspects of the whole. Practicing these limbs simultaneously leads to progressively higher stages of ethics, spirituality, and healing. The first five limbs still the mind and body in preparation for the last three limbs. The eight limbs and their Sanskrit names are as follows (Hartranft, 2003):

1. **Ethical behavior** (*yama*)—nonharming, truthfulness, nonstealing, responsible sexuality, nonacquisitiveness.
2. **Personal behavior** (*niyama*)—purity, commitment, contentment, self-study, and surrender to the whole.
3. **Posture** (*asana*)—physical poses that stretch, condition, and massage the body.
4. **Breath regulation** (*pranayama*)—regulation and refinement of breathing to expand *prana* (life-force) and get rid of toxins.
5. **Sensory inhibition** (*pratyahara*)—temporary withdrawal of the senses from the external environment to the inner self, for example, by closing the eyes and looking inward.

6. **Concentration** (*dharana*)—locking attention on an object or field, such as the breath, mantra, or image.
7. **Meditation** (*dhyana*)—increasingly sustained attention, leading to a profound state of peace and awareness.
8. **Integration** (*samadhi*)—a transcendent state of oneness, wisdom, and ecstasy.

SCIENTIFIC BASIS

Yoga is based on ancient observations, principles, and theories of the mind–body connection. Teachers in India and Tibet passed down this precise knowledge to their students from one generation to the next. Western researchers are beginning to validate many of these health claims. Studies have found that the systematic practice of yoga treats symptoms and/or prevents their onset and recurrence (McCall, 2007). Yoga promotes mindfulness, cognitive skills, and well-being (Galantino, Cannon, Hoelker, Quinn, & Greene, 2008; Khalsa, Rudrauf, et al., 2008; Kiser & Dagnelie, 2008). Poor body alignment and breathing are major factors in health problems. Yoga decreases fatigue and improves physical fitness, balance, strength, flexibility, body alignment, and use of extremities (Chen et al., 2008; Chen & Tseng, 2008; Hart & Tracy, 2008; Sathyaprabha et al., 2008; Tekur, Singphow, Nagendra, & Raghuram, 2008). The vital organs and endocrine glands become rehabilitated and more efficient, and the autonomic nervous system stabilizes (Danucalov, Simoes, Kozasa, & Leite, 2008; Raghuraj & Telles, 2008; Dhungel, Malhotra, Sarkar, & Prajapati, 2008).

Researchers have documented positive effects of yoga on attention deficit hyperactivity disorder, asthma, osteoarthritis, carpal tunnel syndrome, obsessive-compulsive disorder, irritable bowel syndrome, HIV/AIDS, multiple sclerosis, chronic low-back pain, and many other health issues (Lipton, 2008). Yoga has reduced insulin resistance and physiological risk factors for cardiovascular disease; improved mood, well-being, and sleep; decreased sympathetic activation; and enhanced cardiovagal function (Innes, Selfe, & Taylor, 2008). Doing yoga has also decreased blood pressure and stress, and increased energy and well-being (Cohen, Chang, Grady, & Kanaya, 2008; Dvivedi, Dvivedi, Mahajan, Mittal, & Singhal, 2008). Yoga has reduced arterial stiffness, a risk for cardiovascular disease (Duren, Cress, & McCully, 2008), and improved fasting blood glucose, lipid profile, oxidative stress markers, and antioxidant status (Gordon et al., 2008). Depression, binge eating, neuroticism, and pain have all been decreased through yoga (Smith et al., 2008).

INTERVENTION

Each of Patanjali's Eight Limbs is a potential nursing intervention. Nurses can develop yoga practices for healthy adults, children, pregnant women, persons confined to a chair, and individuals with physical challenges (McCall, 2007).

Technique

After assessing each individual's needs, nurses can adapt any of Patanjali's Eight Limbs (Hartranft, 2003) as a nursing intervention. For example, some people may need encouragement to behave with nonviolence and compassion toward self and others (Limb 1). Other individuals may need teaching about cleanliness and nutrition (Limb 2). Nurses can demonstrate yogic poses (Limb 3) and yogic breathing techniques (Limb 4). See Exhibit 8.1 and Exhibit 8.2.

Withdrawal of the senses can help individuals to let go of external stimuli and sleep (Limb 5). Individuals who learn to concentrate and meditate can develop meaning in suffering and motivation to develop optimal health (Limb 6 and Limb 7). By experiencing integration, individuals can experience oneness and joy, even when seriously ill or dying (Limb 8) (see Exhibit 8.3).

Guidelines

The best way to learn yoga is to do it. Books, classes, and audiovisual aids describe guidelines for beginning through advanced levels. Qualified teachers can assist nurses to do yoga and use yoga as a nursing intervention. Some individuals benefit more from individual attention and small yoga studios than from large yoga classes at fitness and recreation centers (McCall, 2007).

Exhibit 8.1

Corpse Pose or Deep Relaxation (Savasana)

1. Lie flat on your back with arms relaxed near your sides, palms up, and head, trunk, and legs straight. If you feel uncomfortable, put a pillow and/or blanket under your head and/or knees.
2. Close your eyes, relax, and let your body sink.
3. Breathe in a circular manner: slowly, evenly, deeply through nostrils, from the abdomen, with the in-breath the same length as the out-breath, and no break in-between.
4. When ready, open your eyes, bend your knees, turn to your right, and get up.

Nurses can use Corpse Pose to encourage deep relaxation and to treat hypertension, anxiety, insomnia, chronic fatigue, and other health problems (Cameron, 2008; McCall, 2007).

Note: Adapted from Cameron (2008) and McCall (2007).

Exhibit 8.2

Alternate Nostril Breathing (*Nadi Shodhana*)

1. Sit comfortably with a straight back; breathe in a circular manner, as described in Exhibit 8.1.
2. Place right thumb on right nostril, ring finger on left nostril, and inhale through both nostrils.
3. Use thumb to close right nostril; exhale slowly through left nostril, and then inhale slowly through left nostril.
4. Use ring finger to close left nostril; exhale slowly through right nostril, and then inhale slowly through right nostril.
5. This sequence constitutes one round; repeat for five more rounds.

Nurses can use this *pranayama* technique to create balance by giving each side of the body equal time and strengthening the breath in the weaker nostril.

Note: Adapted from Cameron (2008) and McCall (2007).

Exhibit 8.3

Meditation

1. Lie in Corpse Pose or sit comfortably with a straight back in a chair or on a meditation cushion; close eyes, relax, look inward, and breathe in a circular manner, as described in Exhibit 8.1.
2. Focus on your breath. As you inhale through your nose, silently count "One." Exhale. On the next in-breath, count, "Two," and so on. When your mind wanders away, bring it back to your breath and start with one again. At 10, go back to 1 again.
3. When you are deeply relaxed and focused, open up to your inner experience; simply observe and let go of whatever arises, without attachment, judgment, or direction.

Measurement of Outcomes

Nurses can determine the effectiveness of yoga by asking individuals how they feel after doing yoga. Most health problems develop over time, and yoga may not alleviate them right away. Minor difficulties often respond quickly, but serious problems require sustained, patient practice. Yoga advocates gradual change. Optimal benefits occur from regular practice. Short-term outcomes are notable, however, including a more relaxed attitude, decreased anxiety, improved balance, and increased musculoskeletal flexibility. Faithful practice produces long-term outcomes of better physical, spiritual, and mental health (McCall, 2007).

Precautions

Complications may result from doing yoga in a harmful manner, such as straining to accomplish poses. Yoga discourages anything unnatural, competitive, or hurtful. To avoid injury, nurses can encourage gentleness, mindfulness, and moderation. Although teachers and other aids can be helpful, individuals must seek their own inner wisdom.

Currently, no licensure is required for yoga teachers. However, Yoga Alliance (http://www.yogaalliance.org/) has developed standards for yoga teachers and yoga schools. The International Association of Yoga Therapists (http://www.iayt.org/) is developing standards for yoga therapists—yoga teachers who treat health issues. The American Council on Exercise (http://www.acefitness.org/findanacepro/default.aspx), the American College of Sports Medicine (http://www.acsm.org//AM/

Template.cfm?Section=Home_Page), and the Aerobic and Fitness Association of America (http://www.afaa.com/) certify that a teacher knows about physiology and biomechanics, but many excellent yoga teachers don't have this certification (Lipton, 2008).

USES

Nurses can use yoga as a separate intervention or as part of an integrated health plan. Exhibit 8.4 lists selected studies documenting the effectiveness of yoga for specific health issues. Yoga can help nurses to become healthier and be a healing presence. By doing yoga themselves and using yoga as an intervention, nurses promote nonreactivity of the mind and inner calmness that embraces (rather than denies) difficult circumstances in a healing manner (Cameron, 2002).

CULTURAL IMPLICATIONS

Yoga benefits people of all cultures in ways that make it a universally healthy way of life. In India, yoga is practiced alongside *ayurveda*, a traditional healing system. For Tibetans, yoga goes hand in hand with traditional Tibetan medicine, which is similar to ayurveda. Tibetan medicine and ayurveda teach practitioners how to develop a healthy body and mind in order to live a yogic life (Cameron, 2002; Frawley, 1999; Ninivaggi, 2008). Millions of people all over the world adapt yoga to their culture. When yoga moved to the U.S., the focus of yoga became physical fitness because of Americans' fascination with youth. Recently Americans have been developing more interest in the deeper dimension of yoga (Lipton, 2008; McCall, 2007).

FUTURE RESEARCH

The U.S. National Center for Complementary and Alternative Medicine at the National Institutes of Health (http://nccam.nih.gov/) is funding clinical trials to study the effects of yoga on everything from insomnia to diabetes, HIV disease, immune function, and chronic obstructive pulmonary disease. Yoga's holistic, integrated approach poses challenges

Exhibit 8.4

Selected Studies Documenting the Effectiveness of Yoga for Specific Health Issues

Anxiety: Agte & Chiplonkar, 2008; Butler et al., 2008.

Cancer: Danhauer, et al., 2008; Duncan, Leis, & Taylor-Brown, 2008; Galantino et al., 2008.

Diabetes: Alexander, Taylor, Innes, Kulbok, & Selfe, 2008; Gordon et al., 2008.

Eating disorders: Scime & Cook-Cottone, 2008.

Epilepsy: Lundgren, Dahl, Yardi, & Melin, 2008; Sathyaprabha et al., 2008.

Heart failure: Pullen et al., 2008.

Maternal labor: Chuntharapat, Petpichetchian, & Hatthakit, 2008.

Migraine headache: Wahbeh, Elsas, & Oken, 2008.

Musculoskeletal conditions: Birdee et al., 2008; Tekur et al., 2008.

Obesity: Cohen et al., 2008.

Older adults' fitness: Chen et al., 2008; Chen & Tseng, 2008.

Perimenopausal and menopausal symptoms: Chattha, Nagarathna, Padmalatha, & Nagendra, 2008; Chattha, Raghuram, Venkatram, & Hongasandra, 2008; Innes et al., 2008.

Premenstrual syndrome: Dvivedi et al., 2008.

Substance abuse: Khalsa, Khalsa, Khalsa, & Khalsa, 2008.

for conducting scientific research because yoga affects body and mind in a manner that may not be reproducible and quantifiable. Teasing out specific aspects of yoga is difficult and may not produce statistically significant results. The lack of standardized practices, variety of yoga styles, small sample sizes, and short periods of study complicate the applicability of research results (Lipton, 2008). Nurses would benefit from well-designed studies that address the following research questions:

1. Which yoga practices are therapeutic for specific health issues?
2. What characterizes individuals who systematically practice yoga?
3. How can individuals be encouraged to do yoga regularly?
4. What are effective strategies for teaching nurses to do yoga?

REFERENCES

Agte, V. V., & Chiplonkar, S. A. (2008). Sudarshan Kriya Yoga for improving antioxidant status and reducing anxiety in adults. *Alternative & Complementary Therapies, 14*(2), 96–100.

Alexander, G. K., Taylor, A. G., Innes, K. E., Kulbok, P., & Selfe, T. K. (2008). Contextualizing the effects of yoga therapy on diabetes management. *Family & Community Health, 31*(3), 228–239.

Birdee, G. S., Legedza, A. T., Saper, R. B., Bertisch, S. M., Eisenberg, D. M., & Phillips, R. S. (2008). Characteristics of yoga users. *Journal of General Internal Medicine, 23*(10), 1653–1658.

Butler, L. D., Waelde, L. C., Hastings, T. A., Chen, X. H., Symons, B., & Marshall, J. (2008). Meditation with yoga, group therapy with hypnosis, and psychoeducation for long-term depressed mood: A randomized pilot trial. *Journal of Clinical Psychology, 64*(7), 806–820.

Cameron, M. (2008). The essence of yoga: Ethics, spirituality, and healing. *Wellnessworks, 3*(1), 18–20.

Cameron, M. E. (2002). *Karma & happiness: A Tibetan odyssey in ethics, spirituality, and healing* (Foreword by His Holiness the Dalai Lama). Minneapolis: Fairview Press.

Cameron, M. E., & Parker, S. A. (2004). The ethical foundation of yoga. *Journal of Professional Nursing, 5,* 275–276.

Chattha, R., Nagarathna, R., Padmalatha, V., & Nagendra, H. R. (2008). Effect of yoga on cognitive functions in climacteric syndrome: A randomised control study. *BJOG: An International Journal of Obstetrics and Gynaecology, 115*(8), 991–1000.

Chattha, R., Raghuram, N., Venkatram, P., & Hongasandra, N. R. (2008). Treating the climacteric symptoms in Indian women with an integrated approach to yoga therapy. *Menopause, 15*(5), 862–870.

Chen, K. M., Chen, M. H., Hong, S. M., Chao, H. C., Lin, H. S., & Li, C. H. (2008). Physical fitness of older adults in senior activity centres after 24-week silver yoga exercises. *Journal of Clinical Nursing, 17*(19), 2634–2646.

Chen, K. M., & Tseng, W. S. (2008). Pilot-testing the effects of a newly-developed silver yoga exercise program for female seniors. *Journal of Nursing Research, 16*(1), 37–46.

Chuntharapat, S., Petpichetchian, W., & Hatthakit, U. (2008). Yoga during pregnancy. *Complementary Therapies in Clinical Practice, 14*(2), 105–115.

Cohen, B. E., Chang, A. A., Grady, D., & Kanaya, A. M. (2008). Restorative yoga in adults with metabolic syndrome. *Metabolic Syndrome & Related Disorders, 6*(3), 223–229.

Danhauer, S. C., Tooze, J. A., Farmer, D. F., Campbell, C. R., McQuellon, R. P., Barrett, R., et al. (2008). Restorative yoga for women with ovarian or breast cancer. *Journal of the Society for Integrative Oncology, 6*(2), 47–58.

Danucalov, M. A., Simoes, R. S., Kozasa, E. H., & Leite, J. R. (2008). Cardiorespiratory and metabolic changes during yoga. *Applied Psychophysiology and Biofeedback, 33*(2), 77–81.

Dhungel, K. U., Malhotra, V., Sarkar, D., & Prajapati, R. (2008). Effect of alternate nostril breathing exercise on cardio respiratory functions. *Nepal Medical College Journal, 10*(1), 25–27.

DiStasio, S. A. (2008). Integrating yoga into cancer care. *Clinical Journal of Oncology Nursing, 12*(1), 125–130.

Duncan, M. D., Leis, A., & Taylor-Brown, J. W. (2008). Impact and outcomes of an Iyengar yoga program in a cancer centre. *Current Oncology, 15*(Suppl. 2, 109), 72–78.

Duren, C. M., Cress, M. E., & McCully, K. K. (2008). The influence of physical activity and yoga on central arterial stiffness. *Dynamic Medicine, 7*, 2.

Dvivedi, J., Dvivedi, S., Mahajan, K. K., Mittal, S., & Singhal, A. (2008). Effect of '61-points relaxation technique' on stress parameters in premenstrual syndrome. *Indian Journal of Physiology & Pharmacology, 52*(1), 69–76.

Frawley, D. (1999). *Yoga and ayurveda.* Twin Lakes, WI: Lotus Press.

Galantino, M. L., Cannon, N., Hoelker, T., Quinn, L., & Greene, L. (2008). Effects of Iyengar yoga on measures of cognition, fatigue, quality of life, flexibility, and balance in breast cancer survivors: A case series. *Rehabilitation Oncology, 26*(1), 18–27.

Gordon, L. A., Morrison, E. Y., McGrowder, D. A., Young, R., Fraser, Y. T., Zamora, E. M., et al. (2008). Effect of exercise therapy on lipid profile and oxidative stress indicators in patients with type 2 diabetes. *BMC Complementary and Alternative Medicine, 8*, 21.

Hart, C. E., & Tracy, B. L. (2008). Yoga as steadiness training: Effects on motor variability in young adults. *Journal of Strength and Conditioning Research, 22*(5), 1659–1669.

Hartranft, C. (2003). *The yoga-sutra of Patanjali.* Boston: Shambhala.

Innes, K. E., Selfe, T. K., & Taylor, A. G. (2008). Menopause, the metabolic syndrome, and mind-body therapies. *Menopause, 15*(5), 1005–1013.

Kabat-Zinn, J. (2005). *Coming to our senses.* New York: Hyperion.

Khalsa, S., Khalsa, G. S., Khalsa, H. K., & Khalsa, M. K. (2008). Evaluation of a residential Kundalini yoga lifestyle pilot program for addiction in India. *Journal of Ethnicity in Substance Abuse, 7*(1), 67–79.

Khalsa, S. S., Rudrauf, D., Damasio, A. R., Davidson, R. J., Lutz, A., & Tranel, D. (2008). Interoceptive awareness in experienced meditators. *Psychophysiology, 45*(4), 671–677.

Kiser, A. K., & Dagnelie, G. (2008). Reported effects of non-traditional treatments and complementary and alternative medicine by retinitis pigmentosa patients. *Clinical & Experimental Optometry, 91*(2), 166–176.

Lipton, L. (2008). Using yoga to treat disease: An evidence-based review. *Journal of the American Academy of Physician Assistants, 21*(2), 34–6, 38, 41.

Lundgren, T., Dahl, J., Yardi, N., & Melin, L. (2008). Acceptance and commitment therapy and yoga for drug-refractory epilepsy. *Epilepsy and Behavior, 13*(1), 102–108.

McCall, T. (2007). *Yoga as medicine.* New York: Bantam Books.

Ninivaggi, F. J. (2008). *Ayurveda.* Westport, CT: Praeger.

Pullen, P. R., Nagamia, S. H., Mehta, P. K., Thompson, W. R., Benardot, D., Hammoud, R., et al. (2008). Effects of yoga on inflammation and exercise capacity in patients with chronic heart failure. *Journal of Cardiac Failure, 14*(5), 407–413.

Raghuraj, P., & Telles, S. (2008). Immediate effect of specific nostril manipulating yoga breathing practices on autonomic and respiratory variables. *Applied Psychophysiology and Biofeedback, 33*(2), 65–75.

Sathyaprabha, T. N., Satishchandra, P., Pradhan, C., Sinha, S., Kaveri, B., Thennarasu, K., et al. (2008). Modulation of cardiac autonomic balance with adjuvant yoga therapy in patients with refractory epilepsy. *Epilepsy & Behavior, 12*(2), 245–252.

Scime, M., & Cook-Cottone, C. (2008). Primary prevention of eating disorders. *International Journal of Eating Disorders, 41*(2), 134–142.

Smith, B. W., Shelley, B. M., Dalen, J., Wiggins, K., Tooley, E., & Bernard, J. (2008). A pilot study comparing the effects of mindfulness-based and cognitive-behavioral stress reduction. *Journal of Alternative and Complementary Medicine, 14*(3), 251–258.

Tekur, P., Singphow, C., Nagendra, H. R., & Raghuram, N. (2008). Effect of short-term intensive yoga program on pain, functional disability and spinal flexibility in chronic low back pain. *Journal of Alternative and Complementary Medicine, 14*(6), 637–644.

Wahbeh, H., Elsas, S. M., & Oken, B. S. (2008). Mind–body interventions. *Neurology, 70*(24), 2321–2328.

9 Biofeedback

MARION GOOD
JACLENE A. ZAUSZNIEWSKI

This chapter provides an overview of biofeedback, its scientific basis, health conditions in which it is useful, and a technique that can be used by nurses trained in its practice.

DEFINITION

Biofeedback is based on holistic self-care perspectives in which the mind and body are not separated and people can learn ways to improve their health and performance. Biofeedback therapists use instruments and teach self-regulation strategies to help people to increase voluntary control over their internal physiological and mental processes. Biofeed-back instruments measure physiological activity such as muscle tension, skin temperature, cardiac activity, and brainwaves and then provide immediate and real-time feedback to the person in the form of visual and/ or auditory signals that increase his/her awareness of his/her internal processes. The biofeedback therapist then teaches the person to change these signals and take a more active role in maintaining the health of his/her mind and body. The holistic and self-care philosophies behind biofeedback and its focus on helping persons gain more control over his/her functioning make the intervention an appropriate one for nurses to use. Over time, the person can learn to maintain these changes without continued use of an instrument (Biofeedback Certification Institute of America, 2000).

SCIENTIFIC BASIS

The following data provide the basis for the use of biofeedback:

- Biofeedback originated from research in the fields of psychophysiology, learning theory, and behavioral theory. It has been used by nurses for decades and is consistent with self-care nursing theories.
- For centuries it was believed that responses such as heart rate were beyond the individual's control. In the 1960s scientists found that the autonomic nervous system (ANS) had an afferent as well as a motor system, and control of ANS functioning was possible with instrumentation and conditioning.
- Heart rate variability (HRV) biofeedback was first studied by Soviet scientists in the 1980s. HRV is the amount of fluctuation from the mean heart rate. It represents the interaction between sympathetic and parasympathetic systems and specifically targets autonomic reactivity. HRV biofeedback is based on the premise that slowed breathing will increase the HRV amplitude, strengthen baroreflexes, and improve ANS functioning (McKee, 2008). HRV is easy to learn and can be used with inexpensive, user-friendly devices, some of which can be used independently in the home.
- Neurofeedback uses electroencephalogram (EEG) feedback that shows the person their real-time patterns in cortical functioning. (Yucha & Montgomery, 2008).
- The model for biofeedback is a skills-acquisition model in which persons determine the relationship between ANS functioning and their voluntary muscle or cognitive/affective activities. They learn skills to control these activities, which are then reinforced by a visual and/or auditory display on the biofeedback instrument. The display informs the person whether control has been achieved, reinforcing learning.

- Behavioral strategies, such as relaxation or muscle strengthening, are often part of biofeedback treatment to modify physiological activity.
- Biofeedback with relaxation strategies can be used to control autonomic responses that affect brain waves, peripheral vascular activity, heart rate, blood glucose, and skin conductance.
- Biofeedback combined with exercise can strengthen muscles weakened by conditions such as chronic pulmonary disease, knee surgery, or age.

INTERVENTION

Nurses are ideal professionals to provide biofeedback because of their knowledge of physiology, psychology, and health and illness states. However, to use biofeedback they need to acquire special information, skills, and equipment. It is recommended that information be gained from classes and workshops available in many locations in the United States. Nurses using biofeedback should become certified by the Biofeedback Certification Institute of America (www.bcia.org), which offers certifications in General Biofeedback, Neurofeedback, and Pelvic Muscle Dysfunction Biofeedback. The Association for Applied Psychophysiology and Biofeedback (AAPB) is an excellent resource for information and can be contacted at 10200 W. 44th Avenue, Wheat Ridge, CO 80033 (303-422-8436).

The Biofeedback Foundation of Europe (BFE) sponsors education, training, and research activities in biofeedback. On their Web site, http://www.bfe.org, BFE lists courses that are approved by BCIA. In more remote areas where hands-on courses are not available, Biofeedback Resources International (BRI) is a company that offers a self-directed online course that meets the didactic requirements for BCIA certification. Face-to-face training programs with hands-on training and mentoring, however, are strongly recommended. Both the BRI and the AAPB Web sites offer biofeedback equipment for sale.

Technique

A biofeedback unit consists of a sensor that monitors the patient's physiological activity and a transducer that converts what is measured into an electronic visual or auditory display to the patient. Frequently measured physiological parameters include muscle depolarization, which is monitored by electromyelogram (EMG), and peripheral temperature.

Biofeedback provides information about changes in a physiological parameter when behavioral treatments such as relaxation or strengthening exercises are used for a health problem. For example, a relaxation tape helps persons relax muscles, whereas the EMG biofeedback instrument informs the learner of progress (i.e., reduced tension in the muscle). Temperature feedback is also used with relaxation. As muscles relax, circulation improves and the fingers and toes become warmer. When exercises are used to strengthen perineal muscles in preventing urinary incontinence, success in contracting the correct muscles may be monitored by a pressure sensor inserted into the vagina. In health conditions exacerbated by stress, biofeedback is often combined with stress-management counseling.

Biofeedback is most frequently used in an office or clinic setting in eight to twelve 30-minute training sessions (McKee, 2008). Prior to beginning training at the initial session, the therapist and patient should decide upon the number of sessions. If the patient has not achieved mastery or control of a function by the end of the agreed-upon number of sessions, the reasons and the need for further sessions should be discussed. Both behavioral and feedback parts of the therapy should be identified to patients.

The first session is devoted to assessing the patient, choosing the appropriate mode of feedback, discussing the roles of the nurse and the patient, and obtaining baseline measurements. Measuring several parameters helps in getting valid baseline data. Because success will be determined by changes from baseline, it is essential that these are accurate and reflect the true status of the parameter being used. The first session will be longer than subsequent ones, perhaps lasting 1 to 2 hours. Behavioral exercises are provided.

The therapist plays a key role in the success of biofeedback. It is helpful for the nurse to have advanced training in relaxation, imagery, and stress-management counseling. Because practice of the behavioral techniques is vital, the nurse who succeeds in motivating patients to practice at home is most likely to have patients who achieve their goals.

The final sessions focus on integration of the learning into the person's life. The patient is connected to the machine, but does not receive feedback while practicing the technique; the nurse monitors the degree of control achieved. Descriptions of stressful situations are provided, and the person is asked to practice the procedure as if in those situations. Final measurements are taken. Follow-up sessions at 1 month and 6 months are advocated.

Guideline for Biofeedback-Assisted Relaxation

A protocol for using biofeedback with cognitive–behavioral interventions for relaxation and stress management is found in Exhibit 9.1. This technique could be used for hypertension, anxiety, asthma, headache, or pain because muscle relaxation improves these conditions. The protocol should be tailored to the patient, condition, and type of feedback.

Various types of relaxation exercises, such as autogenic phrases or systematic relaxation, may be used. To increase patient awareness of the relaxed state versus the state of tension, progressive muscle relaxation with alternate contraction and relaxation may be helpful. Imagery may relax patients by distracting the mind and reducing negative or stressful thoughts. Hypnosis and self-hypnosis also produce an alternative state of mind. Soft music relaxes and distracts and may be used with relaxation or imagery.

It is important to keep the requirements for home practice simple, interesting, and meaningful. Boredom with the same relaxation tape, failure to find a convenient time to practice, and lack of noticeable improvements may decrease adherence to home practice. Changing to a new relaxation technique can revive interest. To integrate new skills into daily life, patients can progress to mini-relaxation and use of cues (thoughts, positions, or activities) to signal relaxation. Other interventions and biofeedback modalities appropriate for adults and children can be found in the literature (Olness & Kohen, 1996; Schwartz & Andrisik, 2003).

Although some patients have multiple symptoms that all require treatment, training should only address one symptom at a time. Other symptoms can be treated sequentially after mastery of the first one is attained. The patient can decide which symptom will be treated first.

Measurement of Outcomes

Feedback parameters that reflect mastery of the behavioral intervention are found in Exhibit 9.2. Frequently used mastery parameters include

Exhibit 9.1

Biofeedback Protocol

1. **Before first session:**
   - Determine health problem for which biofeedback treatment is sought.
   - Ask for physician's name so care can be coordinated. Give information on location, time commitment, and cost.
   - Request a 2-week patient log with medications and the frequency and severity of the health problem (e.g., number, intensity, and time of headaches).
   - Answer questions.

2. **First session:**
   - Interview patient for a health history; include the specific health condition.
   - Assess abilities for carrying out current medical regimen and behavioral intervention. Assess cultural preferences for behavioral treatments.
   - Discuss rationale for biofeedback, type of feedback, and behavioral intervention.
   - Explain that the role of the nurse is to provide ten 50-minute sessions once a week, using the biofeedback instrument to supply physiological information.
   - Explain that the patient is the major factor in the successful use of biofeedback and that it is important to continue to keep a log of the health problem, including home practice sessions. The patient should consult the physician if health problems occur.
   - Explain the procedure. If using frontal muscle tension feedback, apply 3 sensors to the forehead after cleaning the skin with soap and water and applying gel. Set the biofeedback machine and operate according to instructions.
   - Obtain baseline EMG readings of frontal muscle tension for 5 minutes while the patient sits quietly with closed eyes.
   - Instruct the patient to practice taped relaxation instructions for 20 minutes while the EMG sensors are on the forehead. Ask the patient to watch the biofeedback display for information on the decreasing level of muscle tension.
   - Review the 2-week record of the health problem and set mutual goals.
   - Give a tape and instructions for practicing relaxation at home. Provide a log to record practice and responses. Discuss timing, frequency, length, and setting for practice.
   - Discuss self-care for any possible side effects to the behavioral intervention.

3. **Subsequent sessions:**
   - Open the session with a 20-minute review of the health-problem log, stressors, and ways used for coping in the past week; provide counseling for adaptive coping.
   - Apply sensors and earphones and let the patient practice relaxation for 20 minutes while watching the display. Quietly leave the room after the patient masters the technique.
   - Vary relaxation techniques to maintain interest and increase skill.
   - Give instructions for incremental integration of relaxation into daily life. For example, add 30-second mini-relaxation exercises for busy times of the day (e.g., touch thumbs to middle fingers, close eyes, and feel relaxation spreading though the body).

(continued)

Exhibit 9.1 *(continued)*

4. Final session:
- Conduct the session as above; obtain final EMG readings.
- Discuss a plan for ongoing practice and stress management after treatment ends.

heart rate, muscle tension, peripheral temperature, blood pressure, heart rate variability, and EEG neurofeedback. It is important that the nurse be clear about mastery parameters that consist of ongoing feedback to the patient, for learning purposes, and outcome parameters that reflect the desired health improvement. For example, temperature feedback is used in peripheral vascular problems, but health care outcomes may be fewer episodes of painful vasoconstriction. Both EMG feedback and temperature feedback are learning modalities used in persons with diabetes mellitus, tension headache, and chronic pain. Outcomes may include decreased glycoslated hemoglobin, fewer and/or less severe headaches, cessation of urinary incontinence, or relief of pain.

Precautions

Biofeedback should be used cautiously, if at all, in persons with depression psychosis, seizures, and hyperactive conditions. Those with rigid personalities may be unwilling to change their mode of functioning. However, negative reactions may be related to relaxation rather than to biofeedback, and may be avoided by means of patient education and the type of relaxation used (Schwartz & Andrisik, 2003).

Biofeedback-assisted relaxation is expected to lower blood pressure and heart and respiratory rates. Excessive decreases should be avoided in patients with cardiac conditions, hemodynamic instability, or multiple illnesses.

Use of relaxation therapies may also reduce the amount of medication needed to control diabetes mellitus, hypertension, and asthma. This should be discussed with patients and physicians; responses should be carefully monitored. For example, in persons with diabetes there is also the potential for hypoglycemic reactions to occur if patient education is not done and/or adjustments in insulin or diet are not made. Patients should be taught to manage hypoglycemia and blood glucose. The nurse should keep simple carbohydrates, glucagon, and a blood

Exhibit 9.2

Parameters Used for Feedback to Patients

Airway resistance

Blood pressure

Blood volume

Bowel sounds

EEG neurofeedback

EMG muscle feedback

Forced expiratory volume

Galvanic skin response

Gastric pH

Heart rate

Heart rate variability

Peripheral skin temperature

Pneumography

Tidal volume

Tracheal noise

Vagal nerve stimulation

glucose monitor in the office and have the expertise to administer them. Home practice can be timed to avoid low blood glucose (McGrady & Bailey, 2005).

Electric shock is a potential hazard when any electrical equipment is used. Dangerous levels of current flow may arise from equipment malfunction or operator error. The AAPB publishes a list of companies whose products have met their safety code.

Although biofeedback is noninvasive, cost-effective, and very promising in the treatment of many conditions, it is not a miracle intervention. It requires that the therapist be knowledgeable about the health problem, intervention, and medication effects, with a sincere interest in patient outcome. Patient time, attention, and motivation to practice are also necessary for success. To control the condition, ongoing use of the behavioral technique may be needed after biofeedback sessions end. This should be made very clear before training is initiated.

USES

Biofeedback has been used in the treatment of many medical and psychological problems. For example, neurofeedback is used for attention and learning disabilities, seizures, depression, brain injury, substance abuse, and anxiety. HRV biofeedback, another relatively new approach, is possibly efficacious for depressive disorders, asthma, coronary heart disease, and myocardial infarction (Yucha & Montgomery, 2008). The AAPB Web site lists 34 conditions in which biofeedback has been empirically studied resulting in an efficacy rating of 3 (probably efficacious) to 5 (efficacious and specific). Biofeedback has been shown to be efficacious in multiple observational, clinical, and wait-list controlled studies, including replications. A visitor to the Web site can click on the health condition of interest and obtain information on the level of evidence, the reason biofeedback would help this condition, and the supporting evidence.

Yucha and Montgomery (2008) review the efficacy ratings for many disorders that have been treated with biofeedback. The health condition for which the best evidence is available is urinary incontinence in females (Level 5—efficacious and specific). Biofeedback treatment of hypertension in adults, anxiety, and chronic pain are at Level 4 (efficacious), whereas diabetes mellitus, fecal incontinence, and insomnia are at Level 3 (probably efficacious). Other populations that have been treated efficaciously with biofeedback are described in Exhibit 9.3.

Inspection of the PubMed database reveals that nurses have authored biofeedback studies on health problems that are of interest to nurses and commonly seen in nursing care. These problems include labor stress, pelvic floor muscle strength after delivery, poststroke footdrop, chemotherapy, stress in mastectomy, climacteric symptoms, incontinence, blood glucose in diabetes, stress in nurses, pediatric migraine, hemodialysis, overactive bladder, hypertension, movement in hemiplegia, anxiety, and chronic lumbar pain.

Tension Headache

Controlled clinical and follow-up studies have shown that biofeedback reduces tension headaches in adults and children. Tension headaches are caused by prolonged tension in the face, jaws, neck, and shoulders. Muscle tension feedback is used to teach patients to recognize their level of tension and relax the muscles using relaxation therapy. Yucha and Montgomery (2008) found that several meta-analyses reported that biofeedback has a stable medium effect size for migraine and is as good as current medications for both migraine and tension headaches. (Andrasik, 2007; Nestoriuc & Martin, 2007). The effects last for most people as long as they continue to practice the behavioral techniques they have learned.

Fecal Incontinence

A *Cochrane Review* of 11 eligible randomized or quasirandomized trials evaluated biofeedback and/or anal sphincter exercises in 564 adults with fecal incontinence. The limited number of trials and their methodological weaknesses does not allow a definitive assessment of the possible role of anal sphincter exercises and biofeedback therapy in this population (Norton, Cody, & Hosker, 2006). This was supported by other reviews (Yucha & Montgomery, 2008).

Motor Function After Stroke

A second *Cochrane Review* was found, but the 13 trials were small, generally poorly designed, and utilized varying outcome measures. Nevertheless, a small number of individual studies suggested that EMG biofeedback plus standard physiotherapy improved motor power, functional recovery, and gait quality when compared with physiotherapy alone; no combined treatment effect could be found (Woodford & Price, 2007; Yucha & Montgomery, 2008).

Children and Adolescents

Age-appropriate biofeedback can be used to treat many conditions in children and adolescents, such as migraine, hypertension, and fecal incontinence. Biofeedback, combined with self-hypnotherapy, helps them change their thoughts and bring about changes in their bodies (Olness & Kohen, 1996). The authors describe special biofeedback equipment, explanations, and inductions for children, and many imaginative and appealing techniques.

CULTURAL ASPECTS

Biofeedback therapy has been used and studied around the world. There are national biofeedback associations in 15 countries in North and South America, Europe, Asia, the Middle East, and Russia (Biofeedback International Resources, 2008). Although the number of articles published outside the United States cannot be easily estimated, the PubMed database identifies scientific articles about biofeedback that have been written in Japanese, German, Dutch, French, Spanish, Chinese, Norwegian, Finnish, Czech, Hebrew, Korean, Russian, and other languages. Interestingly, many of the articles written in these languages are about urinary and fecal incontinence, whereas articles written in English by authors affiliated with these countries are about biofeedback for a wider variety of disorders. In the Russian language there are dozens of studies on many different health problems. In the Japanese language there are three studies, two on stuttering and one on psychogenic torticollis. Many studies from countries around the world are written in English.

Using their native language, nurses have authored or coauthored research reports on biofeedback for a variety of health problems of interest to nurses. In the Korean language, nurses have reported biofeedback studies of abdominal breathing training for quality of life after mastectomy (Kim et al., 2005), extremity movement in hemiplegic patients (Kim, Kim, & Kang, 2003), and progressive muscle relaxation for stress and climacteric symptoms (Jeong, 2004). In Japanese, nurses reported that combined autogenic relaxation training and biofeedback relieved chronic lumbar pain (Yamazaki, Hoshino, Ito, Matsuo, & Katsura, 1985). In the German language, nurses reported a home biofeedback training program for fecal incontinence in elderly patients (Musial, Hinninghofen, Frieling, & Enck, 2000). In French, nurses wrote that biofeedback and relaxation were used for patients with hypertension (Brassard & Couture, 1993). The knowledge and use of biofeedback and behavioral therapies has spanned many cultures.

FUTURE RESEARCH

There continues to be great need for randomized controlled clinical trials to determine the effectiveness, acceptability, and durability of biofeedback in treating physiological and psychological conditions in adults, children, and minorities around the world. Biofeedback studies of prevalent local health problems are needed in developing countries, but large multicenter studies with similar inclusion criteria, biofeedback protocol, and research methods are needed to show overall efficacy (Yucha, 2002). Nurses can address the following questions:

1. What is the cost of biofeedback treatment for persons in various countries?
2. Are there differences in effects when culturally appropriate behavioral treatments are given along with biofeedback?
3. What are the predictors of improvement in using biofeedback for managing health?

REFERENCES

Andrasik, F. (2007). What does the evidence show? Efficacy of behavioural treatments for recurrent headaches in adults. *Neurological Sciences, 28*(Suppl. 2), S70–S77.

Association for Applied Psychophysiology and Biofeedback (AAPB). Retrieved December 20, 2008, from http://www.aapb.org

Biofeedback Certification Institute of America. Retrieved December 20, 2008, from www.bcia.org/

Biofeedback International Resources (2008). Frequently asked questions. Retrieved from http://biofeedbackinternational.com/faqs.htm.

Brassard, C., & Couture, R. T. (1993). Biofeedback and relaxation for patients with hypertension. *Canadian Nurse, 89*(1), 49–52.

Jeong, I. S. (2004). Effect of progressive muscle relaxation using biofeedback on perceived stress, stress response, immune response and climacteric symptoms of middle-aged women. *Taehan Kanho Hakhoe Chi, 34*(2), 213–224.

Kim, K. S., Kim, K. S., & Kang, J. Y. (2003). Effects of upper extremity exercise training using biofeedback and constraint-induced movement on the upper extremity function of hemiplegic patients. *Taehan Kanho Hakhoe Chi, 33*(5), 591–600.

Kim, K. S., Lee, S. W., Choe, M. A., Yi, M. S., Choi, S., & Kwon, S. H. (2005). Effects of abdominal breathing training using biofeedback on stress, immune response and quality of life in patients with a mastectomy for breast cancer. *Taehan Kanho Hakhoe Chi, 35*(7), 1295–1303.

McGrady A. & Bailey B. (2005). Diabetes mellitus. In M. S. Schwartz & F. Andrisik (Eds.), *Biofeedback: A practitioner's guide* (3rd ed., pp. 727–750). New York: Guilford.

McKee, M. G. (2008). Biofeedback: An overview in the context of heart-brain medicine. *Cleveland Clinic Journal of Medicine, 75*(2), S31–S34.

Musial, F., Hinninghofen, H., Frieling, T., & Enck, P. (2000). Therapy of fecal incontinence in elderly patients: Study of a home biofeedback training program. *Zeitschrift fur Gerontologie und Geriatrie, 33*(6), 447–453.

Nestoriuc, Y., & Martin, A. (2007). Efficacy of biofeedback for migraine: A meta-analysis. *Pain, 128*(1–2), 111–127.

Norton, C., Cody, J. D., & Hosker, G. (2006). Biofeedback and/or sphincter exercises for the treatment of faecal incontinence in adults. *Cochrane Database Systematic Review,* (3), CD002111.

Olness, K., & Kohen, D. P. (1996). *Hypnosis and hypnotherapy with children* (3rd ed.). New York: Guilford.

Schwartz, M. S., & Andrisik, F. (Eds.). (2003). *Biofeedback: A practitioner's guide* (3rd ed.). New York: Guilford.

Woodford, H., & Price, C. (2007, April 18). EMG biofeedback for the recovery of motor function after stroke. *Cochrane Database of Systematic Reviews,* Issue 2, Art. No. CD004585.

Yamazaki, C., Hoshino, N., Ito, C., Matsuo, T., & Katsura, T. (1985). Nursing of a patient with chronic lumbar pain—success with autogenic training combined with biofeedback. *Kango Gijutsu. Japanese Journal of Nursing Art, 31*(5), 628–634.

Yucha, C. B. (2002). Problems inherent in assessing biofeedback efficacy studies. *Applied Psychophysiology and Biofeedback, 27*(1), 99–106.

Yucha, C., & Montgomery, D. (2008). *Evidence-based practice in biofeedback and neurofeedback.* Wheat Ridge, CO: Association for Applied Psychophysiology and Biofeedback.

10 Meditation

MARY JO KREITZER
MARYANNE REILLY-SPONG

INTRODUCTION

Meditation is a self-directed practice for relaxing the body and calming the mind that has been used by people in many cultures since ancient times. It is frequently viewed as a religious practice, although its health benefits have long been recognized. It is a recommended intervention for stress reduction, anxiety and anxiety-related disorders, insomnia, expanding awareness, and overall improvement in well-being. Whereas earlier research studies focused on behavioral outcomes associated with meditation (self-reported changes in anxiety, depression, insomnia, and quality of life), more recent research has documented immunological and neurological changes. Research in the area of meditation for adolescents and children is in the early stages.

The resurgence of interest in meditation has drawn largely upon Eastern religious practices, particularly those of India, China, and Japan. Records substantiate the use of meditation by Hindus in India as early as 1500 B.C. Taoists in China and Buddhists in India and China included meditation as an integral part of their religious life. Zen Buddhists in China and Japan reaffirmed the centrality of meditation and practiced a sitting meditation in which a quiet panoramic awareness of whatever is happening at the time is maintained.

Meditation has also been an important aspect of the Western world and the Judeo-Christian tradition. Christian monks and hermits went to the desert to meditate and meditation remains a key element of monastic life. Contemplation, centering prayer, and praying the rosary (repeating the Hail Mary and other prayers on a circlet of beads) are forms of meditation. West (1979) noted the use of meditation in the American Indian culture, the Kung Zhu/twasi of Africa, and the Native Americans of Alaska of North America. In the United States, the most common forms of meditation are sedentary, although there is an increasing interest in many moving meditations such as the Chinese martial art *tai chi*, the Japanese martial art of *aikido*, and walking meditation in Zen Buddhism. Although specific meditative practices vary considerably, the outcomes are similar for all techniques.

DEFINITIONS

Many definitions of meditation can be identified in the literature. West (1979) defined meditation as an exercise in which the individual focuses attention or awareness on a single object. Welwood's definition (1979) is broader, describing meditation as a technique that allows individuals to investigate the process of their consciousness and experiences and to discover the more basic underlying qualities of their existence as an animate reality. Intense concentration blocks other stimuli, allowing the person to become more aware of self.

Everly and Rosenfeld (1981) divided meditation techniques into four forms: Mental repetition, physical repetition, problem concentration, and visual concentration. In *mental repetition*, the person concentrates on a word or phrase, commonly called a *mantra*. Concentration on breathing is frequently the focus in *physical repetition* techniques; however, dance or other body movements can be the object of concentration. Jogging, for example, allows for concentrating on a physical activity, repetitive breathing, and the sound of one's feet hitting the ground. In samatha Buddhist meditation, the person "watches" or concentrates on the breath entering and flowing from the tip of the nostrils. In *problem-contemplation* techniques, an attempt is made to solve a problem that contains paradoxical components, which Zen terms a *koan*. Finally, *visual concentration* techniques are akin to imagery.

Borysenko (1988) defines meditation simply as any activity that keeps the attention pleasantly anchored in the present moment. It is the way we learn to access the relaxation response. Kabat-Zinn, Wheeler, and colleagues (1998) note that meditation is fundamentally different from relaxation techniques in both methods and objectives. A common but erroneous assumption is that the goal of meditation is to achieve a specific, highly pleasant meditative state akin to deep relaxation. According to these authors, there is no single meditative state and the overall orientation is one of non-striving and non-doing. Kabat-Zinn (2005) emphasizes that meditation is best thought of as a "way of being" rather than a collection of techniques. *Mindfulness* expands our capacity for awareness and for self-knowing. When a mindful state is cultivated, it frees people from routinized thought patterns, senses, and relationships and the destructive mind states and emotions that accompany them. When people are able to escape from highly conditioned, reactive, and habitual thinking, they are able to respond in more effective and authentic ways.

SCIENTIFIC BASIS

An understanding of the scientific basis for meditation is emerging. In 1979, West noted that there were few theoretical explanations for meditation's effectiveness, though various explanations had been proposed, including adaptive regression (Shafii, 1973) and desensitization, in as much as meditating allows the person to deal with unfinished psychic material (Tart, 1971). Everly and Rosenfeld (1981) suggested that the role of the focal device used in meditation is to allow the intuitive, non–ego-centered mode of thought processing to dominate consciousness in place of the normally dominant analytic, ego-centered style. When the left (rational, analytic) hemisphere of the brain is silenced, the intuitive mode produces extraordinary awareness. A positive mood, an experience of unity, an alteration in time-space relationships, an enhanced sense of reality and meaning, and an acceptance of things that seem paradoxical are experienced in this superconscious state. A serious meditator may progress through a continuum from beginning meditation to the superconscious state.

In a report to the National Institutes of Health (1992) on alternative medical systems and practices in the United States, research on meditation was summarized as one of several mind–body interventions. In describing how and why meditation may work, Kenneth Walton, Director of the Neurochemistry Laboratory at Maharishi International University in Fairfield, Iowa, cited the link between and among chronic stress, serotonin metabolism, and the hippocampal regulation of the hypothalamic–pituitary–adrenocortical (HPA) axis.

Brain imaging techniques such as positron emission tomography (PET) and functional magnetic resonance imaging (fMRI) have emerged over the past 20 years and have enabled scientists to study the human brain in action. *Neuroplasticity* refers to the structural and functional changes in the brain that result from training and experience. Research on neuroplasticity has confirmed that the brain is not a static organ; rather, it is designed to respond to changing experiences. Neuroplasticity research, Schwartz reports, has documented the ability of neurons to literally forge new connections, to blaze new paths through the cortex, and even assume new roles (Schwartz & Begley, 2002). Research on mental training through meditation published by Lutz and colleagues has provided the most compelling scientific data thus far on what happens in the brain when people meditate (Lutz, Greischar, Rawlings, Richard, & Davidson, 2004). In a study comparing Tibetan monks with student volunteers, this team of researchers found that meditation is associated with brain changes that allow people to achieve different levels of awareness. Longtime practitioners of meditation were found to have unusually powerful gamma waves and the movement of these waves through the brain was better organized and coordinated than in the students. In a separate randomized trial, Davidson and colleagues (2003) demonstrated that the area of the brain associated with positive emotion, the left anterior cerebrum, showed greater activity in participants who completed an 8-week mindfulness meditation program, and these participants also benefitted from an increase in antibody titers to an influenza vaccine.

INTERVENTION

A wide variety of meditation approaches is described in the literature; however, the following six techniques will be described: mindfulness meditation, transcendental meditation (TM), centering prayer, relaxation response, walking the labyrinth, and breath awareness.

Techniques

Mindfulness Meditation

Mindfulness, awareness, and insight meditation are Western terms used interchangeably to describe the Buddhist practice of *vipassana* meditation. The goal of this meditative practice is to increase insight by becoming a detached observer of the stream of changing thoughts, feelings, drives, and visions until their nature and origin are recognized. The process includes eliciting the relaxation response, centering on breath, and then focusing attention freely from one perception to the next. In this form of meditation, no thoughts or sensations are considered intrusions. When they drift into consciousness, they become the focus of attention (Kutz et al., 1985).

An extension of the practice of mindfulness meditation is what Borysenko (1988) calls "meditation in action" (p. 91). It involves a "be here now" approach that allows life to unfold without the limitation of prejudgment. Mindfulness exercises are carried out during normal, daily activities using this approach. It requires being open to an awareness of the moment as it is and to what the moment could hold. It produces a relaxed state of attentiveness to both the inner world of thoughts and feelings and the outer world of actions and perceptions. Borysenko notes that mindfulness requires a change in attitude: Joy is not sought in finishing an activity, but rather in doing it.

Mindfulness-based stress reduction programs (MBSR) originated with the Stress Reduction Clinic at the University of Massachusetts Medical Center and are currently used in more than 120 clinics, hospitals, and HMOs in the United States and abroad (Kabat-Zinn et al., 1998). It is generally understood that in MBSR instruction, participants receive training in three formal meditation techniques: a body-scan meditation, a sitting meditation, and mindful *hatha* yoga, which involves simple stretches and postures.

Transcendental Meditation

A much-publicized technique, transcendental meditation was developed and introduced into the United States in the early 1960s by the Indian leader Maharishi Mahesh Yogi. It is estimated that there are now well over 2 million practitioners. The concept of TM is relatively simple. Students are given a mantra (a word or sound) to repeat silently over and over again while sitting in a comfortable position. The mantra is selected not for its meaning but strictly for its sound. It is the understanding that this sound alone attracts the mind and leads it effortlessly and naturally to a slightly subtler level of the thinking process. If thoughts other than the mantra come to mind, the student is asked to notice them and return to the mantra. It is suggested that practitioners meditate for 20 minutes in the morning and again in the evening. TM is easily learned and is practiced by people of every age, education, culture, and religion. It is not a philosophy and does not require specific beliefs or changes in behavior or lifestyle (Russel, 1976).

Centering Prayer

Though similar to TM in several respects, centering prayer is based in Christianity and is designed to reduce the obstacles to contemplative prayer and union with God. Thomas Keating (1995), the founder of the centering prayer movement, describes centering prayer as a discipline designed to withdraw our attention from the ordinary flow of thoughts. The understanding is that people tend to identify with their thoughts (the "debris" that floats along the surface of the "river") rather than being in touch with the river itself (the source from which these mental objects are emerging). Keating suggests that, like boats or floating debris, our thoughts and feelings must be resting on something. They are resting, he asserts, on the inner stream of consciousness, which is our participation in God's being. In centering prayer, as with TM, people are encouraged to find a comfortable position, to close their eyes, and to focus on a sacred word. Keating notes that 20 to 30 minutes is the minimum amount of time necessary for most people to establish interior silence and to get beyond their superficial thoughts.

Relaxation Response

The relaxation response incorporates four elements that are common in many of the other relaxation techniques: a quiet environment, a mental device, a passive attitude, and a comfortable position. A quiet environment, which is an element of Benson's technique (1975), eliminates outside stimuli and allows the person to concentrate on the mental device. Some people prefer a church or chapel for meditating, but such a place may not be readily accessible. Playing music while meditating is not advocated because it may draw the person's attention away from the internal processes. People should select the place they wish to use for meditation and continue to use that place. This eliminates adjusting to new surroundings and stimuli each time a person meditates.

Use of a mental device helps shift the mind from logical, externally oriented thought to inner rumination. The purpose of the mental device is to preoccupy oneself with an emotionally neutral, repetitive, and monotonous stimulus. Unlike TM, in which the teacher gives the student a mantra, Benson's technique requires the person to select the mental device that will be used whenever the person meditates. It may be a sound, word, or phrase that is repeated silently or aloud, a phrase or portion of a religious prayer or psalm. Fixation on an object is also sometimes used as the mental device.

Walking the Labyrinth

A labyrinth is a single-path (unicursal) structure that has an unambiguous route to the center and back and is not designed to be difficult to navigate. As a spiritual tool or practice, it is thousands of years old. Labyrinths have been found in many ancient cultures, including Greece, Egypt, China, Peru, Ireland, and Scandinavia. As noted by Curry (2000), the labyrinth has roots that extend into prehistoric times and transcend geographic and cultural boundaries. Walking the labyrinth, for many, is a spiritual and even transformative process that can lead to self-discovery and insight.

Labyrinths are increasingly being installed in public areas such as churches, parks, health care facilities, and businesses but may also be found in private homes. Labyrinths can be made with any substance, including bricks, stones, and grasses. They may be carved into a hillside or painted on a piece of canvas.

When people walk through the labyrinth, they encounter a series of twists and turns as they move to the center and then back out. Sands (2001) describes four phases of walking the labyrinth: crossing the threshold, journeying in, arriving at a resting place, and journeying out. There is no one or preferred way to walk the labyrinth. Some use it as a meditative practice and are open to whatever thoughts or insights emerge. Others may enter the labyrinth with a question that they want to explore.

In spite of a lack of published clinical trials on outcomes related to labyrinths, many hospitals have installed labyrinths believing that they can reduce stress in patients and family members as well as staff. Kaiser-Permanente, a large hospital system on the West Coast of the United States, installed labyrinths at three medical centers.

Breath Awareness

Breathing is common to all meditation techniques, but the use of the breath varies across meditation practices. Some meditation practices, such as Zen Buddhist meditation, direct that the practitioner control the breath. Other practices, such as vipassana, or awareness meditation, prescribe passive breathing that is carefully observed.

Breath awareness can be practiced both as a technique to promote awareness and health, or may be used as needed. According to Kabat-Zinn (1990), continued practice of breath awareness is an anchor for mindfulness, which helps the practitioner to remain in-the-moment, bringing calm and creativity to situations requiring perspective. The practice of breath awareness requires a "beginner's mind," open to observation without attempting to change the breath.

Guidelines. Kabat-Zinn (1990) describes a simple process that can be used to teach breath awareness to patients:

1. Sit or lie in a comfortable position. If sitting, keep a straight spine and let the shoulders drop.
2. Close your eyes if that is comfortable, or gaze ahead without focusing.
3. Focus on your full in-breath and out-breath. Notice the sensation of the breath, especially in the rising and falling abdomen.
4. Don't try to change the breath, just notice the "waves" of your own breathing.
5. When your mind wanders away from the breath (e.g. you notice that you are thinking of something else), just return your focus to the breath.

Kabat-Zinn recommends 15 minutes of breath-awareness practice daily. Some patients may initially have difficulty practicing this technique for even 3 minutes. They may be encouraged to gradually increase the duration of practice. Many experts encourage abdominal breathing, where the breath is inhaled through the nose, and the focus is on the rising and falling of the belly. This form of breathing, as opposed to chest breathing, is more efficient and accomplishes greater air exchange and is associated with calm physiologic states, such as peripheral vessel dilation and hand-warming (Fried, 1990).

Patients in highly anxious states may benefit from pursed-lips breathing (Lorig et al., 2006). Although this is a more active breathing technique, it may help a patient with shortness of breath due to exertion or hyperventilation. In this technique, the patient is taught the basic abdominal breathing technique, focusing on the rising and falling of the belly, but purses her lips, as if whistling, during the exhale. The exhale through pursed lips will take longer than the inhale. An assessment of the individual is needed to determine what might be the most appropriate technique. This requires that nurses have knowledge about various approaches to meditation. A sample script for breath awareness is available at http://takingcharge.csh.umn.edu/therapies.

Measurement of Outcomes

Whereas earlier studies of meditation focused on self-report measures and easy-to-obtain physiologic data (changes in blood pressure, respiratory rate, etc.), there is increased interest in neurobiologic and immune system changes. Lutz and colleagues (2004) documented changes in brain structure and function as a result of prolonged meditation. Robinson, Matthews, and Witek-Janusek (2003), in their study of HIV/AIDS patients, found natural killer cell activity and number increased significantly in the mindfulness-based stress-reduction group compared to a control group. In another study with HIV/AIDS patients, Creswell, Myers, Cole, and Irvin (2008) demonstrated that mindfulness meditation practice buffered declines in CD4+ T lymphocytes. It is likely that future meditation research will continue to attempt to elucidate the mechanism of action as well as outcomes associated with meditation. Another trend in the research is evaluation of patient variables as indicators of response to meditation practice.

To document the efficacy of meditation in a clinical setting, nurses can use blood pressure readings, heart rate, and respiratory rate as indicators of its effectiveness. Measures should not only be taken before and immediately after practicing meditation, but also at other times during the day, and records should be kept to determine whether changes occur over time. Because the person is resting while meditating, it would be expected that the readings would be lower after practice. It is also important that continued follow-up be done to determine whether the effect persists over time.

Precautions

Meditation is not a benign intervention. The nurse must be aware of side effects of the intervention, persons for whom it should not be used, and assessments to be made while the person practices meditation. Careful monitoring of reactions to medications is necessary, as doses may need to be altered. Everly and Rosenfeld (1981) noted problems of overdosage with insulin, sedatives, and cardiovascular medications in people who meditated. Because of the effect meditation can have on the cardiovascular system, blood pressure should be checked before meditation begins. If the systolic pressure is below 90 mm Hg, meditation should not be practiced. Patients should be instructed not to meditate if they become light-headed or dizzy. Also, individuals should not stand immediately after meditating because, frequently, a hypotensive state is reached.

Benson (1975) notes that hallucinations can occur if the person meditates for several hours at a time. Loss of contact with reality is a possibility, and continued assessment is needed to determine whether this is occurring. Lazarus (1976) reported cases of attempted suicide, schizophrenia, and severe depression after the continued practice of meditation. In their review of the application of meditation in psychotherapy, Perez-De-Albeniz and Homes (2000) summarize that patients with a history of psychosis and dissociative states may be particularly at risk for adverse reactions to meditation.

USES

There is a substantial body of research supporting the use of meditation for a wide variety of conditions. Exhibit 10.1 lists conditions for which

Exhibit 10.1

Conditions for Which Meditation Has Been Used

Anxiety (Kabat-Zinn, Massion, et al., 1992; Miller, Fletcher, & Kabat-Zinn, 1995)

Asthma (Wilson, Honsberger, Chin, & Novey, 1975)

Cancer (Carlson, Speca, Patel, & Goodey, 2004; Speca, Carlson, Goodey, & Angen, 2000)

Carotid atherosclerosis (Castillo-Richmond et al., 2000)

Chronic pain (Kabat-Zinn, Lipworth, & Burney, 1985; Kabat-Zinn et al., 1992; Zautra et al., 2008)

Coronary artery disease (Guzzetta, 1980; Zamarra, Schneider, Besseghini, Robinson, & Salerno, 1996)

Depression (Teasdale et al., 2000)

Diagnostic procedures (Frenn, Fehring, & Kartes, 1986)

Drug abuse (Shafii, 1973)

Fibromyalgia (Astin et al., 2003)

Headache (Benson, Klemchuk, & Graham, 1974)

HIV/AIDS (Robinson et al., 2003)

Hypertension (Schneider, Staggers, Alexander, & Sheppard, 1996)

Irritable bowel syndrome (Keefer & Blanchard, 2002)

Menopause (Carmody, Crawford, & Churchill, 2006)

Organ transplantation (Gross et al., 2004; Kreitzer, Gross, Ye, Russas, & Treesak, 2005)

Psoriasis (Kabat-Zinn et al., 1998)

Psychotherapy (Bogart, 1991)

Posttraumatic stress disorder (Simpson et al., 2007)

Sleep disturbance (Winbush, Gross, & Kreitzer, 2007)

it has been used. Use of meditation for patients with chronic pain, hypertension, and anxiety and generalized stress will be discussed.

In addition to being a low-cost intervention with demonstrated efficacy, there are some data that suggest meditative practices may also impact overall use of health care services. In a study comparing 2,000 people who meditated with a group of non-meditators of comparable age, gender, and profession, it was found that over a 5-year period, use of medical services (visits to the doctor and hospitalizations) by the group that meditated was 30 to 87% less than the group of nonmeditators (Orme-Johnson, 1987). The difference was greatest for individuals over 40 years of age.

Conditions/Populations

Chronic Pain

Use of meditation for patients experiencing chronic pain has been well documented, experientially and empirically. Early studies of mindfulness-based stress reduction examined the impact of MBSR on patients with chronic pain. In a study of 51 patients with chronic pain who had been unsuccessfully treated by conventional methods, Kabat-Zinn (1982) reported significant decreases in pain and in the number of medical symptoms reported by patients enrolled in a 10-week training program. Significant reductions in mood disturbances and psychiatric symptomatology were also noted. One methodological limitation of this study was the lack of a comparison or control group.

A larger clinical trial by Kabat-Zinn et al. (1985) examined the impact of mindfulness meditation on 90 chronic pain patients. Statistically significant reductions were reported in present-moment pain, negative body image, inhibition of activity by pain, symptoms, mood disturbance, and psychological symptomatology, including anxiety and depression. A comparison group of chronic pain patients did not show significant improvement on these measures. Improvements reported by the patients who received the 10-week mindfulness meditation training were maintained up to 15 months post-meditation training for all measures except present-moment pain.

A 4-year follow-up of 225 chronic pain patients (Kabat-Zinn, Lipworth, Burney, & Sellers, 1987) enrolled in an 8-week mindfulness meditation training program documented that improvements in physical and psychological status were maintained: 93% of patients reported the present use of at least one of the three meditation practices taught in the initial training.

In a randomized controlled clinical trial of patients with fibromyalgia (Astin et al., 2003), an 8-week mindfulness-based meditation intervention was compared with an education support group. Comparison of outcomes at baseline with those at 8, 16, and 24 weeks indicated that both groups demonstrated statistically significant improvements in pain severity across time. However, there was no difference between the mind–body training group and the education support group control. In a recent randomized comparison of mindfulness meditation to cognitive behavioral therapy for rheumatoid arthritis, patients with the most recurrent depression responded more favorably to meditation (Zautra et al., 2008).

In a 1-year follow-up of relaxation response meditation in patients with irritable bowel syndrome (Keefer & Blanchard, 2002), statistically significant reductions in abdominal pain were found post-course, and these changes were maintained over the long term.

Hypertension

Because of the decreases in blood pressure experienced by persons who had practiced TM, Benson (1975) explored the effectiveness of the relaxation response in persons with hypertension. Statistically significant changes between the experimental and control groups were found in his initial study. Mean systolic pressures decreased from 146 to 137 mmHg, and mean diastolic pressures from 93.5 to 88.9 mmHg in subjects who were taught and who practiced Benson's technique. Blood pressure was not measured immediately after meditation, but readings were taken at random times throughout the day instead. It is hypothesized that meditation counteracts the sympathetic responses of the fight-or-flight reaction to stressors.

A study of hypertensive African Americans (Castillo-Richmond et al., 2000) was designed to measure the impact of a TM program on carotid atherosclerosis. In a randomized controlled trial comparing a TM program with a health education program, groups were matched for teaching format, instructional time, home practice, and expectations of health outcomes. Preliminary findings revealed that the TM program was associated with reduced carotid atherosclerosis. This study is encouraging, given the high incidence of hypertension and cardiovascular disease in the African American population.

In a recent randomized controlled trial, middle school students were randomly assigned to practice a mindful breath awareness exercise or to an education control where equal time was spent discussing cardiovascular health promotion. At a 3-months' posttest, meditators experienced statistically significant decreases in resting and daytime ambulatory systolic pressures, daytime systolic pressure, and daytime ambulatory heart rate (Barnes, Davis, Murzynowski, & Treiber, 2004).

As cited in a major State of the Research Report on Meditation, meta-analysis of two trials of TM compared to Progressive Muscle Relaxation showed that TM produced significantly greater improvements in systolic and diastolic pressures (Ospina et al., 2007).

Anxiety and Generalized Stress

Two studies have examined the effect of a group mindfulness-based meditation program on patients with anxiety disorders. In a study of 22 patients diagnosed with generalized anxiety disorder or panic disorder with or without agoraphobia, Kabat-Zinn and colleagues (1992) reported significant reductions in anxiety and depression. These improvements were maintained at a 3-month follow-up. Another follow-up study of this same patient population at 3 years (Miller, Fletcher, & Kabat-Zinn, 1995) revealed maintenance of the gains reported in the original study on the following measures: anxiety, depression, number and severity of panic attacks, mobility, and fear.

Astin (1997) conducted a study of the effect of an 8-week mindfulness-based stress-reduction program on 28 medical students who were randomized to an experimental group or a nonintervention control group. Participants in the mindfulness meditation training evinced significant reductions in overall psychological symptomatology (depression and anxiety), increases in a perceived sense of control, and higher scores on a measure of spiritual experiences. Astin concluded that mindfulness meditation might serve as a powerful cognitive-behavioral coping strategy for transforming the ways in which people respond to life events.

Grossman and colleagues' meta-analysis of 20 MBSR research studies that utilized standard measures of distress (depression, anxiety, coping) demonstrated that mindfulness meditation benefits a wide range of chronic conditions, with moderate to large effect sizes (Grossman, Niemann, Schmidt, & Wallach, 2004).

The impact of a mindfulness-based stress-reduction program on English- and Spanish-speaking patients cared for in a bilingual inner-city primary care clinic was studied by Roth and Creaser (1997). Data revealed that patients who completed the 8-week training program reported statistically significant decreases in medical and psychological symptoms and improvement in self-esteem. Anecdotal reports of the 79 patients who completed the training program indicated that many experienced changes far more profound than the documented reduction in physical and psychological symptoms. Changes reported included greater peace of mind; more patience; less anger and fewer temper outbursts; better interpersonal communication; more harmonious relationships with family members; improved parenting skills; more restful sleep; decreased use of medications for pain, sleep, and anxiety; decrease or cessation of smoking; weight loss; greater acceptance of aspects of life over which they have no control; greater self-knowledge; and a marked improvement in the overall sense of well-being.

CULTURAL APPLICATIONS

As noted earlier, meditation has its origins in both Eastern and Western cultures and its practice is both secular and religious. No studies have focused specifically on patterns of utilization of meditation among different cultural groups; however, a recent study of the adult population in Hennepin County, Minnesota, includes data on use of complementary healing practices, including the use of "meditation or other relaxation therapies." The SHAPE 2006 (Survey of Health of Adults, the Population and the Environment) project is a health surveillance project that was designed to monitor the health status of adults in Hennepin County (Hennepin County Human Services and Public Health Department, 2008). Data were obtained from over 7,500 adults, including individuals representing six racial and ethnic groups: Black/African American (both U.S.-born and African-born groups), Asian/Pacific Islander, Southeast Asian, Hispanic/Latino and White. In this survey, striking differences were noted in the use of meditation among the various racial and ethnic groups. When asked whether they have used meditation or relaxation during the past 12 months, 15.5% of U.S.-born Black/African Americans responded affirmatively, compared to 4.1% of African-born Black/African Americans. Utilization among other groups was reported as follows: Asian/Pacific Islander (8.2%), Southeast Asian (3.9%), Hispanic/Latino (11.5%), and White (14.8%).

FUTURE RESEARCH

Although nurses are increasingly using meditation in their practice, the research base for its use in nursing is sparse. Much of the current research is being conducted by interdisciplinary teams. Because meditation holds great promise as a therapeutic nursing intervention, nurses should be encouraged to contribute to whatever research is being done. Questions and areas that merit further investigation include:

1. What are the characteristics of people who benefit from meditation? Do people who continue to practice it differ significantly from those who abandon it?
2. How easily generalized are the effects of meditation? Does its use affect areas of the person's life other than those for which it was taught? If the person is taught meditation as a means of decreasing hypertension, is there also an improvement in sleep or other areas?
3. How does meditation differ in process and outcome from other forms of self-regulation such as hypnosis, relaxation, and guided imagery?
4. What are biologic and behavioral outcomes associated with meditation?

WEB SITES

Mind and Life Institute: www.mindandlife.org

Center for Spirituality and Healing, University of Minnesota: http://takingcharge.csh.umn.edu/

REFERENCES

Astin, J. (1997). Stress reduction through mindfulness meditation: Effects of psychological symptomatology, sense of control, and spiritual experiences. *Psychotherapy and Psychosomatics, 66*, 97–106.
Astin, J., Berman, B., Bausell, B., Lee, W., Hochberg, M., & Forys, K. (2003). The efficacy of mindfulness meditation plus Qigong movement therapy in the treatment of fibromyalgia: A randomized controlled trial. *Journal of Rheumatology, 30*, 2257–2262.

Barnes, V. A., Davis, H. C., Murzynowski, J. B. & Treiber, F. A. (2004). Impact of meditation on resting and ambulatory blood pressure and heart rate in youth. *Psychosomatic Medicine, 66,* 909–914.

Benson, H. (1975). *The relaxation response.* New York: Avon.

Benson, H., Klemchuk, H., & Graham, J. (1974). The usefulness of the relaxation response in the therapy of headache. *Headache, 14,* 49–52.

Bogart, G. (1991). Meditation and psychology: A review of the literature. *American Journal of Psychotherapy, 45,* 383–412.

Borysenko, J. (1988). *Minding the body, mending the mind.* New York: Bantam.

Carlson, L., Speca, M., Patel, K., & Goodey, E. (2004). Mindfulness-based stress reduction in relation to quality of life, mood, symptoms of stress and levels of cortisol, dehydroepinandrosterone sulfate (DHEAS) and melatonin in breast and prostate cancer. *Psychoneuroimmunology, 29,* 448–474.

Carmody, J., Crawford, S., & Churchill, L. (2006). A pilot study of mindfulness-based stress reduction for hot flashes. *Menopause: The Journal of The North American Menopause Society, 13*(5), 760–769.

Castillo-Richmond, A., Schneider, R., Alexander, C., Cook, R., Myers, H., Nidich, S., et al. (2000). Effects of stress reduction on carotid atherosclerosis in hypertensive African Americans. *Stroke, 31*(3), 568–573.

Creswell, J. D., Myers, H. F., Cole, S. W., & Irwin, M. R. (2009). Mindfulness meditation training effects on CD4+ T lymphocytes in HIV-1 infected adults: A small randomized controlled trial. *Brain, Behavior, and Immunity, 23*(2), 184–188.

Curry, H. (2000). *The way of the labyrinth.* New York: Penguin Compass.

Davidson, R. J., Kabat-Zinn, J., Schumacher J., Rosenkranz, M., Muller, D., Santorelli, S. F., et al. (2003). Alterations in brain and immune function produced by mindfulness meditation. *Psychosomatic Medicine, 65,* 564–570.

Everly, G., & Rosenfeld, R. (1981). *The nature and treatment of the stress responses.* New York: Plenum.

Frenn, M., Fehring, R., & Kartes, S. (1986). Reducing stress of cardiac catheterization by teaching relaxation. *Dimensions of Critical Care Nursing, 5,* 108–116.

Fried, R. (1990). *The breath connection: How to reduce psychosomatic and stress-related disorders with easy-to-do breathing exercises.* New York: Plenum Press.

Gross, C. R., Kreitzer, M. J., Russas, V., Treesak, C., Frazier, P. A., & Hertz, M. I. (2004). Mindfulness meditation to reduce symptoms after organ transplant: A pilot study. *Advances in Mind–Body Medicine, 20*(2), 20–29.

Grossman P., Niemann, L., Schmidt, S., & Wallach, H. (2004). Mindfulness-based stress reduction and health benefits: A meta-analysis. *Journal of Psychosomatic Research, 57,* 35–43.

Guzzetta, C. E. (1989). Effects of relaxation and music therapy on patients in a coronary care unit with presumptive acute myocardial infarction. *Heart & Lung, 18,* 609–618.

Hennepin County Human Services and Public Health Department. (2008, July). *SHAPE 2006 Adult data book: Survey of the health of all the population and the environment.* Minneapolis, MN: Hennepin County. Retrieved April 26, 2009, from http://www.co.hennepin.mn.us/images/HCInternet/HHandSS/Health/Diseases%20and%20Health%20Conditions/SHAPE/AdultDataBookFinal.pdf

Kabat-Zinn, J. (1982). An outpatient program in behavioral medicine for chronic pain based on the practice of mindfulness meditation. *General Hospital Psychiatry, 4,* 33–47.

Kabat-Zinn, J. (1990). *Full catastrophe living: Using the wisdom of your body and mind to face stress, pain, and illness.* New York: Dell.

Kabat-Zinn, J. (2005). *Coming to our senses: Healing ourselves and the world through mindfulness.* New York: Hyperion.

Kabat-Zinn, J., Lipworth, L., & Burney, R. (1985). The clinical use of mindfulness meditation for the self-regulation of chronic pain. *Journal of Behavioral Medicine, 8*(2), 163–190.

Kabat-Zinn, J., Lipworth, L., Burney, R., & Sellers, W. (1987). Four-year follow-up of a meditation program for the self-regulation of chronic pain: Treatment outcomes and compliance. *Clinical Journal of Pain, 2,* 159–173.

Kabat-Zinn, J., Massion, A. O., Kristeller, J., Peterson, L. G., Fletcher, K. E., Pbert, L., et al. (1992). The effectiveness of a meditation-based stress reduction program in the treatment of anxiety disorders. *American Journal of Psychiatry, 149,* 936–943.

Kabat-Zinn, J., Wheeler, E., Light, T., Skillings, A., Scharf, M. J., Cropley, T. G., et al. (1998). Influence of a mindfulness meditation–based stress reduction intervention on rates of skin clearing in patients with moderate to severe psoriasis undergoing phototherapy (UVB) and photochemo-therapy (PUVA). *Psychosomatic Medicine, 60,* 625–632.

Keating, T. (1995). *Open mind, open heart.* New York: Continuum.

Keefer, L., & Blanchard, E. (2002). A one year follow-up of relaxation response meditation as a treatment for irritable bowel syndrome. *Behavior Research & Therapy, 40,* 541–546.

Kreitzer, M. J., Gross, C. R, Ye, X., Russas, V., & Treesak, C. (2005). Longitudinal impact of mindfulness meditation on illness burden in solid organ transplant recipients: Results of a pilot study. *Progress in Transplantation, 15*(2), 166–172.

Kutz, I., Leserman, J., Dorrington, C., Morrison, C., Borysenko, J., & Benson, H. (1985). Meditation as an adjunct to psychotherapy. *Psychotherapy and Psychosomatics, 43*(4), 209–218.

Lazarus, A. A. (1976). Psychiatric problems precipitated by transcendental meditation. *Psychological Reports, 39,* 601–602.

Lorig, K., Holman, H., Sobel, D., Laurent D., Gonzalez, V., & Minor, M. (2000). *Living a healthy life with chronic conditions: Self-management of heart disease, arthritis, diabetes, asthma, bronchitis, emphysema and others.* Boulder, CO: Bull Publishing.

Lutz, A., Greischar, L., Rawlings, N., Richard, M., & Davidson, R. (2004). Long-term meditators self-induce high amplitude gamma synchrony during mental practice. *Proceedings of the National Academy of Sciences, 101*(46), 16369–16373.

Miller, J. J., Fletcher, K., & Kabat-Zinn, J. (1995). Three-year follow-up and clinical implications of a mindfulness meditation–based stress reduction intervention in the treatment of anxiety disorders. *General Hospital Psychiatry, 17,* 192–200.

National Institutes of Health. (1992). *Alternative medicine: Expanding medical horizons.* Washington, DC: U.S. Government Printing Office.

Orme-Johnson, D. W. (1987). Medical care litigation and the transcendental meditation program. *Psychosomatic Medicine, 49,* 493–507.

Ospina, M. B., Bond, T. K., Karkaheh, M., Tjosvold, L., Vandermeer, B., Liang, Y., et al. (2007, June). *Meditation practices for health: State of the research.* (Evidence Report/Technology Assessment No. 155. Prepared by the University of Alberta Evidence-based Practice Center under Contract No. 290-02-0023. AHRQ Publication No. 07-E010). Rockville, MD: Agency for Healthcare Research and Quality.

Perez-De-Albeniz, A. & Holmes, J. (2000). Meditation: concepts, effects and uses in therapy. *International Journal of Psychotherapy, 5*(1), 49–58.

Robinson, F., Matthews, H., & Witek-Janusek, L. (2003). Psycho-endocrine-immune response to mindfulness-based stress reduction in individuals infected with the human immunodeficiency virus: A quasiexperimental study. *Journal of Alternative and Complementary Medicine, 9*, 683–694.

Roth, B., & Creaser, T. (1997). MBSR: Experience with a bilingual inner-city program. *Nurse Practitioner, 20*, 150–176.

Russel, P. (1976). *The TM technique.* Boston: Routledge and Kegan Paul.

Sands, H. R. (2001). *The healing labyrinth.* New York: Barrons.

Schneider, R. H., Staggers, F., Alexander, C. N., & Sheppard, W. (1996). A randomized controlled trial of stress reduction for hypertension in older African-Americans. *Hypertension, 2*, 820–827.

Schwartz, J., & Begley, S. (2002). *The mind and the brain.* New York: Regan Books.

Shafii, M. (1973). Adaptive and therapeutic aspects of meditation. *International Journal of Psychoanalysis and Psychotherapy, 2*, 431–443.

Simpson, T. L., Kaysen, D., Bowen, S., MacPherson, L. M., Chawla, N., Blume, A., et al. (2007). PTSD symptoms, substance abuse, and Vipassana meditation among incarcerated individuals. *Journal of Traumatic Stress, 20*(3), 239–249.

Speca, M., Carlson, L., Goodey, E., & Angen, M., (2000). A randomized, waitlist controlled clinical trial: The effect of a mindfulness meditation–based stress reduction program on mood and symptoms of stress in cancer outpatients. *Psychosomatic Medicine, 62*, 613–622.

Tart, C. (1971). A psychologist's experiences with transcendental meditation. *Journal of Transpersonal Psychology, 3*, 135–143.

Teasdale, J., Segal, S., Williams, J., Ridgeway, V., Soulsby, J., & Lau, M. (2000). Prevention of relapse/recurrence in major depression by mindfulness-based cognitive therapy. *Journal of Consulting and Clinical Psychology, 68*, 615–625.

Welwood, J. (1979). *The meeting of the ways: Explorations in east/west psychology.* New York: Schocken.

West, M. (1979). The psychosomatics of meditation. *Journal of Psychosomatic Medicine, 24*, 265–273.

Wilson, A. F., Honsberger, R. W., Chin, R. T., & Novey, H. S. (1975). Transcendental meditation and asthma. *Respiration, 32*, 74–78.

Winbush, N. Y., Gross, C. R., & Kreitzer, M. J. (2007). The effects of mindfulness-based stress reduction on sleep disturbance: a systematic review. *Explore, 3*(6), 585–591.

Zamarra, J. W., Schneider, R. H., Besseghini, I., Robinson, D. K., & Salerno, J. W. (1996). Usefulness of the TM program in the treatment of patients with coronary artery disease. *American Journal of Cardiology, 77*, 867–870.

Zautra, A. J., Davis, M. C., Reich, J. W., Nicassio, P., Tennen, H., Finan, P., et al. (2008). Comparison of cognitive behavioral and mindfulness meditation interventions on adaptation to rheumatoid arthritis for patients with and without history of recurrent depression. *Journal of Consulting and Clinical Psychology, 76*(3), 408–421.

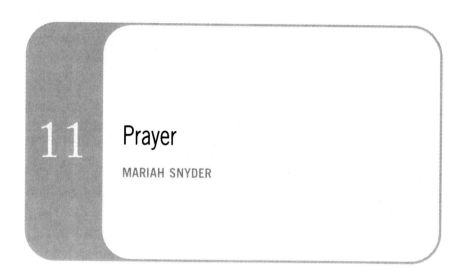

11 Prayer

MARIAH SNYDER

Prayer has been identified as a complementary therapy by the National Center for Complementary and Alternative Medicine (2008). Prayer is ubiquitous, having been used by persons of all cultures throughout time. Findings from a study of African Americans revealed that prayer was used by 60% of the subjects (Brown, Barner, Richards, & Bohman, 2007). In a survey by the National Center for Health Statistics and the National Center for Complementary and Alternative Medicine prayer was the most frequently used complementary therapy by the 31,000 adults contacted. Nearly 50% of the respondents indicated personally using prayer for health reasons, whereas 25% noted others prayed for them (Prayer and Spirituality in Health, 2005).

Some contend that prayer, given its philosophical basis, cannot be studied using randomized clinical trials as the person praying usually seeks to conform to God's will, and God may not always will what the person is specifically requesting (Dusek, Astin, Hibberd, & Krucoff, 2003). However, Roberts, Ahmed, and Hall (2006) suggested that the effects of prayer not dependent on divine intervention may exist and may be studied using randomized clinical trials.

People often equate prayer with religion, yet prayer, like spirituality, transcends religion. Prayer and spirituality acknowledge the existence of a Greater or Supreme Being and we as humans have a connectedness with this Being. Cultural and religious groups have different names for this Higher Being: God, Supreme Being, Mother Earth, Master of the Universe, Creator, Absolute, El, or Great Spirit.

Spirituality, of which prayer is a component, has been a part of nursing for centuries. Religious orders provided much of the hospital care for the sick. Schools of nursing were often sponsored by church-related institutions. The holistic perspective of nursing mandates that nurses assess the spiritual needs of a patient along with the physical, psychological, and social elements. With the increasing cultural diversity in American society it is necessary for nurses to be acquainted with prayer and religious practices found in multiple cultures.

DEFINITION

"Prayer" is from the Latin *precarius*, which means to obtain by begging, and from *precari*, which means to entreat. A simple definition of prayer is the lifting up of the heart and soul to a Supreme Being. According to Nouwen, Christensen, and Laird (2006), "prayer is an attitude of an open heart silently in tune with the Spirit of God, revealing itself in gratitude and contemplation" (p. 62). Prayer, simply, is having a conversation with a loving God.

Prayer and meditation (chapter 10) share many commonalities. Whereas the object of meditation is to focus attention on a word or object so as to become more attentive and aware, the focus of prayer is on communication with a Higher Being. There are many forms of meditation and some of these, such as centering, incorporate prayer.

Many different types of prayer have been described in the literature. Exhibit 11.1 provides a description of types of prayer that are commonly used. Prayer may be done on an individual basis, within a group, or as part of a faith or religious community. In the latter context, prayer often has prescribed words and rituals. Some faith communities, however, are characterized by spontaneity in words and actions, whereas in others silent prayer is primary. Prayer is unique to an individual in that each person establishes his or her relationship with the Absolute or Higher Being.

SCIENTIFIFIC BASIS

As was noted earlier, some suggest that it is oxymoronic to explore the scientific basis of prayer because spirituality and science have a different

Exhibit 11.1

Types of Prayer

Adoration or praise: Acknowledging the greatness of a Higher Being

Colloquial: Communicating informally with Higher Being

Directed: Requesting a specific outcome

Intercessory: Communicating with a Higher Being for another who has a need

Lamentation: Communicating to a Higher Being during bereavement

Nondirected: Requesting the best thing to occur in a given situation

Petition: Asking a Higher Being for a personal request

Ritual: Using set words and/or practices often within a specific religious faith

Thanksgiving: Offering gratitude to a Higher Being for a request or gift received

philosophical perspective. Mueller, Plevak, and Rummans (2001) proposed a number of reasons why persons experience positive results from religious involvement. Spiritual practices such as prayer often engender positive emotions. These emotions in turn help to reduce a person's stress. Persons involved in religious experiences have been shown to have an enhanced immune function. Persons with religious affiliations often have a support system that provides comfort and assistance. Research is needed to validate these hypotheses.

Since the seminal research by Joyce and Welldon (1965), numerous research studies on prayer have been conducted, and findings from many of these studies support the benefits prayer has on health. Byrd (1997) randomized patients who were admitted to a critical care unit into a group who received intercessory prayer by Christians and a control group. All subjects agreed to be in the study but did not know to which group they were assigned. Findings showed that patients in the intercessory prayer group required less ventilatory assistance and fewer antibiotics and diuretics than did patients in the control group. Harris and colleagues (1999) reported that patients in a coronary care unit who received intercessory prayer had an 11% reduction in critical care outcome scores, contrasted with a 4% reduction in the control group. In both of these studies, the length of hospital stay was not affected by prayer. In the MANTRA project, a multicenter study on the effects of intercessory prayer and healing touch with patients undergoing percutaneous corornary interventions, findings showed that patients treated with two-tiered prayer had a 30% lower death rate and rehospital-ization rates at 6 months than did patients in the control group (Emax Health, n.d.).

Studies have also been conducted on the use of prayer with persons having chronic conditions. Sicher, Targ, Moore, and Smith (1998) found that the use of distant healing prayer with persons with AIDS resulted in the experimental group having a lower severity index after 6 months than subjects in the control group. Subjects in the prayer group showed improved mood; however, no differences in CD4+ counts were found between the two groups. In a subsequent study of adults who were HIV-1-positive and who engaged in spiritual activities such as prayer had a reduced risk of death (Fitzpatrick et al., 2007). Konkle-Parker, Erlen, and Dubbert (2008) reported that prayer and spirituality were facilitators of persons with HIV adhering to their medication regimen. Complementary therapies were used by 78% of women who were at an increased risk for breast and ovarian cancer with prayer being one of the most used therapies (Mueller, Mai, Bucher, Peters, Loud, & Greene, 2008)

A number of studies have documented the effectiveness of prayer as a coping strategy. Ai, Dunkle, Peterson, and Bolling (1998) found that patients who prayed following cardiac surgery had a significant decline in depression at 1 year compared to immediately after surgery and that they had less overall distress. The relationship between church attendance and health was examined by Strawbridge, Cohen, Shema, and Kaplan (1997). They found that people who frequently attended church had lower mortality rates than those who attended on an infre-quent basis. Persons who went to church regularly also were more likely to engage in health-promoting behaviors such as exercising and not smoking.

Positive results from prayer have not been found in all of the studies reviewed. In a meta-analysis of studies in which prayer was used as the intervention, Masters and Speilmans (2007) found no evidence that distant intercessory prayer had any impact on health outcomes. Blumenthal and colleagues (2007) reported that prayer, meditation, and church attendance contributed minimally to decreased cardiac mor-bidity in acute myocardial infarction patients who had depression or low levels of social support.

The mechanism of how prayer works, whether intercessory on behalf of others or for oneself, is not known. Dossey (1999) has proposed that prayer is one of a number of nonlocal phenomena, that is, prayer is not constrained by space or time. The person praying does not have to be in proximity to the person being prayed for to be effective. A question about whether the person being prayed for must believe in the efficacy of prayer or be receptive to it for it to be effective has not been explored. In research studies, patients have given consent to be the recipient of prayers. However, in daily life, many prayers are offered for others without their knowledge. Therefore, it is difficult to design studies on prayer that would control for intercessory prayers outside of the research.

INTERVENTION

When prayer is discussed in terms of health, intercessory prayer (that is, prayer for others or for self in relation to a particular problem) is often the type of prayer being used. Less attention has been given to exploring the impact of overall prayerfulness on the lives of individuals.

Assessment

Spiritual assessment should be part of a patient's health history obtained by nurses or other health professionals. Many spiritual assessments include information about the beliefs people hold, how they address the Higher Being, and things that are important to them in order to pray. The Joint Commission (2008) notes the minimal spiritual assessment should obtain information about the faith community or denomination of the patient and what beliefs and spiritual practice, if any, are important to the patient. Examples of other questions that may provide information that is helpful to the health team in planning holistic care are:

- Does the patient use prayer in her/his life?
- How does the patient express his/her spirituality?
- What type of spiritual/religious support does the patient desire? (Joint Commission)

Findings from the spiritual assessment will guide the nurse in deciding if, when, and how to use prayer as an intervention. Persons often find prayer helpful when a diagnosis has been made, during times of high anxiety, prior to and after diagnostic tests and surgery, when giving birth, and when death is imminent. Prayers of thanksgiving should not be forgotten in times of recovery or when the findings from a diagnostic test show no serious condition.

Increased attention is being paid to health professionals praying for their patients (Post, Puchalski, & Larson, 2000). Praying is closely linked to caring for a person. Praying for patients can be as simple as asking God (or the name used for the Higher Being) to bless the patients and families you meet during the day, or it may be a short prayer as one enters a room. (We have little information about the dose of prayer needed for effectiveness. Are long prayers better than short ones?) Remen (2000) commented that caring for the souls of our patients is as important as caring for their bodies.

Technique

If nurses feel comfortable doing so, they can ask if patients would like the nurse to join them in praying. Reading scripture or reading from a holy book is one way to pray with a person. The nurse can create an environment conducive to prayer: playing meditative music, freedom from interruptions, and obtaining books or supplies needed for the person to pray such as a kumalka for a Jewish man or a rosary for a Catholic. Many hospitals, nursing homes, and clinics have a chapel or room for prayer and meditation. The health status of many patients in acute care settings does not allow them to go to a chapel; however, family members may find peace and comfort in this space.

Patients with a religious affiliation may wish to use the formal prayers of their faith tradition. For example, Christians may find the Lord's Prayer comforting. Patients of the Jewish faith may want to read the psalms or have them read to them, and Muslims may choose to read from the Qur'an (Koran). Giving praise to the four directions may be a prayer form that people of Native American ancestry desire to use. Nurses need to respect whatever form or ritual the prayer takes. Exhibit 11.2 provides short prayers from several faith traditions that were obtained from http://www.worldprayers.org. Numerous Web sites provide prayers of many religions that can be shared with patients. A Web site containing Christian prayers and meditations for each day is available at http://www.sacredspace.ie.

Prayer circles or chains exist in many churches and groups. These provide a vehicle for intercessory prayer to be offered for a particular

Exhibit 11.2

Examples of Prayers Used in Several Faith Groups

Islam

In the name of God, the Compassionate, the Merciful.

Say, "It is God, Unique,

God the Ultimate.

God does not reproduce and is not reproduced.

And there is nothing at all equivalent to God."

Qur'an-112:1–4

Hinduism

From the point of Light within the Mind of God

Let light stream forth into the minds of men.

Let Light descend on Earth.

From the point of Love within the Heart of God

Let love stream forth into the hearts of men.

May Krishna return to Earth.

From the centre where the Will of God is known

Let purpose guide the little wills of men—

The purpose which the Masters know and serve.

From the centre which we call the race of men

Let the Plan of Love and Light work out

And may it seal the door where evil dwells.

Let Light and love and Power restore the Plan on Earth.

From *http://www.worldprayers.org* (Retrieved November 10, 2008).

person or family. If nurses are aware of prayer circles, they can ask a patient or family member if he or she would like to have a group include him or her in the prayers being offered.

Measurement of Outcomes

The purpose for which prayer is being used will dictate the outcomes to measure. Because of the mind–body–spirit interactions, nurses may want to include more holistic measures than simply measurement of physiological or psychological status. For example, psychological and spiritual variables that could be measured are contentment, overall well-being, and person's relating that they are more at peace. The effect of prayer may be healing rather than curing an illness that presents a challenge to Western measurement indices.

Precautions

Because of the highly personal nature of faith, spirituality, religious beliefs and practices, it is important for the nurses to assess both the prayer preferences of patients and their own personal beliefs and comfort with using prayer. Knowledge about the beliefs and practices of other faith traditions is imperative in our pluralistic society. Using prayer improperly may offend others, awaken old antipathies, and make patients uncomfortable. Assessment and then offering possibilities is paramount.

Because prayer is to a Supreme Being and the "result" depends on what the Supreme Being determines is best for the person, the outcome is truly outside the person praying. When the outcome is not the one desired by the patient or family, the nurse must be careful not to use such platitudes as "God knows what is best," but rather provide comfort and support.

USES

Prayer has been used with persons having every type of illness, of all age groups, and from all cultures. Exhibit 11.3 lists selected conditions for which studies on the use of prayer have been conducted. The literature also contains many anecdotal accounts about the efficacy of prayer in persons who are ill. In a number of surveys, prayer has been the most frequently used complementary therapy (Barnes, Powell-Griner, McFann, & Nahin, 2002; Brown, Barner, Richards, & Bohman, 2007; King, & Pettigrew, 2004).

CULTURAL ASPECTS

Although prayer can be used separately from a religious context, knowledge about the beliefs and practices of the major religions is helpful.

Exhibit 11.3

Selected Studies Documenting the Effectiveness of Prayer

Acute myocardial infarct (Blumenthal et al., 2007)

Addictive behaviors (Walker, Tonigan, Miller, Comer, & Kahlich, 1997)

Cancer (Mueller et al., 2008; Rezaei, Adib-Hajbaghery, Seyedfatemi, & Hoseini; 2008)

Cardiac conditions (Blumenthal, et al., 2007)

Caregivers (Wilks & Vonk, 2008)

Community-dwelling elderly (Cheung, Wyman, & Halcon, 2007)

Diabetes (Yeh, Eisenberg, Davis, & Phillips, 2002)

Hemodialysis (Walton, 2007)

HIV-1 adults (Fitzpatrick et al., 2007)

Medication adherence (Konkle-Parker, Erlen, & Dubbert, 2008)

Poststroke (Robinson-Smith, 2002)

Reduction of anxiety (Tloczynski & Fritzsch, 2002)

Readers are referred to references such as *World Religions* (Bowker, 2003) that will provide them with information about religious traditions. This knowledge will help the nurse be comfortable in providing spiritual support for patients of diverse cultural and religious backgrounds and not offending a patient by proposing a prayer or ritual that is not part of the person's faith practices.

Muslim Prayer

For patients who are Sunni Muslims, the five mandatory daily prayers must be performed in health and during illness. Shi'ite Muslims offer prayer three times a day. According to al-Shahri and al-Khenaizaan (2005), the five prayer times can be combined into three and modified according to the patient's status. It is traditional for persons to wash or cleanse themselves before praying. Each prayer period takes 5 to 10 minutes and, if possible, the patient is required to face toward the *Ka'abah*. A quiet environment for prayer is desired. Patients may ask to read from the Qur'an. Persons may also find it comforting to hear the Qur'an being sung or chanted on a compact disc or DVD.

Buddhist Prayer

Buddhists, like people who follow other traditions, often pray to some-one or something for the realization of particular goals. Buddhist prayer may consist of asking for something, chanting a mantra, reciting a guru's name, spinning a prayer wheel, or prostrating in front of an altar (Cabezon, 2004). Buddhists may pray out loud or silently, alone or in a group as a joint activity. Typically, though, Buddhist prayer consists of training the mind to heal negative thinking and bring body and mind into harmony, or to send positive energy to someone (Shantideva, 2003). According to Buddhism, this kind of prayer, ordinarily called meditation, awakens inner capacities of strength, compassion, and wisdom (Lewis, 2008). For example, Buddhists do Tonglen meditation to breathe in someone's suffering, and breathe out compassion to the person (Cameron, 2002).

FUTURE RESEARCH

Prayer continues to be a frequently used complementary therapy. In conducting research on prayer, especially using randomized clinical trials, many challenges are encountered. The following are several areas in which research is needed:

1. Most of the reported studies on prayer have been from a Judeo-Christian perspective. Explorations on the impact of prayer on health outcomes need to reflect the many cultures and religions of the world.
2. Few studies have provided specific information about the "dose" of prayer used or of the impact that types of prayer other then intercessory may have on health outcomes. Studies exploring these variables are needed.
3. Study designs that take into account the philosophical basis of prayer and the vast network of persons who may be praying for an individual need to be developed.

REFERENCES

Ai, A. L., Dunkle, R. E., Peterson, C., & Bolling, S. F. (1998). The role of private prayer in psychological recovery among midlife and aged patients following heart surgery. *The Gerontologist, 38,* 591–601.

Al-Shahri, M. Z., & al-Khenaizan, A. (2005). Palliative care for Muslim patients. *Journal of Supportive Oncology, 3,* 432–436.

Barnes, P. M., Powell-Griner, E., McFann, K., & Nahin, R. L. (2005). *CAM at the NIH: Focus on Complementary and Alternative Medicine, 12*(1). Retrieved October 24, 2008, from *http://nccam.nih.gov/news/newslette/2005_winter/prayer.htm*

Blumentahl, J. A., Babyak, M. A., Ironson, G., Thoresen, C., Powell, L., Czajkowski, S., et al. (2007). Spirituality, religion, and clinical outcomes in patients recovering from an acute myocardial infarction. *Psychosomatic Medicine, 69,* 501–508.

Bowker, J. (2003). *World religions.* London: DK Publishing.

Brown, C. M., Barner, J. C., Richards, K. M., & Bohman, T. M. (2007). Patterns of complementary and alternative therapy medicine use in African Americans. *Journal of Complementary & Alternative Medicine, 12,* 751–758.

Byrd, R. C. (1997). Positive therapeutic effects of intercessory prayer in a coronary care unit population. *Southern Medical Journal, 81,* 826–829.

Cabezon, J. (2004). Prayer. In R. E. Buswell (Ed.), *Encyclopedia of Buddhism* (Vol. 2, pp. 671–673). New York: Macmillan.

Cameron, M. E. (2002). *Karma & happiness: A Tibetan odyssey in ethics, spirituality, & healing.* Minneapolis, MN: Fairview Press.

Cheung, D. K., Wyman, J. F., & Halcon, L. L. (2007). Use of complementary and alternative therapies in community-dwelling older adults. *Journal of Alternative & Complementary Medicine, 13,* 997-1006.

Dossey, L. (1999). *Reinventing medicine.* New York: Harper San Francisco.

Dusek, J. A., Astin, J. A., Hibberd, P. L., & Krucoff, M. W. (2003). Healing prayer outcome studies. *Alternative Therapies in Health and Medicine, 9* (Suppl.), A44–A53.

Emax Health. (n.d.) *Results of first multicenter trial of intercessory prayer, healing touch in heart patients.* Retrieved August 8, 2008, from http://www.emaxhealth.com/26/2585.html

Fitzpatrick, A. L., Standish, L. J., Berger, J., Kim, J. G., Calabrese, C., & Polissar, N. (2007). Survival in HIV-1-positive adults practicing psychological or spiritual activities for one year. *Alternative Therapies in Health & Medicine, 13*(5), 18–20, 22–24.

Harris, W. S., Gowda, M., Kolb, J. W., Strychacz, C. P., Vacek, J. L., & Jones, P.G. (1999). A randomized, controlled trial of the effects of remote, intercessory prayer on outcomes in patients admitted to the coronary care unit. *Archives of Internal Medicine, 159,* 2273–2278.

The Joint Commission. (2008). Spiritual assessment. Retrieved August 22, 2008, from *http://www.jointcommission.org/AccreditationPrograms*

Joyce, C. R., & Welldon, R. M. (1965). The objective efficacy of prayer. *Journal of Chronic Disease, 18,* 367–376.

King, M. O., & Pettigrew, A. C. (2004). Complementary and alternative therapy use by older adults in three ethnically diverse populations: A pilot study. *Geriatric Nursing 25*(1), 30–37.

Konkle-Parker, D. J., Erlen, J. A., & Dubbert, P. M. (2008). Barriers and facilitators to medication adherence in a southern minority population with HIV disease. *Journal of the Association of Nurses in AIDS Care, 19,* 98–114.

Lewis, G. R. (2008). *Prayer in Buddhism*. Buddhist Faith Fellowship of Connecticut: Buddhist Prayer. Retrieved October 25, 2008, from *http://buddhistfaith.tripod.com/ pureland_sangha/id41.html*

Masters, K. S., & Spielmans, G. I. (2007). Prayer and health: Review, meta-analysis, and research agenda. *Journal of Behavioral Medicine, 30,* 329–338.

Mueller, P. S., Mai, P. L., Bucher, J., Peters, J. A., Loud, J. T., & Greene, M. H. (2008). Complementary and alternative medicine use among women at increased genetic risk of breast and ovarian cancer. *BMC Complementary & Alternative Medicine, 8,* 17.

Mueller, P. S., Plevak, D. J., & Rummans, T. A. (2001). Religious involvement, spirituality, and medicine: Implications for clinical practice. *Mayo Clinic Proceedings, 76,* 1225–1235.

National Center for Complementary and Alternative Medicine. (2008). *What is CAM?* Retrieved August 21, 2008, from *http://nccam.nih.gov/health/whatiscam*

Nouwen, H., Christensen, M. I., & Laird, R. I. (2006). *Spiritual direction*. New York: HarperCollins.

Post, S. G., Puchalski, C. M., & Larson, D. B. (2000). Physicians and patient spirituality: Professional boundaries, competency, and ethics. *Annals of Internal Medicine, 132,* 578–583.

Prayer and Spirituality in Health: Ancient Practices, Modern Science. (2005). *CAM at the NIH: Focus on Complementary and Alternative Medicine, 12 (1).* Retrieved on October 24, 2008, from http://nccam.nih.gov/neww/newsletter/2005_winter/ prayer.htm

Remen, R. N. (2000). *My grandfather's blessings*. New York: Riverhead Books.

Rezaei, M., Adib-Hajbaghery, M., Seyedfatemi, N., & Hoseini, F. (2008). Prayer in Iranian cancer patients undergoing chemotherapy. *Complementary Therapies in Clinical Practice, 14,* 90–97.

Roberts, L., Ahmed, I., & Hall, S. (2006). Intercessory prayer for the alleviation of ill health. *Cochrane Database of Systematic Reviews 2006.* (4). Retrieved August 21, 2008, from www. Cochrane.org/reviews/en/ab000368.html

Robinson-Smith, G. (2002). Prayer after stroke: Its relationship to quality of life. *Journal of Holistic Nursing, 20,* 352–366.

Sacredspace. (2005). *Daily prayer online*. Retrieved September 27, 2009, from http:// www.sacredspace.ie

Shāntideva. (2003). The way of the bodhisattva: A translation of the Bodhicharyāvatāra (Padmakara Translation Group, Trans.). Boston: Shambhala.

Sicher, F., Targ, E., Moore, D., & Smith, H. S. (1998). A randomized double-blind study of the effect of distant healing in a population with advanced AIDS: Report of a small scale study. *Western Journal of Medicine, 169,* 356–363.

Strawbridge, W. J., Cohen, R. D., Shema, S. J., & Kaplan, G. A. (1997). Frequent attendance at religious services and mortality over 28 years. *American Journal of Public Health, 87,* 957–961.

Tloczynski, J., & Fritzsch, S. (2002). Intercessory prayer in psychological well-being: Using a multiple-baseline, across subjects design. *Psychological Reports, 91,* 731–741.

Walker, S. R., Tonigan, J. S., Miller, W. R., Comer, S., & Kahlich, L. (1997). Intercessory prayer in the treatment of alcohol abuse and dependence: A pilot investigation. *Alternative Therapies in Health and Medicine, 3,* 79–85.

Walton, J. (2007). Prayer warriors: A grounded theory study of American Indians receiving dialysis. *Nephrology Nursing Journal: Journal of the American Nephrology Nurses' Association, 34,* 377–386.

Wilks, S. E, & Vonk, M. E. (2008). Private prayer among Alzheimer's caregivers: mediating burden and resiliency. *Journal of Gerontological Social Work, 50,* 113–131.

World prayers. Retrieved November 15, 2004, from *http://www.worldprayers.org*

Yeh, G. Y., Eisenberg, D. M., Davis, R. B., & Phillips, R. S. (2002). Use of complementary and alternative medicine among persons with diabetes mellitus: Results of a national survey. *American Journal of Public Health, 92,* 1648–1652.

12 Storytelling

MARGARET P. MOSS

The art and science of storytelling is presented in this chapter as a mechanism that can be used in alternative or complementary therapy. Its historical roots in orality (also known as oralism) will be defined and explicated through examples from primary oral cultures. These are cultures that do not have a written language system (Sampson, 1980). In direct contrast, taking the art form into the future, digital storytelling will be explored. Storytelling will then be connected to its use as an alternative method in which to affect the path of one's health in terms of education, prevention, and intervention. Finally, concrete recommendations for health professionals will close out the chapter.

DEFINITIONS

Orality

"The narratives we live and share everyday are our identity as a storied people and make visible what matters most in our lives" (Heliker, 2007, p. 21). Although there are around 3,000 languages in existence today, only 106 have ever been written and less than half of those are said to have "literature" (Edmondson, 1971). Orality is defined as a mostly verbal communication system employed by whole cultures and devoid of the conventions or use of the written word (Olson & Torrance, 1991). The connection of orality or oralism to storytelling is intuitive. Storytelling is as universal in human communication as "the basic orality of language is permanent" (Ong, 1972, p. 7).

Literate societies evolved from oral societies. Each literate individual evolved from an oral beginning (Olson & Torrance, 1991). That is not to say that the formal and informal rules of orality are not as intricate as those in written communication. However, the vast majority of languages have never been translated into a written language (Edmondson, 1971).

The speaker, the process, and the aesthetics of orality are keys to imparting information (Lord, 1960). The rules concerning who speaks and when are defined by the culture. For instance, in some American Indian tribes, certain stories can only be told in the winter, others in the summer. Some words are not to be spoken at certain times of the day or to certain listeners. The process may be as in a prayer, a dance, or a story and can be in front of a large audience, or one-on-one. Aesthetics may involve the use of masks, rattles, costumes, or specific surroundings. Finally, orality uses postural and gestural tools, as well as silence, as paralinguistic features in the transmission of the communication (Tedlock, 1983). "Formulaicness is valued when wisdom is seen as knowledge passed down through generations. Novelty is valued when wisdom is viewed as new information" (Tannen, 1982, p.6). Therefore, anyone wishing to impart information through purposive oral means, such as through storytelling, will need to understand the key components, rules, and assigned power of oralism.

Storytelling

Storytelling is defined as the art or act of telling stories (Story, 2009). A story is "a narrative, either true or fictitious, in prose or verse, designed to interest, amuse, or instruct the hearer or reader; [a] tale." Sociolinguist William Labov (as cited in Sandelowski, 1994) states that a complete story typically is composed of:

- an abstract—what the story is about;
- an orientation—the "who, when, where, and what" of the story;

- the complicating action—the "then-what-happened" part of the story;
- the evaluation—the "so-what" of the story;
- the resolution—the "what-finally-happened" portion of the story;
- the coda—the signal a story is over; and
- the return to the present. (Sandelowski, 1994, p. 25)

It is the instructive nature of storytelling that is of interest for health care as an alternative means to an outcome, namely, improved health. But it must also be understood that lives, including our health are "shaped by the stories we live" (Heliker, 2007, p. 21). Stories have shaped patients' current selves, and it is through stories that nurses can "interest, amuse or instruct" them as listeners. Storytelling has paralleled human endeavors and will continue to evolve through future mechanisms.

Digital Storytelling

Digital storytelling is "the modern expression of the ancient art of storytelling. Digital stories derive their power by weaving images, music, narrative and voice together, thereby giving deep dimension and vivid color to characters, situations, experiences, and insights" (Rule, 2009).

Although technology in digital storytelling provides the processes and aesthetics, it can also present some difficulties. For those cultures with restrictions on word use, the 24-hour, 365-day availability of words via computer technology brings uncertainty. Matching the listener and the teller and their implicit contract is of utmost importance when choosing the type of conveyance.

Storytelling, whether traditional or digital, whether oral or written, serves multiple purposes across the life span and can be used by nurses. Nurses listen to stories whenever patients tell them what is going on in their lives and they tell and retell stories every time they pass on information about patients (Fairbairn & Carson, 2002). Whether it is the person being cared for or the nurse, each person telling the story "is" the story being told (Sandelowski, 1994). It is in the unfolding, intertwining, and connecting that a story becomes my story, your story, or our story. Stories are woven into the threads of life's fabric in our daily lives (Barton, 2004). We are all connected on a deeper or (if you prefer) higher level and storytelling can take us to these levels.

SCIENTIFIC BASIS

Storytelling "is one of the world's most powerful tools for achieving astonishing results" in almost any industry (Guber, 2007, p. 55). Through an implicit contract between the storyteller and the listener (Guber), time is always a necessary ingredient. The storyteller must take the time to fully tell a story through all of its parts, using the necessary gestures, processes, and aesthetics. A story, as a sequence of events with discernable relations between those events and culminating in some conclusion, is a cognitive package (Bergner, 2007) that can be given to the listener. The listener must make time available to be present within the story to "hear" the message and absorb it. Successful transmission will allow the listener to repeat the story to others in some form. Repetition, of course, leads to stronger transmission on both sides.

Effective storytellers will understand their listener(s) and what they already know, what they care about, and what they want to hear (Guber, 2007). The great storyteller will guide the story through essential elements based on the listener's understanding that the story is larger than the teller (Guber).

American Indian Exemplar

The Zuni Indians of New Mexico use storytelling through all parts of their lives. It is used casually and formally. It is used in secular and sacred telling. The teller can be a priest, a *kiva* group, a grandmother, or another person. A *kiva* is a "medicine (i.e., priestly) society" to which males are initiated as youths and remain as men to carry out the work of the *kiva* (Moss, 2000). The purpose of the dances they perform can be solely to "heal" listeners from sickness. Through word of mouth, the news may spread that a Rain Dance is called. Unlike what Hollywood portrays, this dance calls listeners to one of the small plazas (flat dirt squares) in the village where they can receive needed healing prayers.

Time is part of the contract. The listener arrives at a loosely determined time and waits. The dancers and lead teller arrive some time later. The teller knows why the listeners are there: The contract is intact. There is respectful listening and targeted telling. The telling is in the form of prayer, song, and dance. The team is in full regalia, with masks and dress from centuries of performances. A formula is employed in the telling. It can take hours. The teller(s), the process, and the aesthetics all come together in dance, silence, and singing to heal the listener.

INTERVENTION

Bergner (2007) writes about the "staying power of stories," which has obvious benefits when delivering therapeutic messages. He tells of stories that patients have recounted as far back as 8 years earlier.

Technique

Stories in therapy draw from the general culture of the patient, integrate common knowledge sequences, and therefore do not require the acquisition of new knowledge to participate (Bergner, 2007). Code words can then be used to recall the entire story for the patient at later dates. Stories can be targeted to specific diagnoses in increasing meaning for the patient. This allows taking away aspects that do not apply and bringing in aspects that may be unique to the patient.

Guidelines

The following guideline sequence has been presented in the literature for storytelling in therapy: present the story, elaborate as needed to increase understanding, and then discuss application to this particular patient situation (Bergner, 2007). In some cultures, there are situations in which reality can be "spoken into being." Again, often these are strongest in oral cultures. However, even in the dominant culture in the United States people will shush a person if they speak about death, cancer, or some bad thing happening.

In primarily oral cultures, such as traditional indigenous societies, it would be difficult to explain advance directives or informed consent in the manner in which they are presented in Western medical facilities. This applies whether in caring for a patient or in conducting research. As an example, it may be the task of a health care provider to tell a traditional American Indian elder from the Southwest that he/she could die, or lose a leg, or get an infection if the suggested traditional treatments were completed. The patient would perceive harm in even "hearing" this message. He/she certainly would not want to review or sign a consent form that contained these facts. In this case, one would be wise to use a hypothetical story instead. The harm would be taken away from the patient and, instead, the teller would describe to the listener "facts" about "another" person in a similar situation, drawing from cultural norms and common knowledge and ask the listener whether the hypothetical person would be willing to go through the procedure.

Using the above guidelines, there would be elaboration as needed in a context familiar to the patient. For instance, one might describe the following:

> Mr. Vigil was an elderly pueblo man who had diabetes. He had had it for 20 years and lived fairly comfortably with his family on the pueblo and saw his doctor regularly. There came a time when Mr. Vigil's leg began to bother him more and more. He tried several things with his doctor to increase blood flow and promote nerve health. Even though he did what he could for his health, it became apparent that he may have to lose the leg to continue living and being with his family. The doctor told him that he would still be able to participate in ceremonies and get around after the surgery with the use of a prosthetic leg and physical therapy. Mr. Vigil was worried. What do you think he was worried about? What do you think he might have decided? What questions would you ask if you were Mr. Vigil?

The use of vignettes such as the preceding one has been introduced in research as well as in practice.

When using stories as an intervention, one should use the ideas of orality, where repetition, setting, aesthetics, and process are important in the transmission of information. Implementing these will assist the listener in retaining the information.

Suggestions for Implementing Storytelling

Suggestions for health care practitioners, educators, or researchers contemplating using storytelling include:

- **Learn the difference between orality and literacy:**
  - ◆ It is much more than that one group reads and the other writes.
  - ◆ A whole system of rules for use of each exist.
  - ◆ Each uses differing paths to arrive at the desired outcomes.
  - ◆ Orality and literacy may be used separately or together.

■ **Understand the parts and mechanisms for telling the story:**
  ◆ The right person tells the right patient the right set of "facts" at the right time, in the right way and the right place.
■ **Understand differences in response to storytelling by age and culture:**
  ◆ Younger *and* older patients may be more attuned to traditional, oral, face-to-face storytelling.
  ◆ The teenage through middle-adult patient may be more open and attuned to digital storytelling techniques.
  ◆ Using vignettes and anecdotes in the third person takes the pressure off of the listener.
■ **Use technology as appropriate:**
  ◆ Certain cultures may *not* access the computer for fear of encountering a word deemed inappropriate at certain times or to certain people.
  ◆ Interactive media can be used with almost all persons *if geared specifically to* their age, culture, and level of technological proficiency.

Measurement of Outcomes

A variety of tools can be used to measure outcomes of storytelling. Depending on the purpose for which storytelling is being used, instruments that measure anxiety, depression, social isolation, spirituality, caring, and sense of well-being may be appropriate. Qualitative research methods may also be used to measure the effectiveness or changes brought about through storytelling, including increased understanding of the information.

Precautions

Those using storytelling need to be prepared to deal with the strong emotions stories may evoke. Health professionals should be ready to assist and support the participants, as diverse reactions can occur. A list of available resources for making referrals for follow-up will be helpful. Only persons trained in psychotherapy should utilize storytelling with people who have psychological problems. The health sciences represent disciplines that attempt to understand humans from their various perspectives and philosophies, but these disciplines have grown so specialized in their jargon that the message to the patient may easily be lost (Evans, 2007). The use of storytelling in common vernacular can be an antidote to this loss of message.

USES

The use of storytelling in health care settings, health care research, and teaching is unlimited. This section will share some examples of the use of storytelling. Nurses can use storytelling in multiple situations across the life span for a variety of purposes. Stories can be used in family therapy and can assist members to tap into the flow of meaning of the past, present, and future, and help patients open up possibilities for making meaning and healing (Roberts, 1994).

Older Persons: Practice

To increase the reciprocity of care between nursing home staff and residents, *story sharing* has been used as an intervention strategy. To lessen the almost totally task-oriented nature of caring, the use of story sharing has been shown to increase the quality of life of residents in six different nursing homes (Heliker, 2007). Through story sharing, the staff was encouraged to come to know the patients, their backgrounds, interests, and likes. Active listening and expressions of concern are key. It is a mutual process in which each learns about the other and trust and shared experiences become evident. The intervention suggested by Heliker used three 1-hour sessions between six nurse aides and a facilitator. In Session 1, staff learn about confidentiality, respectful and attentive listening, and role playing. In Session 2, staff bring an object that holds personal meaning for themselves, to better understand the residents and what few possessions residents may have with them and the monumental meaning of these possessions. In Session 3, staff learn about "sharing informs care" practices. Both residents and aides reported being in a better relationship with each other, which can be seen as a "best practice" in the care of older, frail adults (Heliker).

Older Persons: Education

"Many older adults were raised in an era when learning occurred primarily through reading, discussion, and retelling stories" (Cangelosi &

Sorrell, 2008, p. 19). Often it is through storytelling, whether formal or informal, that otherwise missed information will be shared. Many elderly parents detail numerous topics and events until they hit upon pertinent information in describing their current problem. Unless this "wandering" is not only allowed but encouraged, especially with older patients, crucial data needed for their care will be missed. When questions requiring only *yes* and *no* answers are asked and are hurried in encounters with elderly persons, older persons will not be able to share information with the health care professional that is vital to their health story. Probing questions require time, patience, and empathy. In addition, older persons will need time to *hear* and process what the health care provider is telling them. One strategy is to share health information in a group setting allowing for support from others in the group (Cangelosi & Sorrell). But by using storytelling as an intervention for teaching older persons, unique learning needs will be met (Cangelosi & Sorrell).

Digital Storytelling

Digital storytelling may be an effective way to educate younger people, whether in the classroom or in patient education, in this world of ever changing technology. Visual and audio media may stimulate deeper learning in this population, which is largely familiar and comfortable with the use of technology (Sandars, Murray, & Pellow, 2008). Sandars and colleagues have used digital storytelling with medical students. As a guideline, they suggest the following 12-step sequence of events for digital storytelling:

1. Decide on the topic of the story.
2. Write the story.
3. Collect a variety of multimedia to create a story.
4. Select which to use to create the story.
5. Create the story.
6. Present the digital story.
7. Encourage reflection at each stage of the project.
8. Avoid being too ambitious.
9. Provide adequate technical support.
10. Develop a relevant assessment framework.
11. Embed it within existing teaching and learning approaches.
12. Persuade others of its value.

Here, building the story encourages active learning and constant reflection for the teller. This process could be used with other populations such as patient groups. Although the storyteller is in many ways the learner in this situation, the same orality notions are in play. The storyteller, the process, and the aesthetics are of great import. Here, rather than regalia, video and audio supply the aesthetics.

CULTURAL APPLICATIONS

In many indigenous societies, especially when they are described as primary oral cultures, Western health practices will be seen as the alternative and complementary modalities (Moss, 2000). This is important, as the practitioner—or here, the storyteller—must understand that to a patient coming from a primary oral culture, storytelling is already seen as primary to their well-being. There have been a number of health-related studies that use storytelling in various cultures (Crawford O'Brien, 2008; Finucane & McMullen, 2008; Inglebret, Jones, & Pavel, 2008; Larkey, & Gonzalez, 2007; Leeman, Skelly, Burns, Carlson, & Soward, 2008).

In a narrative analysis of 115 stories of women of African descent, Banks-Wallace (2002) found storytelling useful for learning more about the historical and contextual factors affecting the well-being of these women. The major functions storytelling served were: contextual grounding, bonding with others, validating and affirming experiences, venting and catharsis, resisting oppression, and educating others.

Rogers (2004) found storytelling at the heart of 11 Pacific Northwest African American widows, 55 years of age and older, who described their experience of bereavement after their husbands' deaths. During the interviews, the widows took on various mannerisms and speech patterns of persons who were part of the story. These included changed tones, mimicking the voices of those involved, and use of hands, body language, and facial expressions. Nurses should be aware of storytelling as a means to gain in-depth understanding and cultural insight into African American experience.

Culturally appropriate communication methods, such as storytelling, have been found to be effective in health-promotion activities. The *talking circle* is one format in which the art of storytelling occurs. Indigenous Ojibwa and Cree women healers use talking circles as instruments of healing and storytelling in their everyday traditional practice (Struthers, 1999). Storytelling was preferred as a natural pattern of communication for Yakima Indians to learn about health promotion related to cervical cancer prevention (Strickland, Squeoch, & Chrisman, 1999).

FUTURE RESEARCH

Technology will certainly play a larger role in storytelling in the future. However, the orality of storytelling with which we are familiar will always be retained. Therefore, integrating future trends will keep the modality in line with evolving human endeavors. Wyatt and Hauenstein (2008) explore "how technology and storytelling can be joined to promote positive health outcomes" (p.142). They recognize that, although storytelling is widely used to teach children in the classroom, it has been minimally used in the health arena as a teaching–learning tool. With advances in technology—and its ubiquitous presence—interactive, digital storytelling tools may provide one mechanism to help enhance health promotion.

Explorations are needed to determine the efficacy of vignettes in both research and practice, particularly with persons from other cultures and with elders. Triangulation of qualitative and quantitative measures will provide a more complete examination of a patient's reflection, understanding, and outcomes. Specific questions that require exploration include:

1. What are strategies to use to help nurses become more comfortable using storytelling as an intervention?
2. What are some ways in which vignettes can be used with persons from diverse cultures and age groups?

REFERENCES

Banks-Wallace, J. (2002). Talk that talk: Storytelling and analysis rooted in African American oral tradition. *Qualitative Health Research, 12*(3), 410–426.

Barton, S. S. (2004). Narrative inquiry: Locating Aboriginal epistemology in a relational methodology. *Journal of Advanced Nursing, 45*(5), 519–526.

Bergner, R. M. (2007). Therapeutic storytelling revisited. *American Journal of Psychotherapy, 61*(2), 149–162.

Cangelosi, P. R., & Sorrell, J. M. (2008). Storytelling as an educational strategy for older adults with chronic illness. *Journal of Psychosocial Nursing and Mental Health Services, 46*(7), 19–22.

Crawford O'Brien, S. (Ed.). (2008). *Religion and healing in Native America: Pathways for renewal.* Westport, CT: Praeger.

Edmondson, M. E. (1971). *Lore: An introduction to the science of folklore and literature.* New York: Holt, Rinehart, & Winston.

Evans, J. (2007). The science of storytelling. *Astrobiology, 7*(4), 710–711.

Fairbairn, G. J., & Carson, A. M. (2002). Writing about nursing research: A storytelling approach. *Nurse Researcher, 10*(1), 7–14.

Finucane, M. L., & McMullen, C. K. (2008). Making diabetes self-management education culturally relevant for Filipino Americans in Hawaii. *Diabetes Educator, 34*(5), 841–853.

Guber, P. (2007). The four truths of the storyteller. *Harvard Business Review, 85*(12), 52–59, 142.

Heliker, D. (2007). Story sharing: Restoring the reciprocity of caring in long-term care. *Journal of Psychosocial Nursing and Mental Health Services, 45*(7), 20–23.

Inglebret, E., Jones, C., & Pavel, D. M. (2008). Integrating American Indian/Alaska native culture into shared storybook intervention. *Language, Speech, and Hearing Services in Schools, 39*(4), 521–527.

Larkey, L. K., & Gonzalez, J. (2007). Storytelling for promoting colorectal cancer prevention and early detection among Latinos. *Patient Education and Counseling, 67*(3), 272–278. DOI:10.1016/j.pec.2007.04.003.

Leeman, J., Skelly, A. H., Burns, D., Carlson, J., & Soward, A. (2008). Tailoring a diabetes self-care intervention for use with older, rural African American women. *Diabetes Educator, 34*(2), 310–317.

Lord, A. (1960). *The singer of tales* (2nd ed.). Cambridge, MA: Harvard University Press.

Moss, M. P. (2000). *Zuni elders: Ethnography of American Indian aging.* Unpublished dissertation, University of Texas Health Science Center at Houston. Available at: http://digitalcommons.library.tmc.edu/dissertations/AAI9974591/

Olson, D. R., & Torrance, N. (Eds.). (1991). *Literacy and orality.* Cambridge, UK: Cambridge University Press.

Ong, W. J. (2002). *Orality and literacy.* New York: Routledge.

Roberts, J. (1994). *Tales and transformations: Stories in families and family therapy.* New York: Norton.

Rogers, L. S. (2004). Meaning of bereavement among older African American widows. *Geriatric Nursing, 25*(1), 10–16.

Rule, L. (2009). *Digital storytelling.* Retrieved January 9, 2009, from http://electronic portfolios.com/digistory

Sampson, G. (1980). *Schools of linguistics.* Stanford, CA: Stanford University Press.

Sandars, J., Murray, C., & Pellow, A. (2008). Twelve tips for using digital storytelling to promote reflective learning by medical students. *Medical Teacher, 30*(8), 774–777.

Sandelowski, M. (1994). We are the stories we tell: Narrative knowing in nursing practice. *Journal of Holistic Nursing, 12*(1), 23–33.

Story. (2009). *Dictionary.com.* Retrieved February 28, 2009, from: http://dictionary.ref erence.com/search?q=story&db=luna

Strickland, C. J., Squeoch, M. D., & Chrisman, N. J. (1999). Health promotion in cervical cancer prevention among the Yakima Indian women of the Wa'Shat Longhouse. *Journal of Transcultural Nursing, 10*(3), 190–196.

Struthers, R. (1999). *The lived experience of Ojibwa and Cree women healers.* Unpublished dissertation, University of Minnesota, Minneapolis.

Tannen, D. (Ed.). (1982). *Spoken and written language: Exploring orality and literacy.* New York: Ablex Publishing.

Tedlock, D. (1983). *The spoken word and the work of interpretation.* Philadelphia: University of Pennsylvania Press.

Wyatt, T. H., & Hauenstein, E. (2008). Enhancing children's health through digital story. *Computers, Informatics, Nursing: CIN, 26*(3), 142–148; quiz, 149–150.

13 Journaling

MARIAH SNYDER

Journal writing is one of a group of therapies that provide an opportunity for persons to reflect on and analyze their lives and the events and people surrounding them and to get in touch with their feelings. Memoirs, life review, and storytelling are other interventions that utilize a similar scientific basis. All of these therapies require the person to be engaged in reflecting upon and analyzing her/his life and experiences.

From the beginning of history, people have recorded the events of their lives, first in pictures and then in words. Reeve Lindbergh states:

> To write as honestly as I can in my journals about my everyday life and the thoughts and feelings I have as I go along is an old tenacious yearning, maybe due [to] an early discomfort with the oddly intangible[enormities] of my family history. Or perhaps this effort is just something else my mother left to me; her belief that writing is the way to make life as perceptible as life can be perceived. (2008, p. 80)

Although much anecdotal evidence exists about the beneficial effects of journaling, research on the use of journals is sparse. However, results of studies revealing the positive outcomes of journaling have been published (Esterling, L'Abate, Murray, & Pennebaker, 1999; Petrie, Fontanilla, Tomas, Booth, & Pennebaker, 2004; Smith, Anderson-Hanley, Langrock, & Compas, 2005). In nursing, research has been related primarily to journaling as an educational tool.

DEFINITION

The terms journaling, diary, and expressive writing are often used interchangeably. Diaries focus on the recording of events and encounters; journals serve as a tool for recording the process of one's life (Cortright, 2008). Events and experiences are noted in journals, with emphasis on the person's reflections about these events and the personal meaning assigned to them. In journal writing, interplay between the conscious and unconscious often occurs. Forms of expressive writing, such as poetry and stories, are methods a person may use to explore inner feelings and thoughts. The term *journaling* will be used in this chapter to encompass writing for therapeutic purposes.

SCIENTIFIC BASIS

Journaling is a holistic therapy because it involves all aspects of a person—physical (muscular movements), mental (thought processes), emotional (getting in touch with or expressing feelings), and spiritual (finding meaning). Through journal recordings, people are able to connect with the continuity of their lives and thus enhance wholeness. Writing may also aid persons in identifying unconscious ideas and emotions that may be influencing their behaviors and lives. Awareness of these is furthered as persons reflect on specific events, thoughts, or feelings while recording them, link them with past feelings and meanings, and consider present and future implications.

Progoff (1975), a Jungian psychologist who developed a systematized method for journaling called "the intensive journal," noted that this transpsychological approach provided active strategies that enable persons to draw upon their inherent resources to become whole. Through journaling, Progoff maintained, people become more self-reliant as they develop their inner strengths and draw upon these when faced with problems and challenges such as stress or illness.

Journaling provides an opportunity for catharsis about highly emotional events (Pennebaker, 1997). Unlike merely venting one's feelings, journaling furnishes the avenue for a person to explore causes and solutions and gain insights. A participant in a study by Pennebaker noted:

> Although I have not talked with anyone about what I wrote, I was finally able to deal with it, work through the pain instead of trying to block it out. Now it doesn't hurt to think about it. (p. 38)

Inhibiting expression of emotions may result in increased autonomic activity that may have long-lasting harmful effects on the body, such as precipitating hypertension. Therapies that will assist the person in venting feelings in a healthy manner may help to improve a person's health. Ulrich and Lutgendorf (2002) reported that students who journaled about cognitive and emotional aspects of a stressful event developed a greater awareness of the positive aspects of the event, as compared with students who wrote only about the associated emotions or about overall events. Further support for the efficacy of writing about traumatic events was documented in a second study in which persons with HIV infections wrote about emotional topics versus neutral topics; journaling about emotional topics resulted in a heightened immune function (Petrie, Fontanilla, Thomas, Booth, & Pennebaker, 2004). Letter writing was found by Rancour and Brauer (2003) to help women adjust to altered body image following recurrent breast cancer.

Esterling and colleagues (1999) proposed three hypotheses for why journaling may be helpful in bringing about positive physical and emotional outcomes when someone writes about a traumatic event:

1. Journaling allows the person to access multiple aspects of the event, including its significance and meaning.
2. Journaling makes the event more readily accessible. People can recall more dimensions of the event and, as they deal with it over time, the event becomes more automatic and thus less effort is needed to process events about the trauma.
3. Journaling transfers feelings into language. Applying a label to an emotion may help to reduce its intensity.

INTERVENTION

Various techniques for journaling exist, such as free-flowing writing, topical or focused journaling, and creative writing. The length of time

Exhibit 13.1

Guidelines for Journaling

Date entries.

Write for a specified length of time each day.

Have a specific place to write that is private and where interruptions will not occur; you may wish to light a candle or play music to provide a pleasant environment.

Use a pen.

Do not erase or black out words.

Make entries in a notebook specific to journaling; if desired, personalize the notebook with pictures, drawings, colored markers.

What you write is personal and you do not need to share what is written unless you wish to do so.

journaling is carried out (weeks, months, or years) will depend on the specific purpose of the journaling. Sometimes people initially write during a stressful situation or transition in their lives, but become "hooked" and continue writing after the initial event has ended.

Some general guidelines for journaling or writing are found in Exhibit 13.1. What is most important for journaling is for the person to be honest with self when writing. Knowing that the content is private, and to be shared only if the writer so desires, allows the person to write about difficult feelings. If, on the other hand, they know that what they are writing has to be shared, often an internal censor is activated that may deter them from writing their true feelings.

Entries are made in a special notebook. This may be an expensive book designed exclusively for journaling or an inexpensive spiral notebook. Plain notebooks can be personalized by pasting pictures on the cover or using pictures and colored markers throughout the notebook. Since pencil recordings fade over time, a pen should be used as the person may want to re-read past entries. Some may prefer to use word processing for journaling. If this type of recording is done, strategies are needed to maintain privacy.

When to write and for how long are questions each person needs to answer. Pennebaker (1997) recommended journaling sessions of 15 to 30 minutes. Journaling needs to be the servant and not the master. Establishing a specific time of day to make entries is helpful. Some find early morning a good time to write, when (as has been suggested) information in the unconscious seems to be closest to the surface. Others prefer to do journaling in the evening, to resolve pent-up anger or troublesome events of the day before retiring.

Techniques

Free-Flow Journaling

This is the most common type of journaling. Cortright (2008) suggested writing quickly and allowing words to just fall onto the page, without attention to grammar, punctuation, or spelling. The main goal is to put one's thoughts and feelings "on paper." Journaling provides a vehicle to uncover the wisdom one already possesses and the feelings that have been dormant. Sometimes a person will write pages and pages on one topic or event. At other times, one's mind flits from topic to topic. The latter may happen when one is highly distressed, and concentrating on one topic is difficult. There is no right or wrong way to journal. The main goal is to put words into written form and then reflect on them. One suggestion is, upon finishing the day's entry, to re-read it and then jot down an "insight line" about what your entry is "telling" you (Cortright).

Dialogue Writing

This type of journaling allows a person to see an event or situation from two perspectives (Progoff, 1975). Free-flow writing is like a monologue, whereas dialogue journaling allows the person to view the situation from two perspectives. Dialogue writing may help persons to resolve conflicts and to see the perspective of another person. One young woman who had been adopted as an infant and who was unable to find her birth mother used dialogue journaling to have a conversation with her mother and begin to resolve the anger she had toward her birth mother. Dialogue journaling can also be used for dialoguing with one's feelings.

Topical Journaling

This type of journaling focuses on a specific event or situation. The focus can be the person's illness or that of a family member. Persons

Exhibit 13.2

Online Resources About Journaling

Conversations Within: Journal Writing & Inner Dialog; www.journal-writing.com

Journal for You: www.journalforyou.com

Writing the Journey: http://www.writingthejourney.com

---

are asked to write about their feelings, how the illness will affect or has affected their lives, and fears they have about the treatment or outcome. The author has used topical writing at a corrections facility. A theme is used for each session. For example, at a session near Memorial Day, the theme was remembering. Women were instructed to remember someone who had meant a great deal to them and how this person had contributed to their life. Other topics proposed for journaling were happy memories and then haunting memories. Topical writing is often helpful for persons who have difficulty concentrating because it is more directed than free-flowing journaling.

Creative Writing

Some people may be more comfortable writing in story form or in poetry rather than focusing on specific events or emotions in their lives. This type of writing can assist persons to uncover deeper thoughts or emotions in a safe manner, as a story may have characters saying things that the person would feel uncomfortable attributing to him- or herself. Stories allow for feelings to be seen initially in the people in the story and then as they relate to oneself. Pictures may be used as an initiator of a story.

Some persons like to do free-flowing journaling in a poetic form. This type of writing allows the person to be creative and still explore feelings. Using short lines and spreading the content over a page makes it easier to examine thoughts and emotions.

A number of Web sites provide helpful information about journaling. Some of these are noted in Exhibit 13.2.

Measurement of Outcomes

Many outcomes for journal writing may not be immediately discernable. Some of the possible areas to measure are improvement in self-esteem, reduction in anxiety, and acceptance of a chronic condition. Because journaling is very personal, it may be difficult for the nurse to evaluate specific outcomes, but patients doing journaling can report changes that have occurred. Also, unless patients share their journals, nurses are not aware of the content or focus of the journaling. In some studies using journaling, content analysis has been carried out on journal entries to determine themes (DiNapoli, 2004).

Precautions

Fear that others will find and read journal entries is a common concern and may deter persons from being open in expressing themselves in a journal. A concern expressed at a corrections facility was that the journals would be confiscated and used in court. Care needs to be taken if persons appear to be extremely introspective or scrupulous, as journaling may deepen this inward focus.

USES

Journaling has been used to achieve a variety of outcomes. Exhibit 13.3 lists some of the medical conditions for which journaling has been used. In persons newly diagnosed with a chronic illness, journaling about their perspectives on how the illness will affect their lives may help them uncover fears that could then be discussed with a health professional. Journaling also provides an avenue for persons to identify hidden resources or strengths they may possess that will assist them in living with a chronic illness. Writing positive affirmations and then reading the statements may help them gain confidence in their abilities to manage the chronic condition. Pennebaker and associates have used journaling to help persons deal with stressful events including, losses. Another group of researchers (Rancour & Brauer, 2003) used journaling to assist patients with cancer adjust to changes in their body image.

Research and anecdotal evidence support the use of journaling to improve well-being. DiNapoli (2004) found that journaling assisted adolescent girls with a smoking history to lessen their use of tobacco. Ulrich and Lutgendorf (2002) reported that journaling about stressful events resulted in positive growth and health outcomes. Journaling helped elderly patients adapt to changes occurring with aging (Caplan, Haslett, & Burelson, 2005).

Exhibit 13.3

Uses of Journaling

Assist with transitions (Rancour & Brauer, 2003)

Decrease anxiety (Ulrich & Lutgendorf, 2002)

Decrease depression (Smith, Anderson-Hanley, Langrock, & Compas, 2005)

Decrease use of tobacco (DiNapoli, 2004)

Improve community problem solving (Aronson, Wallis, O'Campo, Whitehead, & Schafer, 2006)

Improve well-being (Ulrich & Lutgendorf, 2002; Richards, Beal, Seagal, & Pennebaker, 2000)

Increase creativity (Senn, 2001)

Personal growth (Wagoner & Wijekumar, 2004)

Spiritual growth (Chittister, 2004)

Although not specifically journaling, diaries have been used in intensive care units (Storlie, Lind, & Viotti, 2003). Nurses and families kept a record of the patients' stays. These were then used in a follow-up program to help patients gain an understanding of their time in the intensive care unit, including dreams and times when the patient was confused or unconscious. The program has proven valuable for patients and staff.

Journal writing has also been used extensively to help people develop spiritually. Chittister (2004) related how journaling on quotations or sayings of others helped her gain new perspectives. Journaling may also be helpful in praying. The act of writing helps keep a person centered on conversation with God. As suggested by Chittister, a scriptural passage or one from a holy book may be the stimulus for using journaling to pray.

CULTURAL ASPECTS

Although journaling is a therapy that many persons find helpful, others, particularly persons from oral-based cultures, may find it daunting to reflect on one's thoughts and experiences in writing. Painting and other forms of art may be an alternative mechanism that can be used to express feelings. The author recalls observing a dementia unit and seeing one resident with angry facial expressions who was pacing rapidly up and down the hall. During an art project this resident chose dark colors and made heavy strokes on the paper. Thus, he seemed to be able to express in art what he was unable to express verbally.

The Hmong culture has been a nonoral culture. The embroidery pieces of art created by Hmong women depict the history of the Hmong. This representational embroidery or "story cloths," are used by members, especially women, to convey experiences of the Hmong and their history to future generations (Arkenberg, 2007).

FUTURE RESEARCH

Research on the efficacy of journaling is in its infancy. Few findings exist to guide clinicians in its use with patients. Some areas in which research is needed are:

1. Many cultures around the world are oral-based and hence journaling may be unknown. Explorations on the use of journaling with persons from various cultures are needed.
2. Technology offers numerous possibilities for ways to journal, especially with the growing number of laptop computers and Blackberries. Few studies have explored the use of technology as a means for journaling.
3. Ethical and legal implications for journaling need exploration and need to be resolved, especially for persons who are incarcerated. Fears about their journals being "used against them" often inhibits persons from expressing feelings about their experiences.

REFERENCES

Arkenberg, R. (2007). Hmong story cloths. *SchoolArts: The Art Magazine for Teachers,* 107(2), 32–33.

Aronson, R. E., Wallis, A. B., O'Campo, P. J., Whitehead, T. L., & Schafer, P. (2006). Ethnographically informed community evaluation: a framework and approach for evaluating community-based initiatives. *Maternal and Child Health Journal, 11,* 97–109.

Caplan, S. E., Haslett, B. J., & Burelson, B. R. (2005). Telling it like it is: The adaptive function of narratives in coping with loss in later life. *Health Communication, 17,* 233–251.

Chittister, J. (2004). *Called to question.* Lanham: Sheed & Ward.

Cortright, S. M. (2008). *Journaling: A tool for your spirit.* Retrieved September 3, 2008, from http://www.journalforyou.com/full_article.php?article_id=7

DiNapoli, P. P. (2004). The lived experience of adolescent girls' relationship with tobacco. *Issues in Comprehensive Pediatric Nursing, 27,* 19–26.

Esterling, B. A., L'Abate, L., Murray, E. J., & Pennebaker, J. W. (1999). Empirical foundations for writing in prevention and psychotherapy: Mental and physical health outcomes. *Clinical Psychology Review, 19,* 79–96.

Lindbergh, R. (2008). *Forward from here.* New York: Simon & Schuster.

Pennebaker, J. W. (1997). *Opening up: The healing power of expressing emotions.* New York: Guilford.

Petrie, K. J., Fontanilla, I., Thomas, M. G., Booth, R. J., & Pennebaker, J. W. (2004). Effect of written emotional expression on immune function in patients with human immunosufficiency virus infection: A randomized trial. *Psychosomatic Medicine, 66,* 272–275.

Progoff, I. (1975). *At a journal workshop.* New York: Dialogue House Library.

Rancour, P., & Brauer, K. (2003). Use of letter writing as a means of integrating body image: A case study. *Oncology Nursing Forum, 30,* 841–846.

Richards, J. M., Beal, W. E., Seagal, J. D., & Pennebaker, J. W. (2000). Effects of disclosure of traumatic events on illness behavior among psychiatric prison inmates. *Journal of Abnormal Psychology, 109,* 156–160.

Senn, L.C. (2001). *The many faces of journaling: Topics and techniques for personal journal writing.* St. Louis: Pen Central Press.

Smith, S., Anderson-Hanley, C., Langrock, A., & Compas, B. (2005). The effects of journaling for women with newly diagnosed breast cancer. *Psycho-Oncology, 14,* 1075–1082.

Storlie, S. L., Lind, R., & Viotti, I. (2003). Using diaries in intensive care: A method for following up patients. *Connect: The World of Critical Care Nursing, 2*(4), 103–108.

Ulrich, P. M., & Lutgendorf, S. K. (2002). Journaling about stressful events: Effects of cognitive processing and emotional expression. *Annals of Behavior Medicine, 24,* 244–250.

Wagoner, D., & Wijekumar, K. (2004). Improving self-awareness of nutrition and life style practices through on-line journaling. *Journal of Nutrition Education & Behavior, 36,* 22–213.

14 Animal-Assisted Therapy

SUSAN O'CONNER-VON

The domestication of animals began over 12,000 years ago and continues today as animals play a significant role in human life (Lindsay, 2000). Much of the knowledge known about the animal–human bond was anecdotal in nature until recently (Pavlides, 2008). Research examining the use of animals as a complementary or alternative therapy is based on studies about pet ownership. It is evident, with approximately 60% of households in the United States owning a pet, that pets play an important role in people's lives (American Veterinary Medical Association, 2007a). Pets can help provide companionship, facilitate exercise, promote feelings of security, be a source of consistency and a comfort to touch (Katcher & Friedmann, 1980). The healing power of pets is "their capacity to make the atmosphere safe for emotions, the spiritual side of healing; whatever you are feeling, you can express it around your pet and not be judged" (Becker, 2002, p. 80).

In a comparative study examining the impact of pet ownership in childhood on young adults' social characteristics and professional choices, those who owned a pet in childhood retrospectively rated their pet higher than television, relatives, and neighbors in terms of social support received during childhood (Vizek, Arambasic, Kerestes, Kuterovac & Vlahovic-Stetic, 2001). The sample comprised 356 college students at a mean age of 21 years (68% women, 32% men). A total of

74% of the sample had pets (mostly dogs) during childhood and were found to be more empathetic and expressed more altruistic attitudes than those students who did not own a pet in childhood. Moreover, those students who had a pet in childhood were more likely to choose a career in the helping professions.

The role that animals play in healing environments was first documented in records from ninth-century Belgium where animals were used with persons with physical disabilities, followed by eighteenth-century England where animals were used with persons with mental illness (Bustad & Hines, 1984; Pavlides, 2008). Florence Nightingale wrote of the connection between animals and health in 1860 by suggesting that pets were perfect companions for the sick, especially those persons with chronic health conditions (Nightingale, 1859/1992).

The 1970s launched the beginning of widespread interest in the interaction between animals and humans in the health care setting. In 1976, Elaine Smith, an American registered nurse, observed the benefits of pets in the health care setting while working in England. She noticed how patients reacted positively to the visits of a chaplain and his golden retriever. Upon returning to the United States, Smith introduced the concept of pet therapy into health care settings and founded Therapy Dogs International (Therapy Dogs International, 2006). In 1977, the Delta Foundation was established to study the human–animal bond and the potential use of animal-assisted therapy (AAT). Scientific research in this area began in the 1980s, with a focus on the establishment of professional standards and guidelines in the 1990s (Fine, 2006)

DEFINITIONS

Animal-Assisted Therapy

Animal-assisted therapy (AAT) is defined as a goal-directed intervention that utilizes the human–animal bond as an integral part of the treatment process (Delta Society, 1996). Although a variety of animal species and breeds are involved in AAT, such as cats, birds, rabbits, horses, and dolphins, it seems dogs account for the highest percentage of animals used for AAT (Hart, 2000).

Some key features of AAT are that (a) specific goals and objectives are set for each patient, (b) progress is measured, and (c) interactions are documented. The goals are designed by a nurse, occupational therapist, physical therapist, physician, or other health care professional who uses AAT in the treatment process (Hart, 2000). A physical goal would include, for example, improved mobility by walking with a dog. Examples of cognitive goals include improved verbal expression (via normal interaction with the animal) and improved short- and long-term memory (via recalling the animal's name and last visit). Examples of social goals include improved social skills and building rapport with others through the animal.

Finally, one example of an emotional goal would be improved motivation shown by getting dressed or walking to see the animal.

Animal-Assisted Activity

Animal-assisted activity (AAA) is defined as the use of the animal–human bond to promote activities to improve a patient's quality of life; however, the activity is not directed by a health professional and is not evaluated (Delta Society, 1996).

Some key features of AAA are that (a) specific goals and objectives are not planned for each patient, (b) visit activities are spontaneous and last as long as needed, and (c) interactions are not necessarily documented. AAAs are less formal and provide human and animal contact for recreation and education.

SERVICE ANIMAL

A service animal is defined in the Americans with Disabilities Act of 1990 as any animal trained to do work for the benefit of a person with a physical or emotional disability (Duncan & Allen, 2000). Service or guide animals are trained specifically for the service they are providing, for example, sight, sound, movement, or support. Once service animals are certified, they have federally approved access to accompany their owner anywhere. Although there is increased awareness and acceptance of therapy dogs in health care and public settings, therapy dogs do not receive federal protection or the same rights as service dogs who assist persons with physical or emotional disabilities.

SCIENTIFIC BASIS

Many research studies indicate that there are physical and/or psychological benefits derived from human–animal bonds. Most of the research that has examined the benefits of AAT has focused on an animal's ability to attenuate a person's response to stress. When a person becomes stressed, the sympathetic nervous system releases a cascade of hormones. Stress reduction strategies, such as petting an animal, can assist in reducing the build-up of these stress hormones (Wolff & Frishman, 2005).

PHYSICAL CONDITIONS

The research examining the impact of AAT on physical conditions has concentrated on several areas of health care, including cardiovascular disease, seizure disorders, and dementia.

Cardiovascular Disease

The study of the relationship between pets and their positive health effects on a human's cardiovascular system dates back to 1929 (Wolff & Frishman, 2005). Several studies demonstrated the effect of pet ownership on survival after myocardial infarction. Friedmann, Katcher, Lynch, and Thomas (1980) conducted the seminal longitudinal study examining the effect of pet ownership on survival for 92 patients after myocardial infarction. Only 5% of the subjects who owned pets died within one year after hospitalization, whereas 28% of those who were not pet owners died during the same interval.

Another study by Friedmann and Thomas (1995), examining pet ownership and one-year survival after myocardial infarction, included the severity of cardiac disease. For the 368 patients in the study, disease severity and pet ownership were found to positively affect survival, whereas marital status and living situations did not.

In the Cardiac Arrhythmia Suppressions Trial (CAST) by Friedmann and Thomas (2003), the investigators examined the effect of owning a pet on heart rate variability (HRV) for patients after recovery from a myocardial infarction. As a noninvasive method of showing risk assessment after myocardial infarction, a depressed HRV predicts cardiac complications and increased mortality. Pet owners in this study had a higher HRV, thus supporting the hypothesis that survival differences between pet owners and non–pet owners were due to differences in the autonomic modulation of the heart, therefore providing long-term cardiac benefits and increased survival rates.

To determine the effects of AAT on hemodynamic measures and state anxiety, 76 patients with advanced heart failure were randomized to (a) a 12-minute AAT session with a therapy dog; (b) a 12-minute visit with a volunteer; or (c) the control group, which included usual care (Cole, Gawlinski, Steers, & Kotlerman, 2007). Data were collected at baseline, at 8 minutes, and at 16 minutes. The results revealed that, compared with the control group, the AAT group had significantly greater decreases in systolic pulmonary artery pressure during and after the AAT intervention and significantly greater decreases in pulmonary capillary wedge pressures during and after the AAT intervention. Moreover, after the intervention, the AAT group had the greatest decrease in state anxiety compared with the other two groups.

Seizure Disorders

The use of animals as an important component of the treatment plan for persons with epilepsy was first documented in 1867 in Germany (Fontaine, 2005). Over the last 2 decades, a number of studies have examined the value of dogs in the care of patients with seizure disorders. A survey of 122 families who had a child with epilepsy reported that, of those living with a dog, 15% of the dogs could predict seizure onset at least 80% of the time (Kirton, Wirrell, Zhang, & Hamiwka, 2004). In addition, 50% of the dogs exhibited behaviors that were protective of the child, such as lying on top of the child during a seizure or pushing the child away from stairs.

Dementia

For over two decades, research has supported the use of AAT with patients with degenerative cognitive disorders. For patients with dementia, interacting with an animal can improve short-term memory and communication (Tyberg & Frishman, 2008) and trigger long-term memory (Laun, 2003). The presence of a therapy dog can decrease agitation and aggression, while increasing social behaviors among patients with dementia (Filan & Llewellyn-Jones, 2006). Indeed, the presence of fish aquariums in a chronic care facility was associated with increased weights and improved nutritional status among 62 patients with Alzheimer's disease (Edwards & Beck, 2002). A study specifically examining problem behaviors in patients with dementia found significantly fewer problem behaviors after placement of a dog in the health care facility (McCabe, Baun, Speich, & Agrawal, 2002).

PSYCHOLOGICAL CONDITIONS

The use of animals for treatment of persons with mental conditions dates back to 1792 in York, England. The goal was to lessen the use of medications and physical restraints by helping residents learn self-control through the care of animals (Fontaine, 2000). Since the 1960's, a number of studies have been conducted to examine the effects of AAT for patients hospitalized on psychiatric wards. AAT can promote feelings of safety and comfort along with a nonevaluative external focus for patients who are not fearful of animals or have a negative attitude toward them (Odendaal, 2000). Specifically, elderly patients with schizophrenia who were exposed to AAT showed improvements in communication, in interpersonal contact with others, and in activities of daily living (Barak, Savorai, Mavashev, & Beni, 2001).

INTERVENTION

AAT has been shown to be a successful intervention for patients of all ages with a variety of physical and psychological conditions.

Guidelines

Selecting an animal for AAT requires careful screening and extensive training (American Veterinary Medical Association, 2007b; Granger & Kogan, 2006).

AAT requires that the animal and handler work together as a team. To provide safe and effective AAT, the AAT team should abide by set standards of practice for AAA and AAT. Examples of Standards of Practice (Delta Society, 1996) for the handler include that he/she: (a) demonstrate appropriate treatment of people and animals; (b) use appropriate social skills; (c) act as the animal's advocate; (d) read the animal's cues; and (e) maintain confidentiality.

AAT Training

Most national therapy dog organizations require the Canine Good Citizen Test (American Kennel Club [AKC], 2003) as a basic skills require-

Exhibit 14.1

Canine Good Citizen Test

Ten Required Exercises

1. Accepting a friendly stranger
2. Sitting politely for petting
3. Appearance and grooming
4. Walking with a loose leash
5. Walking through a crowd
6. Sit and stay on command, staying in place
7. Coming when called
8. Reacting politely to another dog
9. Reacting to distraction without panic or aggression
10. Supervised separation without fear or agitation

Note: From American Kennel Club (2003).

ment for acceptance into a therapy dog training program. The Canine Good Citizen test, developed by the American Kennel Club, is a certification program that tests dogs in everyday situations and requires a dog to have mastered a basic set of skills (Exhibit 14.1).

Most national therapy dog organizations build upon the AKC Canine Good Citizen test in their training programs. Additional requirements may include didactic content for the human partner to address the theory and research supporting AAT, standards of practice, and ethical considerations. The animal partner receives training in simulated health care settings that include such activities as (1) learning how to leave an object alone, such as food or medication, (2) being bumped while walking in a crowded space, (3) being comfortable around hospital equipment such as wheelchairs or walkers, and (4) receiving petting from several people at once.

Measurement of Outcomes

Positive patient outcomes can be dependent on the qualifications and experience of the AAT team. Frequent communication is essential between the AAT team and the health care professionals or therapists involved in the patient's treatment plan (American Veterinary Medical Association, 2007b).

Precautions

Although research supports the positive benefits and the safety of AAT for patients with various health conditions (Tyberg & Frishman, 2008), the potential risks, such as disease transmission, allergies and bites, must be taken into consideration (Beck, 2000).

The major concern for health care facilities is the transmission of infectious diseases.

These potential risks can be decreased by using trained and registered AAT teams along with enforcing standard hand hygiene before and after every visit. Guidelines from the Centers for Disease Control recommend that animals used for AAT be clean, healthy, fully vaccinated, groomed, and free of parasites (Centers for Disease Control, 2003).

To prevent possible risks, a mechanism must be in place for regularly scheduled examinations and preventative care by a veterinarian to assess the physical and behavioral health and well-being of the animal. Results of these examinations must be shared with the appropriate animal regulatory agency and AAT organizations on an annual basis (American Veterinary Medical Association, 2007c).

A comprehensive review specifically examining the potential health risks of animals in the health care setting found that the potential benefits far outweighed the insignificant risks (Brodie, Biley, & Shewring, 2002).

USES

In addition to the types of interventions already mentioned, the variety of ways and settings in which AAT can be used is virtually limitless. One only has to be creative in the design of the intervention. The following is a partial list of additional ways AAT can be utilized and populations in which AAT has been studied (see Exhibit 14.2).

Cultural Applications

There is great diversity in culturally held attitudes about animals, especially pets, both between cultures and within them (Brown, 1985). To understand the diversity of attitudes about animals, it is important to consider the evolution of the domestication of animals and their role

Exhibit 14.2

Populations in Which Animals and Animal-Assisted Therapy Have Been Studied

Adult patients with heart failure (Cole, Gawlinski, Steer, & Kotlerman, 2007)

Adult patients undergoing electroconvulsive therapy (Barker, Pandurangi, & Best, 2003)

Children with acute postoperative pain (Sobo, Eng, & Kassity-Krich, 2006)

Children with cancer (Gagnon et al., 2004)

Children with special health care needs (Gasalberti, 2006)

Children with pervasive developmental disorders (Martin & Farnum, 2002)

Children undergoing dental procedures (Havener et al., 2001)

Elderly patients with Alzeheimer's disease and agitation (Churchill, Safaoui, McCabe & Baun, 1999)

Elderly patients with schizophrenia (Barak, Savorai, Mavashev & Beni, 2001)

Female abuse survivors (Porter-Wenzlaff, 2007)

Lonely elderly adults in long-term care facilities (Banks & Banks, 2002)

Men with aphasia (Macauley, 2006)

Older adults with dementia (Richeson, 2003)

Patients with Alzheimer's disease and nutritional deficits (Edwards & Beck, 2002)

Patients in a rehabilitation facility using psychoactive medications (Lust, Ryan-Haddad, Coover, & Snell, 2007)

---

in society (Young, 1985). Historically, only royalty and the wealthy were able to keep companion animals. Also significant is the influence of religious beliefs; for example, in some religions, cows are considered to be sacred and dogs are considered to be unclean (Brown, 1985).

Before implementing AAT, it is important to be aware of and consider the influence of cultural and personal attitudes about animals. Although one cannot stereotype a person's view of animals based on their ethnic or cultural background, it is important to be aware of the possibility of cultural differences. For example, Koreans in their native country rarely have cats or dogs as pets, because they have been viewed for a long time as a source of food (Chandler, 2005). In contrast, European Americans have integrated cats and dogs into their family system as pets for hundreds of years. Native Americans, on the other hand, may allow their cats and dogs to roam freely, and members of their community share in caring for the animals. Moreover, these animals may never be spayed or neutered, out of respect for the animal's purpose and spirit (Chandler, 2005).

The interest in AAT has grown around the world, following the United States. The Animals Asia Foundation introduced the Dr. Dog program in Hong Kong, China, Philippines, Japan, India, and Taiwan, with over 300 dogs visiting hospitals and schools. In Japan, the Companion Animal Partnership Program was developed by the Japan Animal Hospital Association in 1986. It is the most well-known AAT program and the largest in Japan (ZENOAQ, 2009), with AAT teams visiting schools, nursing homes, and hospitals (Nagata, 2008). In fact, multiple studies examining the impact of AAT and AAA on elders have been conducted in Japan (Kanamori et al., 2001; Kawamura, Niiyama, & Niiyama, 2009; Mano, Uchizono, & Nishimuta, 2003).

In India, Saraswathi Kendra, in collaboration with the Blue Cross of India, pioneered the use of AAT for children with autism beginning in 1996; in 2001, Dr. Dog AAT programs were introduced in schools and nursing homes (Krishna, 2009).

FUTURE RESEARCH

Most research to date supports AAT as making a significant contribution to quality of life for patients of all ages and a variety of physical and psychological health conditions; however, most studies tend to have small sample sizes and lack adequate control groups (Fine, 2006). Studies are needed to examine the physiological mechanisms contributing to the positive effects of AAT on specific conditions, as well as the duration and frequency of AAT needed to provide maximum improvements. For example, because cardiovascular disease is the leading cause of death in the United States, the role of AAT within cardiovascular disease prevention programs needs to be examined. Further research is needed to help identify which patients would most benefit from AAT.

Additional research is needed to examine the relationships between the AAT team, patients, and staff in creating a healing environment that can be transformational for both patients and staff in various health care settings (Zborowsky & Kreitzer, 2008). More research is needed to examine the ethical use, potential fatigue, and health care needs of animals used for AAT. Nurses can take the lead in advocating for the appropriate use of AAT in their health care setting. Additional resources to assist in the implementation of AAT are listed in the bibliography (Exhibit 14.3).

WEB SITES

American Hippotherapy Association

This organization promotes the use of the movement of a horse as a treatment strategy in physical, occupational, and speech therapy sessions for people living with disabilities.
http://www.americanhippotherapyassociation.org/

American Veterinary Medical Association

Established in 1863, members of the American Medical Veterinary Association (AVMA) recognize and promote the importance of the human–animal bond through clinical practice, service, and research. This Web site includes guidelines for Animal-Assisted Activity, Animal-Assisted Therapy, and Resident Animal Programs, including key definitions, guiding principles, preventive medical and behavioral strategies, and wellness guidelines.
http://www.avma.org/issues/policy/animal_assisted_guidelines.a sp

CENSHARE: Center to Study Human–Animal Relationships and Environments

CENSHARE is a diverse group of people from the University of Minnesota and surrounding community dedicated to studying and improving human-animal relationships and environments. Its mission and vision include education, research, and service. CENSHARE is a nonprofit organization relying on external sponsorship to continue its activities.
http://www.censhare.umn.edu/

Delta Society

Delta Society's mission is to improve human health through service and therapy animals. Delta Pet Partners volunteers visit hospitals and hospices with their animals to provide comfort to people in need.
http://www.deltasociety.org/

Dog Programs

This site contains a wide range of therapy dog seminars and services throughout the United States designed for health professionals and educators.
http://www.dogprograms.com/

Michigan State University's Human–Animal Bond Initiative

The MSU College of Nursing, in collaboration with veterinarians and animal behaviorists, developed the Human–Animal Bond Initiative. Their goal is to better understand the interactions between humans and animals and to better assess how animals enrich our lives.
www.nursing.msu.edu/habi

Paws4Therapy

Paws4Therapy specializes in bringing AAT to the acute care hospital setting.
http://www.paws4therapy.com/

Therapet

Therapet assists with the establishment of AAT programs throughout the United States and provides education for health care professionals, along with AAT training and evaluation of animal and human volunteers.
http://www.therapet.org/

Therapy Dogs International, Inc.

Therapy Dogs International, Inc. (TDI) is the oldest registry for therapy dogs in the United States. Founded in 1976 by Elaine Smith, an American registered nurse, who observed the benefits of pets in the health care setting during a visit to England.
http://www.tdi-dog.org

Exhibit 14.3

Additional Resources

Barker, S. (Fall 2004). Pet project. *Cure,* 52–56.

Bouchard, F., Landry, M., Belles-Isles, M., & Gagnon, J. (2004). A magical dream: A pilot project in animal-assisted therapy in pediatric oncology. *Canadian Oncology Nursing Journal, 14*(1), 14–17.

Cangelosi, P., & Embrey, C. (2006). The healing power of dogs: Cocoa's Story. *Journal of Psychosocial Nursing, 44*(1), 17–20.

Eaglin, V. (2008). Attitudes and perceptions of nurses in training and psychiatry and pediatric residents towards animal-assisted interventions. *Hawaii Medical Journal, 67*(2), 45–47.

Geisler, A. (2004). Companion animals in palliative care: Stories from the bedside. *American Journal of Hospice & Palliative Care, 21*(4), 285–288.

Halm, M. (2008). The healing power of the human-animal connection. *American Journal of Critical Care, 17*(4), 373–376.

Horowitz, S. (2008). The human-animal bond: Health implications across the lifespan. *Alternative and Complementary Therapies, 14*(5), 251–256.

Johnson, R., Odendaal, J., & Meadows, R. (2002). Animal-assisted interventions research. *Western Journal of Nursing Research, 24*(4), 422–440.

Kilmer, K. (2008, May). Get involved in pet therapy programs. *Healthcare Traveler,* 8–10.

Lally, R. (2007). The sounds of healing. *ONS Connect, 22*(2), 8–12.

Laun, L. (2003). Benefits of pet therapy in dementia. *Home Healthcare Nurse, 21*(1), 49–52.

Lavoie-Vaughan, N. (2003). Pet project: Four-legged caregivers benefit patients and staff. *Nursing Spectrum Midwest Edition, 4*(4), 8–10.

McKenney, C., & Johnson, R. (2008). Unleash the healing power of pet therapy. *American Nurse Today, 3*(5), 29–31.

Mullet, S. (2008). A helping paw. *RN,* 39–42. Retrieved January 14, 2009, from *www.rnweb.com*

Niksa, E. (2007). The use of animal-assisted therapy in psychiatric nursing. *Journal of Psychosocial Nursing, 45*(6), 56–58.

Schetchikova, N. (2008, August). Animal attraction. *American Chiropractic Association News,* 26–27.

ACKNOWLEDGMENTS

The author wishes to acknowledge the work of Jennifer Jorgenson, who wrote the chapter in the previous edition, which served as a foundation for the present chapter.

The author gratefully thanks her therapy dog, Libby, for showing her the true value of AAT.

REFERENCES

American Kennel Club. (2003). *AKC Canine good citizen program participant's handbook.* Raleigh, NC: American Kennel Club.

American Veterinary Medical Association. (2007a). *U.S. pet ownership.* Retrieved March 15, 2009, from *www.avma.org/reference/marketstats/ownership*

American Veterinary Medical Association. (2007b). *Guidelines for animal-assisted activity and therapy programs.* Schaumberg, IL: Author.

American Veterinary Medical Association. (2007c). Wellness guidelines for animals used in animal-assisted activity, animal-assisted therapy, and resident animal programs. Schaumberg, IL: Author.

Banks, M., & Banks, W. (2002). The effects of animal-assisted therapy on loneliness in an elderly population in long-term care facilities. *Journal of Gerontology, 57*(7), 428–432.

Barak, Y., Savorai, O., Mavashev, S., & Beni, A. (2001). Animal-assisted therapy for elderly schizophrenic patients: A one-year controlled trial. *American Journal of Geriatric Psychiatry, 9*(4), 439–442.

Barker, S., Pandurangi, A., & Best, A. (2003). Effects of animal-assisted therapy on patients' anxiety, fear, and depression before ECT. *Journal of ECT, 19*(1), 38–44.

Beck, A. (2000). The use of animals to benefit humans: Animal-assisted therapy. In A. Fine (Ed.), *Handbook of animal-assisted therapy* (pp. 21–40). New York: Academic Press.

Becker, M. (2002). *The healing power of pets: Harnessing the amazing ability of pets to make and keep people happy and healthy.* New York: Hyperion.

Brodie, S., Biley, F., & Shewring, M. (2002). An exploration of the potential risks associated with using pet therapy in healthcare settings. *Journal of Clinical Nursing, 11*(4), 444–456.

Brown, D. (1985). Cultural attitudes towards pets. *Veterinary Clinics of North America: Small Animal Practice, 15*(2), 311–317.

Bustad, L., & Hines, L. (1984). Historical perspectives of the human-animal bond. In L. Bustad & L. Hinds (Eds.), *The pet connection: Its influence on our health quality of life.* Minneapolis, MN: University of Minnesota Press.

Centers for Disease Control. (2003). Guidelines for environmental infection control in healthcare facilities. *MMWR Recommendations & Reports, 52*(RR-10), 1–42.

Chandler, C. (2005). *Animal assisted therapy in counseling.* New York: CRC Press.

Churchill, M., Safaoui, J., McCabe, B., & Baun, M. (1999). Using a therapy dog to alleviate the agitation and desocialization of people with Alzheimer's disease. *Journal of Psychosocial Nursing and Mental Health Services, 37*(4), 16–22.

Cole, K., Gawlinski, A., Steers, N., & Kotlerman, J. (2007). Animal-assisted therapy in patients hospitalized with heart failure. *American Journal of Critical Care, 16*(6), 575–585.

Delta Society. (1996). *Standards of practice for animal-assisted activities and animal-assisted therapy.* Renton, WA: Author.

Duncan, S., & Allen, K. (2000). Service animals and their roles in enhancing independence, quality of life, and employment for people with disabilities. In A. Fine (Ed.), *Handbook on animal-assisted therapy: Theoretical foundations and guidelines for practice* (pp. 303–323). New York: Academic Press.

Edwards, N., & Beck, A. (2002). Animal assisted therapy and nutrition in Alzheimer's disease. *Western Journal of Nursing Research, 24*(6), 697–612.

Filan, S., & Llewellyn-Jones, R. (2006). Animal-assisted therapy for dementia: A review of the literature. *Intelligence Psychogeriatric, 18*(4), 597–611.

Fine, A. (2006). *Handbook on animal-assisted therapy: Theoretical foundations and guidelines for practice* (2nd ed.). New York: Academic Press.

Fontaine, K. (2000). *Healing practices: Alternative therapies for nursing.* Upper Saddle River, NJ: Prentice Hall.

Fontaine, K. (2005). *Complementary and alternative therapies for nursing practice.* Upper Saddle River, NJ: Pearson Prentice Hall.

Friedmann, E., Katcher, A., Lynch, J., & Thomas, S. (1980). Animal companions and one-year survival of patients after discharge from a coronary care unit. *Public Health Reports, 95*(4), 307–312.

Friedmann, E., & Thomas, S. (1995). Pet ownership, social support, and one-year survival after acute myocardial infarction in the Cardiac Arrhythmia Suppression Trial (CAST). *American Journal of Cardiology, 76,* 1213–1217.

Friedmann, E., & Thomas, S. (2003). Relationship between pet ownership and heart rate variability in patients with healed myocardial infarcts. *American Journal of Cardiology, 91,* 718–721.

Gagnon, J., Bouchard, F., Landry, M., Belles-Isles, M., Fortier, M., & Fillion, L. (2004). Implementing a hospital-based therapy program for children with cancer: A descriptive study. *Canadian Oncology Nursing Journal, 14,* 217–222.

Gasalberti, D. (2006). Alternative therapies for children and youth with special health care needs. *Journal of Pediatric Health Care, 20*(2), 133–136.

Granger, B., & Kogan, L. (2006). Characteristics of animal-assisted therapy/activity in specialized settings. In A. Fine (Ed.), *Handbook on animal-assisted therapy: Theoretical foundations and guidelines for practice* (pp. 263–285). New York: Academic Press.

Hart, L. (2000). Methods, standards, guidelines, and considerations in selecting animals for animal-assisted therapy. In A. Fine (Ed.), *Handbook on animal-assisted therapy: Theoretical foundations and guidelines for practice* (pp. 81–97). New York: Academic Press.

Havener, L., Gentes, L., Thaler, B., Megel, M., Baun, M., Driscoll, F., et al. (2001). The effects of a companion animal on distress in children undergoing dental procedures. *Issues in Comprehensive Pediatric Nursing, 24*(2), 137–152.

Kanamori, M., Suzuki, M., Yamamoto, K., Kanda, M., Matsui, Y., Kozima, E., et al. (2001). A day care program and evaluation of animal-assisted therapy for the elderly with senile dementia. *American Journal of Alzheimer's Disease & Other Dementias, 16*(4), 234–239.

Katcher, A., & Friedmann, E. (1980). Potential health value of pet ownership. *Compendium of Continuing Education for the Practicing Veterinarian, 2*(2), 117–121.

Kawamura, N., Niiyama, M., & Niiyama, H. (2009). Animal-assisted activity experiences of institutionalized Japanese older adults. *Journal of Psychosocial Nursing, 47*(1), 41–47.

Kirton, A., Wirrell, E., Zhang, J., & Hamiwka, L. (2004). Seizure alerting and response behaviors in dogs living with epileptic children. *Neurology, 62*(12), 2303–2305.

Krishna, N. (2009). *Dr. Dog—A programme for children with autism.* Retrieved April 1, 2009, from the Institute for Remedial Intervention Services Web site: http://www.autismindia.com

Laun, L. (2003). Benefits of pet therapy in dementia. *Home Healthcare Nurse, 21*(1), 49–52.

Lindsay, S. (2000). *Handbook of applied dog training and behavior: Adaptation and Learning.* Ames, IA: Iowa State.

Lust, E., Ryan-Haddad, A., Coover, K., & Snell, J. (2007). Measuring clinical outcomes of animal-assisted therapy: Impact on resident medication usage. *Consultant Pharmacist, 22*(7), 580–585.

Macauley, B. (2006). Animal-assisted therapy for persons with aphasia: A pilot study. *Journal of Rehabilitation Research & Development, 43*(3), 357–366.

Mano, M., Uchizono, M., & Nishimura, T. (2003). A trial of dog-assisted therapy for elderly people with Alzheimer's disease. *Journal of Japanese Society for Dementia Care, 2,* 150–157.

Martin, F., & Farnum, J. (2002). Animal-assisted therapy for children with pervasive developmental disorders. *Western Journal of Nursing Research, 24*(6), 657–670.

McCabe, B., Baun, M., Speich, D., & Agrawal, S. (2002). Resident dog in the Alzheimer's special care unit. *Western Journal of Nursing Research, 24*(6), 684–696.

Nagata, K. (2008). Seniors benefiting from animal therapy. Retrieved April 1, 2009, from The Japan Times Online: *http://www.japantimes.co*

Nightingale, F. (1992). *Notes on nursing.* Philadelphia: J. B. Lippincott. (Originally published in 1859)

Odendaal, J. (2000). Animal-assisted therapy: Magic or medicine? *Journal of Psychosomatic Research, 49,* 275–280.

Pavlides, M. (2008). *Animal-assisted interventions for individuals with autism.* Philadelphia: Jessica Kingsley.

Porter-Wenzlaff, L. (2007). Finding their voice: Developing emotional, cognitive, and behavioral congruence in female abuse survivors through equine facilitated therapy. *Explore, 3*(5), 529–534.

Richeson, N. (2003). Effects of animal-assisted therapy on agitated behaviors and social interactions of older adults with dementia. *American Journal of Alzheimers Disorders and Other Dementias, 18*(6), 353–358.

Sobo, E., Eng, B., & Kassity-Krich, N. (2006). Canine visitation (pet) therapy: Pilot data on decreases in child pain perception. *Journal of Holistic Nursing, 24*(1), 51–57.

Therapy Dogs International. (2006). *Associate member's guide* (8th ed.). Flanders, NJ: Author.

Tyberg, A., & Frishman, W. (2008). Animal-assisted therapy. In M. Weintraub, R. Mamtani, & M. Micozzi (Eds.), *Complementary and integrative medicine in pain management* (pp. 115–123). New York: Springer Publishing Company.

Vizek, V., Arambasic, L., Kerestes, G., Kuterovac, G., & Vlahovic-Stetic, V. (2001). Pet ownership in childhood and socio-emotional characteristics, work values and professional choices in early adulthood. *Anthrozoos, 14*(4), 224–231.

Wolff, A., & Frishman, W. (2005). Animal-assisted therapy and cardiovascular disease. In W. Frishman, M. Weintraub, & M. Micozzi (Eds.), *Complementary and integrative therapies for cardiovascular disease* (pp. 362–368). St. Louis, MO: Elsevier Mosby.

Young, M. (1985). The evolution of domestic pets and companion animals. *Veterinary Clinics of North America: Small Animal Practice, 15*(2), 297–309.

Zborowsky, T., & Kreitzer, M. (2008). Creating optimal healing environments in a health care setting. *Minnesota Medicine, 91*(3), 35–38.

ZENOAQ. (2009, March). *Therapy animals in Japan.* Retrieved April 1, 2009, from http://www.zenoaq.jp/html

Energy and Biofield Therapies

PART III

OVERVIEW

Therapies in this category use energy originating in or near the body as well as energy coming from other sources. The concept of energy and its use is universal. Most cultures have a word to describe energy: *qi* (pronounced *chee*) is a basic element of traditional Chinese medicine (TCM); *ki* is the Japanese word for it; in India it is *prana*; the Dakota Indian word is *ton*; and the Lakota Indians term it *waken*. Scientists and consumers tend to have the greatest skepticism about the efficacy of energy therapies, primarily because of the difficulty in measuring such "personal" energy.

Therapies based on energy are not new to nursing. Krieger began investigations of therapeutic touch in the 1960s. *Healing touch,* a term used to encompass a large variety of techniques, is used by nurses around the globe. Healing touch techniques may or may not involve actual physical touching of the body. The nurse seeks to bring energy into the patient or to balance the energy within the person. Although nonnurses also use these therapies, nurses remain the leaders in research on and use of healing touch techniques. An energy therapy originating in Japan, *Reiki,* is becoming more widely used in the United States.

Acupressure and reflexology focus on the *qi*, which is transmitted through the seven meridians that are the basis of TCM. Many insurance companies now reimburse for the administration of acupuncture, another TCM therapy.

Use of bioelectromagnetic therapies is also increasing. These therapies, based on the use of electromagnetic fields, utilize magnets, crystals, transcutaneous nerve stimulation, and pulsed fields. Transcutaneous electrical nerve stimulation (TENS) has been used for several decades in the management of pain.

Light therapy and sound energy therapies are also included in the category of energy therapy. Use of light for treating seasonal affective disorder has received considerable media attention. Sound energy includes vibrational therapies, use of wind chimes, and the voice. Although music could be classified in this category, we have elected to discuss it under the umbrella of mind–body–spirit therapies.

Research on energy therapies is increasing. Development of appropriate research designs and of measurements that can detect changes in energy fields is occurring. Kirlian photography, aura imaging, and gas exchange are some of the methods being used to measure outcomes from energy studies. Solid studies will help to decrease the skepticism about these therapies that persists in both professional and lay circles.

15 Light Therapy

NILOUFAR HADIDI

This chapter provides a definition and overview of light therapy, its history, cultural applications, and scientific basis. It further expands on the use of light therapy to treat seasonal affective disorders and identifies other health conditions for which light therapy could be therapeutic. Techniques that could be used by nurses educated in its practice, precautions, and recommendations for future research are provided.

DEFINITION

Unfortunately, the definition of bright light therapy differs across studies due to a lack of acceptable dosing standards. In their meta-analysis, Golden and colleagues define criteria for bright light treatment for seasonal affective disorder as "a minimum of 4 days of at least 3,000 lux-hours (e.g., 1,500 lux for 2 hours or 3,000 lux for 1 hour)"(Golden et al., 2005, p. 657). In this chapter, light therapy as used in the treatment of seasonal affective disorder is described.

Seasonal affective disorder (SAD) is a mood disorder that occurs more frequently in the dark winter months and disappears spontaneously in spring. However, it has been found to occur with less frequency in summer, and can occur repeatedly year after year. According to the *Diagnostic and Statistical Manual of Mental Disorders,* 4th edition (*DSM-*

IV), SAD is categorized as an indicator of major depression; patients with SAD experience episodes of major depression that tend to recur at specific times of the year (American Psychiatric Association, 1994).

These seasonal episodes may take the form of major depressive or bipolar disorders. Many symptoms of SAD are similar to symptoms of nonseasonal depressive episodes: Low mood (often without prominent diurnal variation), loss of interest, anhedonia, anergia, poor motivation, low libido, anxiety, irritability, and social withdrawal (Eagles, 2004). More than half of patients with SAD experience an increase in sleep duration with poor quality. Further, about the same number of patients experience increases in appetite and weight gain and have cravings for carbohydrates and chocolate (Eagles). Symptoms often start in autumn and winter, peak between December and February, and then subside during spring and summer.

Prevalence rates of SAD have been estimated to be between 0.4 and 2.9% in the general population, and these patients experience significant morbidity and impairment in psychosocial function (Westrin & Lam, 2007). SAD is reported to be more prevalent in women than men and among younger age groups (MacCosbe, 2005). The exact causes of SAD are unknown, but research has demonstrated that reduced sunlight may disrupt the circadian rhythm that is responsible for the body's internal clock (Edery, 2000). The disruption of this cycle may lead to depression.

History of Light Therapy

Since the beginning of time, people have realized the healing power of light. The history of light therapy goes back to ancient Egypt, in which sunlight was used for medical treatments. Healing temples were built with colored crystals built into stone walls so that they were aligned with the sun's rays. People would lie down on benches and their bodies would be immersed with pure or colored lights (Curtis-King, 2008). Later, Hippocrates described the use of sunlight to cure various medical disorders. Although ancient Romans and Arab physicians had no scientific explanation for light therapy at the time, they knew that the healing power of light was helpful for medical treatments (Curtis-King, 2008).

In the early 1980s, researchers discovered that specialized bright light (20 times brighter than normal indoor light), was the most effective treatment for winter depression (Kripke, 1998a). Now research is confirming that this light is effective in improving the symptoms of nonseasonal depression as well (Kripke, 1998b).

SCIENTIFIC BASIS

Research has demonstrated that individuals with SAD are positively affected by light (Partonen & Lönnqvist, 2000; Yamada, Martin-Iverson, Daimon, Tsujimoto, & Takahashi, 1995). Light plays an important role in secretion of melatonin, as well as serotonin.

Melatonin is a natural hormone produced by the pineal gland, a pea-sized structure located at the center of the brain. It is an important nighttime hormone, which has a role in the circadian rhythm, signaling our body to get prepared for sleep. However, overproduction during the day can cause depressive symptoms (Brzezinski, 1997)

Lewy and colleagues (1995) report that taking melatonin supplements and exposure to bright light may change the circadian rhythm and melatonin secretion (Lewy et al., 1995). The authors suggest that light therapy and melatonin administration could be helpful for winter depression, jet lag, and shift work.

INTERVENTION

Technique

The recommended device for provision of light therapy is a fluorescent light box that produces light intensities of greater than 2,500 lux (Westrin & Lam, 2007). Lux is a unit of illumination intensity that corrects for the phototopic spectral sensitivity of the human eye. To better understand the concept of lux, indoor evening room light is usually less than 100 lux, whereas a brightly lit office is less than 500 lux. In contrast, outdoor light is much brighter: a cloudy grey winter day is around 4,000 lux and a sunny day can be 50,000 to 100,000 lux or more (Westrin & Lam, 2007). In a review of studies of light therapy, an average dosage of 2,500 lux daily for one week was superior to placebo in improving depression as measured by Hamilton Depression Rating Scale (HAM-D). Depression decreased by 50% or more when administered in the early morning (53%) than in the evening (38%)

or at midday (32%). All three times were reported to be significantly more effective than control group receiving dim light (11%) (Terman et al., 1989).

It is recommended that patients diagnosed with SAD start light therapy in the fall. For the light therapy to be effective, the light must enter the eyes; however, the person should not be looking at the light directly. Therapy is most effective in the morning, starting with 15-minute time blocks and gradually increasing to 2 hours with 2,500 lux intensity (Mayo Clinic, 2008).

The light enters the eye, and is transmitted with nerve impulses to the pineal gland which controls melatonin secretion. Patients often report relief of depressive symptoms in 3 to 4 days. The time of the day is also an important consideration in light therapy. Often, light therapy is administered in the early morning upon arising. In the meta-analysis of the application of light therapy research by Terman and colleagues (1989), it was concluded that early morning exposure was more effective, when compared with other times of the day.

It is often recommended that individuals with SAD should exercise outdoors during daylight as much as possible (Eagles, 2004). Social contact should be continued, and it is helpful to sufferers of SAD if family and friends have some knowledge of this condition and what to expect.

Light Therapy or Antidepressant?

It has been suggested that the more individuals visibly have SAD, characterized by hypersomnia, carbohydrate carving, and weight gain, the more they would benefit from light therapy rather than from antide-pressants (Eagles, 2004). Further, often people have a preference for natural light therapy over pharmacologic antidepressants (Eagles).

Measurement of Outcomes

Several clinical, placebo-controlled studies have been done using light therapy to treat depression. These studies confirm that light is not only as effective as other methods, it causes no long-term side effects. A meta-analysis of randomized controlled trials of bright light therapy for treatment of SAD suggests that light therapy is effective, with effect sizes equivalent to those of antidepressant pharmacology trials (Golden et al., 2005). However, it must be noted that the authors indicated that most of the studies that met their selection criteria for the meta-analysis did not meet the recognized criteria for rigorous clinical trials.

Another meta-analysis of literature (studies published between January 1975 and July 2003) on phototherapy (either bright light or dawn simulation) suggested that bright light therapy is an effective treatment for SAD (Terman, 2006). The outcome measurement was SAD remission rates as measured by established selfreport depression instruments.

Precautions

The major contradictions for the use of light therapy are retinal disease or diseases that may involve the retina, such as diabetes; it is also contraindicated for those taking photosensitizing medications, such as lithium, phenothiazine antipsychotics, melatonin, and St. John's wort (Reme, Rol, Grothmann, Kaase, & Terman, 1996). An ophthalmologic examination is often recommended for these high-risk patients before starting light therapy.

It is possible to buy a light therapy box over-the-counter without a physician's prescription, but one must know that not all light therapy boxes being sold have been tested for safety and effectiveness. That is why it is crucial to consult with one's health care provider before buying one.

USES

Other uses of light therapy have been reported, including treatment of nonseasonal depressive disorders, acne vulgaris, delayed sleep phase syndrome, and psoriasis. Light therapy for treatment of sleep problems in older adults has been suggested by several studies. As humans age, sleep patterns change; most commonly, with advancing age, persons have difficulty falling sleep, staying asleep, have early-morning awakenings, and difficulty falling back to sleep (Dennis & Montgomery, 2008). Severe sleep disturbances may lead to depression and cognitive impairments (Ford & Kamerow, 1989). Lack of sleep can impair memory, disrupt metabolism, and hasten death (Davenport, 2002). In a study by Campbell and colleagues (1993) on 16 men and women between the ages of 62 and 81 with sleep disturbance who were exposed to bright light therapy, investigators found substantial positive changes in sleep quality as a result of therapy. Waking time within sleep was reduced by an hour, and sleep efficiency improved from 77.5 to 90% without altering time spent in bed.

It has been suggested that light therapy may be an effective therapy for improving sleep patterns of individuals with dementia (Mishima et al., 2007). To determine whether high-intensity ambient light in public areas of long-term care facilities would improve sleep patterns and circadian rhythms of persons with dementia, Sloane and colleagues (2007) conducted a study in geriatric units on 66 older adults with dementia. Results suggested that bright light had a modest but measurable salutary effect on sleep in this population. Further, the investigators concluded that ambient light may be preferable to stationary devices such as light boxes for elderly persons with dementia in long-term care settings. However, a critical review of literature by Shinmi and colleagues on bright light therapy suggests that, due to methodological issues, the impact of bright light on sleep and behavior in dementia patients is inconclusive (Shinmi, Hae, & Sook, 2003).

CULTURAL APPLICATIONS

The ancient Chinese knew of the healing power of natural light. The Chinese principles of Feng Shui are not only based on the principle of the right placement of certain natural elements, but also the use of light to bring a sense of balance and harmony to our lives with good "Chi" or "life giving energy" (Curtis-King, 2008).

The traditional Chinese medicine (TCM) term Qi or "life force flow" implies that there are energetic pathways in the body, similar to the concepts underlying the application of acupuncture (Brooke, 2007). However, instead of needles, "colorpuncture" uses a pen torch that is fitted with interchangeable glass rods to focus light on specific points on the skin. With each treatment, a prescribed pattern of colors in a certain sequence is used to get to the root of the illness. It is believed in the framework of TCM that disease is an indication that the body is out of balance. Thus, the precise targeted light treatments can release emotional trauma and bring the body back to a balanced state (Brooke).

FUTURE RESEARCH

Future research should focus on light therapy as preventive strategy for SAD as well as other conditions such as nonseasonal affective disorder, bipolar disorder, premenopausal syndrome, and premenstrual depression.

There have been successful preliminary studies focused on the impact of melatonin in treatment of severe postoperative delirium unresponsive to antipsychotics or benzodiazepines (Hanania & Kitain, 2002). It would be interesting to investigate whether light therapy would have a similar impact on reducing the incidence or severity of postoperative delirium.

REFERENCES

American Psychiatric Association, Task Force on DSM-IV. (1994). *Diagnostic and statistical manual of mental disorders* (4th ed.). Washington, DC: American Psychiatric Press.

Brooke, P. (2007). The power of light. Retrieved October 29, 2008, from http://poweroflight.nfshost.com/

Brzezinski, A. (1997). Melatonin in humans. *New England Journal of Medicine, 336,* 3, 186–195.

Campbell, S. S., Dawson, D., & Anderson, M. W. (1993). Alleviation of sleep maintenance insomnia with timed exposure to bright light. *Journal of American Geriatrics Society, 41*(8), 829–36.

Curtis-King, L. (2008). The healing power of incoherent polarized light. *Light and Colour, 144.*

Davenport, R. J. (2002, July 31). Up all night. *Science of Aging Knowledge Environment, 30,* 104. Retrieved October 2008, from http://sageke.sciencemag.org/cgi/content/abstract/sageke;2002/30/nw104

Dennis, J., & Montgomery, P. (2008). Bright light therapy for sleep problems in adults aged 60+. *Cochrane Library,* Issue 4.

Eagles, J. M. (2004). Light therapy and the management of winter depression. *Advances in Psychiatric Treatment, 10,* 233–240.

Edery, I., (2000). Circadian rhythms in a nutshell. *Physiological Genomics, 3,* 59–74.

Ford, D. E., & Kamerow, D. B. (1989). Epidemiologic study of sleep disturbances and psychiatric disorders. *Journal of the American Medical Association, 262,* 1479–1484.

Golden, R. N., Gaynes, B. N., Esktrom, R. D., Hamer, R. M., Jacobson, F. M., Suppes, T., et al. (2005). The efficacy of light therapy in the treatment of mood disorders: A review and meta-analysis of the evidence. *American Journal of Psychiatry, 162,* 656–662.

Hanania, M., & Kitain, E. (2002). Melatonin for treatment and prevention of postoperative delirium. *Anesthesia and Analgesia, 94,* 338–339.

Kripke, D. F. (1998a). Light therapy and depression. *Journal of Affective Disorders,* 62(3), 221–223.

Kripke, D. F. (1998b). Light treatment for nonseasonal major depression: Are we ready? In Lam, R.W. (Ed.), *Seasonal affective disorder and beyond* (pp. 159–172). Washington, DC: American Psychiatric Press.

Lewy, A. J., Sack, R. L., Blood, M. L., Bauer, V. K., Cutler, N. L., Thomas, K. H.(1995) Melatonin marks circadian phase position and resets the endogenous circadian pacemaker in humans. *Ciba Foundation Symposium, 183,* 303–317.

MacCosbe, P. E. (2005). Recognizing SAD in the clinical setting: An interview with Paul E. MacCosbe, PharmD, FCP. *Medscape Nurses.* Retrieved September, 28 2008, from http://www.medscape.com/viewarticle/507103

Mayo Clinic. (2008, October). *Light therapy.* MayoClinic.com. Retrieved April 22, 2008, from http://www.mayoclinic.com/health/light-therapy/MY00195

Mishima, K., Okawa, M., Hishikawa, Y., Hozumi, S., Hori, H., & Takahashi, K. (2007). Morning bright light therapy for sleep and behavior disorders in elderly patients with dementia. *Acta Psychiatrica Scandinavica, 89*(1), 1–7.

Partonen, T., & Lönnqvist, J. (2000). Bright light improves vitality and alleviates distress in healthy people. *Journal of Affect Disorder, 57,* 55–61.

Reme, C. E., Rol, P., Grothmann, K., Kaase, H., & Terman, M. (1996). Bright light therapy in focus: Lamp emission spectra and ocular safety. *International Journal of Technology Assessment in Health Care, 4,* 403–413.

Shinmi, K., Hae, H. S., Sook, J. Y. (2003). The effect of bright light on sleep and behavior in dementia: An analytic review. *Geriatric Nursing, 24*(4), 239–243.

Sloane, P. D., Williams, C. S., Mitchell, C. M., Preisser, J. S., Wood, W., Barrick, A. L., et al. (2007). High-intensity environmental light in dementia: Effect on sleep and activity. *Journal of the American Geriatrics Society, 55*(10), 1524–1533.

Terman, M., Terman, J. S., Quitkin, F. M., McGrath, P. J., Stewart, J. W., Rafferty, B. (1989). Light therapy for seasonal affective disorder: A review of efficacy. *Neuropsychopharmacology, 2,* 1–22.

Terman, M. (2006). Review: Light therapy is an effective treatment for seasonal affective disorder. *Evidence Based Mental Health, 9,* 21.

Yamada, N., Martin-Iverson, M. T., Daimon, K., Tsujimoto, T., & Takahashi, S. (1995). Clinical and chronobiological effects of light therapy on nonseasonal affective disorders. *Biological Psychiatry, 37,* 866–73.

Westrin, A., & Lam, R. W. (2007). Seasonal affective disorder: A clinical update. *Annals of Clinical Psychiatry, 19*(4), 239–246.

Wikipedia. (2009, February). Dawn simulation. *Wikipedia, The Free Encyclopedia.* Retrieved April 24, 2008, from *http://en.wikipedia.org/wiki/Dawn_simulation*

Wikipedia. (2009, June). Light therapy. *Wikipedia, The Free Encyclopedia.* Retrieved October 2008, from http://en.wikipedia.org/wiki/Light_therapy

16 Magnet Therapy

CORJENA K. CHEUNG

Magnets have been used for healing purposes for centuries in many countries such as China, Egypt, Greece, and India. It is mentioned in the oldest medical text ever found, the Yellow Emperor's *Classic of Internal Medicine* in 2000 B.C., as well as in the ancient Hindu scriptures, the *Vedas* (Whitaker & Adderly, 1998). Magnet therapy was popular in the United States in the 18th century, where it was used for treating many ailments of the body, especially in some rural areas where few doctors were available. The introduction of antibiotics, cortisone, and other medications resulted in magnet therapy losing its allure. Since the 1960s, there has been a resurgence of interest in magnet therapy by health professionals (Whitaker & Adderly). Currently, magnets have been marketed for a wide range of diseases and conditions, such as soft tissue or muscle sprains, arthritis, respiratory problems, high blood pressure, circulatory problems, stress, and pain (National Center for Complementary and Alternative Medicine [NCCAM], 2008). A recent Google search for the term *magnet therapy* yielded over 1,810,000 links, most of which were commercial advertisements. The modern magnet therapy industry's total sales are estimated at $500 million per year in the United States and $5 billion globally (Winemiller, Billow, Laskowski, & Harmsen, 2005).

Today, energy healing remains a debatable subject in the scientific community. The scientific literature on magnet therapy, although it has yielded conflicting findings in the limited studies, is slowing increasing. Scientists are trying to understand the healing power of magnets, and whether, how, and why magnets work on certain health problems.

DEFINITION

According to the classification of the National Center of Complementary and Alternative Medicine (NCCAM), magnet therapy is classified under the category of energy therapies. Energy therapies operate on the principle that health can be influenced by the subtle realignment of a person's "vital energy"—energy that is innate to all living beings and that, when disordered or blocked, can create disease (Kaptchuk, 1996).

Magnet therapy is the use of magnets that are applied to different parts of the body for specific therapeutic purposes. The term *magnet* comes from the legend of a Greek shepherd, Magnes, who about 2,500 years ago discovered mysterious iron deposits attracted to the nails of his sandals while walking in an area near Mount Ida in Turkey. These deposits, which were known to the ancients as lodestones or live-stones, are now known as magnetite (magnetic oxide, Fe_3O_4) (Macklis, 1993).

SCIENTIFIC BASIS

The Earth's magnetic field and the body's bioenergetic field exist. Magnet therapy is based on the premise that all living things exist in a magnetic field (the Earth), and that the human body exists in and generates a magnetic field that has healing powers. For centuries, the effects of magnets and low-frequency electromagnetic fields on biological processes have been investigated and debated. The application of magnets is believed to restore the balance or flow of electromagnetic energy so as to restore health (Hinman, 2002). However, the mechanism of action is still not fully understood.

According to Oschman (1998), each of the great systems in the body—the musculoskeletal system, the digestive system, the circulatory system, the nervous system, the skin—is composed of connective tissues that have important roles in communication and regulation. The extracellular, cellular, and nuclear matrices throughout the body form an interconnected solid-state network called a "living matrix." Because the main structural components are helical piezoelectric semiconductors, the living matrix generates energetic vibrations, absorbs them from the environment, and conducts a variety of energetic signals from place to place. There are many energetic systems in the living body and many ways of influencing them. The Western concept of "energy" is similar to the concepts "Qi" in traditional Chinese medicine and "Prana" in the Hindu system of traditional medicine (Ayurveda).

Scientists suggest that magnetic fields can influence important biologic processes in the following ways: decrease the firing rate of certain neurons, particularly c-type chronic pain neurons; change the rate of enzyme-mediated reactions, which may play a role in inflammatory cascades and free radical generation; modulate intracellular signaling by affecting the functioning of calcium channels in cell membranes; and cause small changes in blood flow (Wolsko et al., 2004). The *Mayo Clinic Health Letter* reports that magnets may also work by blocking pain signals to the brain (Second Opinion, 1998). Yet another theory, the Hall effect, has been suggested. The Hall effect refers to positively and negatively charged ions in the bloodstream that become activated by a magnetic field and generate heat-causing vasoconstriction and an increased blood and oxygen supply to the affected area (Whitaker & Adderly, 1998).

INTERVENTION

Types of Therapeutic Magnets

A permanent (or static) magnet is either a natural or artificially made magnet that produces magnetic force by the movements of electrons in the atoms of the material that make up the magnet, such as iron or nickel. These materials can be ordered to all lie in one direction (referred to as "north" or "south"). Therefore one large magnetic field can be created where similar poles repel one another and opposing poles attract (Lawrence, Rosch, & Plowden, 1998). The poles are thought to have different effects on the human body. The northern pole is considered negative magnetic energy and is suggested to calm and normalize the body; the southern pole is made up of positive magnetic energy and is believed to be responsible for disordering and overstimulating the biological system (Arizona Unipole Magnetics, 2008a, 2008b). Permanent magnets can be unipolar (one pole of the magnet faces or touches the skin) or bipolar (both poles face or touch the skin, sometimes in repeating patterns). They have magnetic fields that do not change.

There are a number of permanent magnets available commercially, in various shapes and forms, for therapeutic purposes. The three most common forms of permanent magnets are plastiform magnets, neodymium magnetic discs, and ceramic magnets. Plastiform magnets are flexible, rubberized magnetic rolls that can be wrapped around an affected extremity or lie along the full length of the spine. Neodymium magnetic discs are lightweight and can be used on the face and on various acupuncture points. Ceramic magnets can be made in any shape and size (Beattie, 2004). Typically, permanent magnets are placed directly on the skin or inside clothing or other materials that come into close contact with the body.

Electromagnets are magnets produced by electric current passing through a cylindrical coil of wire, also known as a time-varying magnetic field. The magnetic strength is directly proportional to the strength of the electric current. When the electric current is discontinued, the wire loses its magnetism. Pulsed electromagnetism is the process by which alternating electromagnetic fields are delivered in a time-varying manner. The electromagnetic field is primarily used in hospitals, in clinics, and in clinical trials. Its use is under the supervision of a health care provider. Medicare has approved the coverage of electromagnetic therapy for wound treatment (Medlearn Matters, 2004).

Two other electromagnets being used in clinical settings are the magnetic molecular energizer (MME) and transcranial magnetic stimulation (TMS). MME, which acts as a catalyst to improve chemical reactions occurring in the human body, is commonly used for neurological and neuromuscular ailments. MME treatment is currently considered to be experimental by the United States Food and Drug Administration (FDA). TMS, a neurological technique for inducing motor movement by direct magnetic stimulation of the brain's motor cortex, is most often used as a diagnostic tool (NCCAM, 2008). TMS has been explored for treating depression in psychiatric settings (George et al., 1999) and is now being explored for treating migraines (Eads, 2008). The FDA has recently approved TMS treatment for depression (CBS News, 2008).

Repetitive TMS is also available for depression treatment in Canada, Australia, New Zealand, Israel, and the European Union (Miller, 2006).

Strength of Magnets

The strength of a magnet is measured in units referred to as gauss (G), which represents "the number of lines of magnetic force passing through an area of 1 square centimeter" (Whitaker & Adderly, 1998, p. 15). Currently, the Earth's magnetic field is estimated to be about 0.5 G, whereas a refrigerator magnet ranges from 35 to 200 G. Magnets used for pain intervention usually measure from 400 to 5,000 G (Eccles, 2005; Magnetic field therapy, 2003); and magnetic resonance imaging (MRI) machines used to diagnose medical conditions produce up to 200,000 G (Ratterman, Secrest, Norwood, & Ch'ien, 2002). Manufacturers are not required to mark the strength of magnets on their products, so the G of a magnet must be checked against the weight a magnet can lift, with 1 kg equivalent to approximately 600 G (Whitaker & Adderly). Although it is important to determine the correct strength of a magnet for a therapeutic effect, some practitioners believe that the right choice of polarity (north or south pole) is crucial (Bonlie, 2008). However, the issue of polarity remains controversial.

Methods and Duration of Application

Exhibit 16.1 lists various ways in which magnets can be applied to the human body. Generally, it is safe to apply permanent magnets for a long period of time. The time of application largely depends on the type and nature of the disease, the age of the individual, and the strength of the magnet. It is thought that large magnets of more than 2,000 G should be used for short periods of time ranging from several seconds to about 60 minutes for one application (Beattie, 2004).

Measurement of Outcomes

The type of measurement used to determine the effectiveness of a magnet therapy depends on the purpose of the intervention. A variety of outcome measures has been used. For instance, the progression of bone healing has been objectively measured by using X-rays, bone mineral density, and calcium content in bone. Pain relief or stress

Exhibit 16.1

Methods of Application of Magnets

Mode	Applications
Local	Magnets are placed directly on the skin over affected parts
Acu-Site	Local applications with use of acupuncture points
General	Used for whole body or ailments affecting larger body parts
Internal	Magnetic water (ionized water) is ingested
Remote	Wearing magnetic jewelry to treat an ailment remote from the point of application such as a magnetic bracelet for stimulating the thymus gland to boost the immune system

reduction has been measured by an individual's subjective report on a pain/stress rating scale. The improvement of a sleep disorder can be detected by using polysomnography, a diagnostic test that records a number of physiologic variables during sleep. Two objective measurements that have been used to indicate the change of magnetic field in the body are:

1. The superconducting quantum interference device (SQUID), a sensitive magnetometer for mapping the magnetic fields around the human body, can be used to detect an increase or decrease in the biomagnetic field of the body (Oschman, 1997).
2. Kirlian photography is a tool that provides photographs, video, or computer images of energy flow. It introduces a high frequency, high voltage, ultra low current to the object being photographed. This influx of electrical energy amplifies as it travels through the object and makes visible the biological and energetic exchange (Cope, 1980).

USES

Use of electromagnets for diagnostic and intervention purposes requires administration by health professionals. However, many persons use magnets without their being prescribed by health professionals. They use commercially available magnets in the form of wraps, belts, mattresses, and jewelry. Magnets can be purchased in stores and online.

In Japan, therapeutic magnets are licensed as medical devices (Consumer Health Reviews, 2002). Although the FDA has not approved the marketing of magnets with claims of benefits to health such as relieving arthritis pain, a 1999 survey indicated that the permanent magnet was the second most frequently used complementary and alternative medicine (CAM) therapy used by arthritis patients, after chiropractic (Rao et al., 1999).

Acu-magnet therapy is one of the therapies that is commonly practiced in China and Japan. Recent studies on placing magnets on acupuncture sites revealed positive outcomes. A systematic review on acu-magnet therapy using six electronic databases (PubMed, AMED, ScienceDirect College Edition, China Academic Journals, Acubriefs, and the in-house Journal Article Index maintained by the Oregon College of Oriental Medicine Library) was conducted (Colbert et al., 2008). A total of 42 studies met the inclusion criteria. Studies included 32 different clinical conditions ranging from musculoskeletal problems to insomnia in 6,453 patients from 1986 to 2007. A variety of magnetic devices, dosing regimens, and control devices were used. The review reported that 37 of 42 studies (88%) found therapeutic benefit from using acu-magnet therapy, particularly for the management of diabetes (Chen, 2002; Ma & Wei, 1999) and insomnia (Suen, Wong, & Lueng, 2002; Suen, Wong, Leung, & Ip, 2003).

Common Health Conditions Treated With Magnetic Therapy

Pain, inflammatory disorders, and wound healing are three conditions in which magnet therapy has been most frequently used. Additional uses of magnets are noted in Exhibit 16.2.

Pain

Although articles and books contain testimonials to support the efficacy of magnets on pain, little support has been established from science. Findings from systematic reviews of static magnets for pain relief have been contradictory. One review indicated 11 out of 15 (73.3%) studies found a positive effect of static magnets in achieving analgesia for

Exhibit 16.2

Conditions in Which Magnets Have Been Used for Treatment

Bone and wound healing (Henry, Concannon, Yee, 2008; Saltzman, Lightfoot, & Amendola, 2004)

Depression (George et al., 1999; Miller, 2006)

Menopause (Brockie, 2008)

Inflammatory disorders (Johnson, Waite, & Nindl, 2004; Sutbeyaz, Sezer, & Koseoglu, 2006; Wolsko et al., 2004)

Migraine (Eads, 2008)

Pain (Birkner, 2004; Hinman, Ford, & Heyl, 2002; Smania et al., 2003)

a wide variety of pain (neuropathic, inflammatory, musculoskeletal, fibromyalgic, rheumatic, and post-surgical) (Eccles, 2005). Based on nine randomized placebo-controlled trials, another recent systematic review and meta-analysis suggested static magnets offer no significant effects on pain reduction (Pittler, Brown, & Ernst, 2007). Positive and negative studies were spread across magnet strengths. Ideal magnet strength and treatment duration for pain reduction remain unclear. Trials of electromagnets yielded more consistent results. Brown, Parker, Ling, and Wan (2000) found that a majority of female patients with chronic refractory pelvic pain reported a 50% reduction in pain ratings after 4 weeks of treatment with pulsating magnets. Other clinical trials also reported that electromagnets significantly reduced musculoskeletal pain (Jacobson et al., 2001; Pipitone & Scott, 2001; Smania et al., 2003; Thuile & Walzl, 2002).

Inflammatory Disorders

Alfano and associates (2001) reported a significant decrease in pain and tender points and an increase in functional status in patients with fibromyalgia who had magnet therapy versus placebo and control groups. The study also found that unipolar mattress pads were more effective in reducing pain than bipolar pads. Colbert, Markov, Banerji, and Pilla (1999) reported significant improvement in pain and physical function in patients with fibromyalgia who slept for a 4-month period on a mattress pad containing 1100-G unidirectional magnets.

Four recent randomized controlled trials (RCT) applied pulsed electromagnetic field (PEMF) to the treatment of knee osteoarthritis (OA); cervical spine OA, and temporomandibular joint (TMJ) disorder were reviewed. The first (knee) OA study, which included 83 patients, found significant improvements in pain and stiffness in the patients under age 65 (Thamsborg et al., 2005). The second (knee) OA study (N = 36) found reduced impairment in activities of daily living and improved knee function (Nicolakis et al., 2002). The third (cervical spine) OA study (N = 34) found significant improvements in neck pain and disability among the experimental but not the sham-treatment control group (Sutbeyaz, Sezer, & Koseoglu, 2006). In a study of persons with TMJ, however, the PEMF had no specific treatment effects (Peroz et al., 2004). Although results of these studies are promising, their number is limited, and thus no generalizations can be made about their use in improving inflammatory symptoms.

Wound and Bone Healing

A recent RCT was conducted to determine the effects of static magnets on wound healing. Standardized wounds were created in the backs of 33 rats. Wounds in the magnet group healed in an average of 15.3 days, significantly faster than those in either sham group (20.9 days, $p =$ .006) or control group (20.3 days, $p < .0001$) (Henry, Concannon, & Yee, 2008). Pulsating electromagnetic therapy for fracture "non-unions" was granted the "safe and effective" classification by the FDA in 1979 (Horowitz, 2000). However, two recent systematic reviews with a total of five RCTs reported that there were no statistically significant differences between the healing rates of venous leg ulcers or pressure ulcers in people treated with electromagnetic therapy (Ravaghi, Flemming, Cullum, & Olyaee, 2006; Olyaee, Flemming, Cullum, & Ravaghi, 2006). More research is needed to support the use of magnet therapy in wound and bone healing.

Precautions

There are some precautions regarding the placement of magnets. Magnets should not be placed over: (a) the heart, as it may cause arrhythmia;

(b) the carotid artery, as it may cause lightheadedness and dizziness; (c) the stomach within 60 minutes after a meal, as it may interfere with the normal contraction of the digestive tract; (d) any open wounds with active bleeding, as it may increase bleeding; or (e) any transdermal drug-delivery system or patch, as it may increase the amount of drug circulating in the body (Magnetic Field Therapy, 2003). Magnets should not be used with pregnant women or people with pacemakers or defibrillating regulators. Strong magnets are not recommended for small children.

CULTURAL ASPECTS

A therapy that has some similarities to magnets is crystal healing. This is true in both the underlying mechanism of action and in the skepticism that exists about its efficacy. In the eastern cultures, people have used amulets, magical stones, and gems throughout history. The earliest records of crystal healing have been traced to Ancient Egypt. India's Ayurvedic records and traditional Chinese medicine also claim healing with the use of crystals, dating to 5,000 years ago (Medindia, 2008). Crystal healing has been used in many different cultures, including the Hopi Indians of Arizona and the Hawaiian islanders, some of whom still use them. The Chinese attribute extensive healing powers to jade and wear it as a charm against evil or injury. Many Asians believe that emerald will strengthen the memory and increase intelligence (Gardner, 2006).

Crystal healing is a form of healing that uses crystals or gemstones. Crystals have been found to carry vibration that activates certain energy centers within our electromagnetic system and releasing and clearing negative energy. By clearing out the bad spiritual energy, the physical ailment is alleviated (Medindia, 2008). Crystals are used for physical, mental, emotional, and spiritual healing. Believers in crystal healing may carry crystals around with them, believing that they impart healing powers to them wherever they go, or that they have positive vibrations that attract positive events and interactions with others. Additionally, crystals can be worn, placed next to a person's bed as they sleep, and in some cases placed around a person's bathing site.

Some crystal healers suggest placing crystals on specific areas of the body, called *chakras*. *Chakra* is a Hindu term meaning spiritual energy. The theory is that crystals or gemstones carry vibration and direct the flow of energy to the person in a particular part of the body; by placing these vibrational rates within the aura, the aura's vibrational rates will change to restore balance and achieve healing (Bondar & Bondar, 2008).

FUTURE RESEARCH

Claims of positive results from magnet therapies vary greatly, depending upon the condition for which they were used. Findings from Western research about the effectiveness of magnets are inconclusive. The variations in the findings may be attributed to the subjective nature of many of the outcome measures used, the inability to control the etiology and severity of the pathological condition, and variation in the types of magnets and treatment parameters. Because anecdotal reports are regarded as being an unreliable source of evidence, many in the scientific and medical communities consider magnet therapy a fraud and quackery. Conducting controlled, scientific experiments on permanent magnet therapy is challenging because participants can notice if a metal device is magnetized or not. However, as there is little evidence that the application of magnets is harmful, it is reasonable to encourage the practice if a patient experiences symptom relief from their use, especially if the use of magnets can reduce the patient's consumption of medications. Continued efforts are needed to enhance our knowledge about the use of magnet therapy. Questions for further knowledge development include:

1. What is the scientific evidence for the different effects obtained from the north pole and the south pole in magnet therapy?
2. What roles do individual (high vs. low vitality) and environmental (northern vs. southern hemisphere) factors play on the effects of magnet therapy?
3. What are appropriate methodologies for studying the effects of magnet therapies, particularly the use of sham controls?
4. What are the long-term effects of magnet therapy?

REFERENCES

Alfano, A., Taylor, A., Foresman, P., Dunkl, P., McConnell, G., Conaway, M., et al. (2001). Static magnetic fields for treatment of fibromyalgia: A randomized controlled trial. *Journal of Alternative & Complementary Medicine, 7*(1), 53–64.

Arizona Unipole Magnetics. (2008a). *Effects of magnetic energy on living metabolic systems.* Retrieved October 28, 2008, from http://www.azunimags.com/polarity.html

Arizona Unipole Magnetics. (2008b). *Importance of polarity.* Retrieved October 28, 2008, from http://www.azunimags.com/polarity.html

Beattie, A. (2004). *Magnet therapy.* New York: Barnes and Noble.

Birkner, K. (2004). Stop pain with magnets. *Health Educator Reports,* 1–6.

Bondar, T., & Bondar, N. (2008). Crystal healing for the emotions and the mind. *Positive Health,* 19–23.

Bonlie, D. (2008, October). *Magnet and health.* Paper presented at the 9th Annual International Iridology and Integrative Healthcare Congress.

Brockie, S. (2008). Alternative approaches to the menopause. *Practice Nursing, 19*(4), 172–176.

Brown, C., Parker, N., Ling, F., & Wan, J. (2000). Effect of magnet on chronic pelvic pain. *Obstetric & Gynecology, 1*(95), S29.

CBS News (2008). *Magnet device aims to treat depression.* Retrieved on October 26, 2008, from http://www.cbsnews.com/stories/2008/10/21/health/main4535599.shtml?source=RSSattr=Health_4535599

Chen, Y. (2002). Magnets on ears helped diabetics. *American Journal of Chinese Medicine, 30*(1), 183–185.

Colbert, A., Markov, M., Banerji, M., & Pilla, A. (1999). Magnetic mattress pad use in patients with fibromyalgia: A randomized double-blind study. *Journal of Back and Musculoskeletal Rehabilitation, 13,* 19–31.

Colbert, A. Cleaver, J., Brown, K., Harling, N., Hwang, Y., Schiffke, H., et al. (2008). Magnets applied to acupuncture points as therapy—A literature review. *Acupuncture in Medicine, 26*(3), 160–170.

Consumer Health Reviews (2002). *Magnet therapy.* Retrieved on October 28, 2008, from http://www.consumerhealthreviews.com/articles/MagneticTherapy/Magnet-Therapy.htm

Cope, F. (1980). Magnetoelectric charge states of matter-energy. A second approximation. Part VII. *Physiological Chemistry & Physics, 12*(4), 349–355.

Eads, S. (2008). News notes. Migraines and magnetic pulses. *Massage & Bodywork, 23*(5), 19.

Eccles, N. K. (2005). A critical review of randomized controlled trials of static magnets for pain relief. *Journal of Alternative & Complementary Medicine, 11*(3), 495–509.

Gardner, J. (2006). *Vibrational healing through the chakras with light, color, sound, crystals and aromatherapy.* Berkeley, CA: The Crossing Press.

George, M., Nahas, Z., Kozel, F., Goldman, J., Molloy, M., & Oliver, N. (1999). Improvement of depression following transcranial magnetic stimulation. *Current Psychiatry Reports, 1*(2), 114–124.

Henry, S., Concannon, M., & Yee, G. (2008). The effect of magnetic fields on wound healing: Experimental study and review of the literature. *Eplasty, 8,* 40.

Hinman, M. (2002). Therapeutic use of magnets: A review of recent research. *Physical Therapy Review, 7*(1), 33–43.

Hinman, M., Ford, J., & Heyl, H. (2002). Effects of static magnets on chronic knee pain and physical function: A double-blind study. *Alternative Therapies in Health & Medicine, 8*(4), 50–55.

Horowitz, S. (2000). Update on magnet therapy. *Alternative and Complementary Therapies, 12*, 325–330.

Jacobson, J., Gorman, R., Yamanashi, W., Saxena, B., & Clayton, L. (2001). Low-amplitude, extremely low frequency magnetic fields for the treatment of osteoarthritic knees: A double-blind clinical study. *Alternative Therapies in Health and Medicine, 7*(5), 54–69.

Johnson, M., Waite, L., & Nindl, G. (2004). Noninvasive treatment of inflammation using electromagnetic fields: Current and emerging therapeutic potential. *Biomedical Sciences Instrumentation, 40*, 469–474.

Kaptchuk, T. (1996). Historical context of the concept of vitalism in complementary and alternative medicine. In M. Micozzi (Ed.), *Fundamentals of complementary and alternative medicine* (p. 35). New York: Churchill Livingstone.

Lawrence, R., Rosch, P., & Plowden, J. (1998). *Magnet therapy: The pain cure alternative.* Roseville, CA: Prima.

Ma, R., & Wei, Z. (1999). The analysis of 30 patients with diabetes mellitus remedied with magnetic therapy. *Chinese Journal of Convalescent Medicine, 8*(3), 9–10.

Macklis, R. (1993). Magnetic healing, quackery, and the debate about the health effects of electromagnetic fields. *Annals of Internal Medicine, 18*(5), 376–382.

Magnetic field therapy. (2003). Retrieved January 20, 2005, from http://www.chclibrary.-org/micromed/00055750.html

Medindia. (2008). *Crystal healing.* Retrieved on November 24, 2008, from http://www.medindia.net/AlternativeMedicine

Medlearn Matters. (2004). *Electrical stimulation and electromagnetic therapy for the treatment of wounds.* Retrieved November 24, 2008, from http://www.cms.hhs.gov/medlearn/matters/mmarticles/2004/mm3149.pdf

Miller, M. (2006, December 11). Minds and magnets. *Newsweek,* pp. 61–64.

National Center for Complementary and Alternative Medicine. (2008). *Questions and answers about using magnets to treat pain.* Retrieved November 24, 2008, from http://www.nccam.nih.gov/health/magnet/magnet.htm

Nicolakis, P. Kollmitzer, J., Crevenna, R., Bittner, C., Erdogmus, C., & Nicolakis, J. (2002). Pulsed magnetic filed therapy for osteoarthritis of the knee—a double blind sham-controlled trial. *Wiener Klinische Wochenschrift, 114*(15–16), 678–684.

Olyaee, M., Flemming, K., Cullum, N., & Ravaghi, H. (2006). Electromagnetic therapy for treating pressure ulcers. *Cochrane Database of Systematic Reviews, 2.*

Oschman, J. (1997). What is healing energy? Part 2: Measuring the field of life energy. *Journal of Bodywork & Movement Therapies, 1*(2), 117–121.

Oschman, J. (1998). What is healing energy? Part 6: Conclusions: Is energy medicine the medicine of the future? *Journal of Bodywork & Movement Therapies, 2*(1), 46–59.

Peroz, I., Chun, Y., Karageorgi, G., Schwerin, C., Bernhardt, O., Roulet, J., et al. (2004). A multi-center clinical center trial on the use of pulsed electromagnetic fields in the treatment of temporomandibular disorders. *Journal of Prosthetic Dentistry, 91*(2), 180–187.

Pipitone, N., & Scott, D. (2001). Magnetic pulse treatment for knee osteoarthritis: A randomized, double-blind, placebo-controlled study. *Current Medical Research and Opinion, 17*(3), 190–196.

Pittler, M., Brown, E., & Ernst, E. (2007). Static magnets for reducing pain: Systematic review and meta-analysis of randomized trials. *Canadian Medical Association Journal, 177*(7), 736–742.

Rao, J., Mihaliak, K., Kroenke, K., Bradley, J., Tierney, W., & Weinberger, M. (1999). Use of complementary therapies for arthritis among patients of rheumatologists. *Annals of Internal Medicine, 131*(6), 409–416.

Ratterman, R., Secrest, J., Norwood, B., & Ch'ien, A. (2002). Magnet therapy: What's the attraction? *Journal of the American Academy of Nurse Practitioners, 14*(8), 347–353.

Ravaghi, H., Flemming, K., Cullum, N., Olyaee, M. (2006). Electromagnetic therapy for treating venous leg ulcers. *Cochrane Database of Systematic Reviews, 2*.

Saltzman, C., Lightfoot, A., & Amendola, A. (2004). PEMF as treatment for delayed healing of foot and ankle arthrodesis. *Foot and Ankle International, 25*(11), 771–773.

Second opinion. (1998, August). *Mayo Clinic Health Letter, 16*(8), 8.

Smania, N., Corato, E., Fiaschi, A., Pietropoli, P., Aglioti, S., & Tinazzi, M. (2003). Therapeutic effects of peripheral repetitive magnetic stimulation on myofascial pain syndrome. *Clinical Neurophysiology, 114*(2), 350–358.

Suen, L., Wong, T., & Leung, A. (2002). Effectiveness of auricular therapy on sleep promotion in the elderly. *American Journal of Chinese Medicine, 30*(4), 429–449.

Suen, L., Wong, T., Leung, A., & Ip, W. (2003). The long-term effects of auricular therapy nursing magnetic pearls on elderly with insomnia. *Complementary Therapy Medicine, 11*(2), 85–92.

Sutbeyaz, S., Sezer, N., & Koseoglu, G. (2006). The effect of pulsed electromagnetic fields in the treatment of cervical osteoarthritis: A randomized, double-blind, sham-controlled trial. *Rheumatology International, 26*(4), 320–324.

Thamsborg, G., Florescu, A., Oturai, P., Fallentin, E., Tritsaris, K., & Dissing, S. (2005). Treatment of knee osteoarthritis with pulsed electromagnetic fields: A randomized, double-blind, placebo-controlled study. *Osteoarthritis Cartilage, 13*(7), 575–581.

Thuile, C., & Walzl, M. (2002). Evaluation of electromagnetic fields in the treatment of pain in patients with lumbar radiculopathy or the whiplash syndrome. *NeuroRehabilitation, 17*(1), 63–67.

Whitaker, J.,& Adderly, B. (1998). *The pain breakthrough: The power of magnet*. Toronto, Ontario: Little, Brown.

Winemiller, M., Billow, R., Laskowski, E., & Harmsen, W. (2005). Effect of magnetic vs. sham-magnetic insoles on nonspecific foot pain in the workplace: A randomized, double-blind, placebo-controlled trial. *Mayo Clinic Proceedings, 80*(9), 1138–1145.

Wolsko, P., Eisenberg, D., Simon, L., Davis, R., Walleczek, J., Mayo-Smith, M., et al. (2004). Double-blind placebo-controlled trial of static magnets for the treatment of OA of the knee. *Alternative Therapies in Health & Medicine, 10*(2), 36–43.

17 Healing Touch

ALEXA W. UMBREIT

All cultures, both ancient and modern, have developed some form of touch therapy as part of people's desire to heal and care for one another. The oldest written evidence of the use of touch to enhance healing comes from Asia more than 5,000 years ago (Jackson & Keegan, 2009; Hover-Kramer, Mentgen, & Scandrett-Hibdon, 1996; Krieger, 1979). This therapeutic use of the hands has been passed on from generation to generation as a tool for healing. However, philosophical and cultural differences have influenced the way touch has been used throughout the world. The Eastern viewpoint has based its touch-healing practices on energy channels (called meridians), energy fields (auras), and energy centers (*chakras*). Expert practitioners in energetic touch therapies use their hands to influence this flow of energy to promote balance and healing. The Western viewpoint focuses on physiological changes that occur at the cellular level from touch therapies that are believed to influence healing. A blending of both Eastern and Western techniques has led to an explosion of a wide variety of touch therapies (Jackson & Keegan). Nursing has used touch throughout its history and today's nurses are integrating many touch techniques into their practice. One of these therapies is Healing Touch, which now boasts more than 100,000 persons who have been trained worldwide during the past 19 years (Healing Touch Program, 2008a, 2008b, 2008c).

DEFINITION

Healing Touch (HT) is a type of complementary therapy that uses gentle touch and energy-based techniques to influence and support the human energy system within the body (energy centers) and surrounding the body (energy fields) (Healing Touch International, 2008; Healing Touch Program, 2008a, 2008b, 2008c). HT is classified as an energy medicine therapy by the National Institutes of Health, National Center for Complementary and Alternative Medicine (NCCAM, 2007). Based on a holistic view of health and illness, HT focuses on creating an energetic balance of the whole body at the physical, emotional, mental, and spiritual levels rather than on dysfunctional parts of the body. Through this process of balancing the energy system and therefore opening up energy blockages, an environment is created that is conducive to self-healing. Through the interaction of the energy fields between practitioner and client, the use of the HT practitioner's hands, an intention focusing on the client's highest good, and a centering process, noninvasive HT techniques specific for the client's needs are used to create this energetic balance (Umbreit, 2000). Krieger (1979) describes the centering process as a meditation in which one eliminates all distractions and concentrates on that place of quietude within which one can feel truly integrated, unified, and focused. Finding this "place of quietude within" is achieved by many through deep belly breathing, prayer, meditation, or any other technique that slows one down, calms the mind, and accesses a deeper spirit of compassion and strength. To be centered is to be fully present with another person or situation, engaged with heart and mind, deeper feelings, and thoughts. The centered state of mind is maintained throughout the HT treatment.

Umbreit (2000) describes the role of the HT practitioner as observation, assessment, and repatterning of the client's energy field, which is disrupted when there is disease, illness, psychological stressors, and pain. Practitioners describe these disruptions in the energy field as blockages, leaks, imbalances, or congestion. The goal of the HT practitioner is to open up these blockages, seal the leaks, rebalance the energy field to symmetry, and release congestion.

HT evolved from the pioneering work of the therapeutic touch (TT) community which started in 1970 by a nurse, Dr. Dolores Krieger, and Dora Kunz, a natural intuitive healer who assisted many physicians with perplexing patient cases. Together they established TT, described as a "contemporary interpretation of several ancient healing practices...[consisting of learning] skills for consciously directing or sensitively modulating human energies" (Krieger, 1993, p. 11). The practice is based on the assumption that humans are complex energy fields and the potential exists to enhance the natural healing potential in another (Therapeutic Touch, 2008). In health care, TT philosophy, practice, and research have become the base for many newer energetic modalities, including HT.

The HT curriculum, started in 1989 and endorsed by the American Holistic Nurses' Association, involves a formal educational program that teaches techniques including interventions described by Brugh Joy (1979) and Alice Bailey (1984), concepts presented by Rosalyn Bruyere (1989) and Barbara Brennan (1986), and original techniques developed by the founder of HT, Janet Mentgen, and her students (Scandrett-Hibdon, 1996). The six-level HT educational curriculum in energy-based practice moves from beginning to advanced practice, certification, and instructor level. Advanced practice requires at least 105 hours of workshop instruction plus a 1-year course of study, as well as work in case studies, mentoring, ethics, client–practitioner relationships, establishment of a practice, and integration of activities within the health community (Healing Touch Program, 2008a, 2008b, 2008c). After this, students may apply for certification. Instructor status requires more education and mentoring. The HT coursework is open to nurses, physicians, body therapists, counselors, psychotherapists, other health care professionals, and individuals desiring an in-depth understanding and practice of healing work using touch and energy-based concepts (Mentgen, Bulbrook, Hutchison, Wardell, & Komitor, 2007).

SCIENTIFIC BASIS

The nursing profession has long been described as dedicated to the art and science of human caring. Rogers (1990) and Watson (1985) have written extensively about caring as a central quality of the nursing profession, along with nursing's concern for the promotion of health and well-being, taking into account the individual's constant interaction with the environment. It was this concern that led nurse theorist Rogers to develop her concepts of the nature of individuals as energy fields in constant interplay with the surrounding environment (Hover-Kramer et al., 1996). Rogers' theoretical framework postulates that all living things are composed of energy, and there is a continual exchange of energy between them, as they strive toward the goal of balance and universal order. Using the hands, intention, and centering, the HT practitioner assesses the client's energy field and helps direct it to a more open, symmetrical pattern that enhances the client's ability to self-heal. The nursing diagnosis used for HT and other biofield therapies is defined as an "Energy Field Disturbance state in which disruption of the flow of energy surrounding a person's being results in a disharmony of the boyd, mind, and/or spirit" (Carpenito-Moyot, 2006, p. 8).

It is still not clear how energy field modalities, including HT, influence the energy patterns of a recipient or how recipients utilize the energy to enhance their self-healing processes, but the effects of energy-based healing interactions are measurable and significant (Hover-Kramer, 2002). The fields of physics, engineering, biology, and physiology continue to research this area of energy exchange in an attempt to explain what occurs during an energetic interaction (Feinstein & Eden, 2008; Forbes, Rust, & Becker, 2004; Oschman, 2000; Stouffer, Kaiser, Pitman, & Rolf, 1998).

Oschman reports that various energy therapies actually stimulate tissue healing by the production of pulsating electromagnetic fields that induce currents to flow within the body's tissue. It is proposed that these currents are generated via the heartbeat and move throughout the circulatory system and the "living matrix," which Oschman describes as an informational nervous system of the body where electron movement occurs, producing these waves (Oschman, 2008; McCraty, Atkinson, Tomasino, & Tiller, 1998). He states that the heart generates the body's largest electromagnetic field, which can be measured in the space around the body using the superconducting quantum interference device (SQUID). The SQUID has been used to measure these biomagnetic fields emanating from the hands of energy field practitioners who use therapeutic touch, qi gong, yoga, and meditation. It has been found that low electromagnetic frequencies (a coherent pattern) can be emitted from a trained energy healer's hands at a rate needed for tissue healing, which has the possibility to convert a stalled healing process to active repair by restoring coherence to the tissue (Oschman).

Other instruments have been invented to directly measure the human energy field (e.g., Kirlian photography, gaseous discharge visualization, and polycontrast interference) but these instruments are not consistently accurate (Duerden, 2004). Eschiti (2007) states, "[u]ntil science is able to provide accurate, direct measurement of the human energy field, research will need to be conducted by measuring possible effects on the field in an indirect manner" (p. 10).

The concept of energy systems as part of the human interactive environment and healing has been part of many cultures for centuries. Ancient East Indian traditions speak of a universal energy (*prana*) that flows and activates the life force (*kundalini*) (Hover-Kramer et al., 1996). In China, Japan, and Thailand, the basic life energy is called *chi, qi,* or *ki.* The Egyptians called it *ankh* and the Polynesians refer to it as *mana.* Many other cultures throughout the world have equivalent terms for describing human energies (Hover-Kramer, 2002). The common principle is that an imbalance in this energy force can result in illness.

It is unknown precisely how symptoms are managed by HT interventions. What have been observed are changes in outcomes being measured in the nursing research. It may be postulated that because energy fields are in constant interaction within and outside the physical body, internal mechanisms are stimulated by this movement of energy (Umbreit, 2000). However, any explanations given for energy healing remain theoretical, due to limited experimental data and difficulty using traditional scientific analysis because paradoxical findings often coexist (Engebretson & Wardell, 2002).

Studies specific to HT interventions have focused on managing the symptoms of pain, anxiety, and stress; decreasing the side effects of cancer treatments; promoting faster postprocedural recovery; improving mental health; using HT with the elderly to improve pain, appetite, sleep, behavior patterns, and functional abilities; increasing relaxation; and promoting a sense of well-being (Bulbrook, 2000; Cook, Guerrerio, & Slater, 2004; Dowd, Kolcaba, Steiner, & Fashinpaur, 2007; Geddes, 2002; Hutchison, 1999; Krucoff et al., 2001, 2005; MacIntyre et al., 2008; Maville, Bowen, & Benham, 2008; Post-White, Kinney, Savik, Gau, Wilcox, & Lerner, 2003; Scandrett-Hibdon, Hardy, & Mentgen, 1999; Seskevich, Crater, Lane, & Krucoff, 2004; Silva, 1996; Umbreit, 1997, 2000; Wang & Hermann, 2006; Wardell, 2000, 2008; Wardell, Rintala, Tan, & Duan, 2006; Wardell & Weymouth, 2004; Wilkinson et al., 2002).

In pediatrics, two small research studies have been completed (Speel, 2002; Verret, 2000) and two more are in progress (Wardell,

2008) that examine various outcomes. As of September 2008, there were 91 completed HT studies and 33 in progress (Wardell, 2008).

A proposed model of how HT may promote positive changes in client symptoms follows. A trained HT practitioner sends coherent energy waves from his or her hands to the client. This affects the incoherent energy patterns that cause disease or imbalance in the client's energy field and body. Due to a resonant effect, the incoherent energy pattern shifts to a healthier, coherent pattern affecting the client's circulatory, endocrine, and nervous systems, and/or other unidentified mechanisms, promoting positive client responses with the potential to restore optimal health. In other words, the HT practitioner moves and repatterns a client's energy field, promoting a more open and symmetric pattern to enhance the client's perceived sense of well-being. This movement of energy may stimulate physiological, neurochemical, and psychological changes that promote positive impacts on pain, anxiety, wound healing, immune system function, depression, and sense of well-being.

INTERVENTION

Techniques

Nearly 30 HT techniques are taught in the HT curriculum, from the simple to the complex. The HT practitioner determines which to use after an assessment of the client's expressed needs, symptoms presented, and results of an energy field hand scan. They range from localized to full-body techniques. Table 17.1 lists several basic techniques, along with indications and brief descriptions of the procedures. These techniques, which treat a wide range of client symptoms, should be practiced in a supervised setting with an instructor before working with a client.

Most of the HT techniques involve two basic types of hand gestures (called magnetic passes) that are described in terms of "hands in motion" (used to clear congestion or density from the energy field) or "hands still" (used to re-establish energy flow and balance) (Mentgen et al., 2007). In the hands-in-motion gestures, the hands make gentle brushing or combing motions, usually downward and outward, to remove congested energy from the field. The hands remain relaxed, palms facing downward toward the patient, between 1 and 6 inches above the skin or clothing. The hand strokes may be slow and sweeping or short and

Table 17.1

BASIC HEALING TOUCH TECHNIQUES

TECHNIQUES	INDICATIONS	BRIEF DESCRIPTION OF PROCEDURE
Full Body Techniques		
Basic healing touch (HT) sequence	Promote relaxation. Reduce pain. Lower anxiety, tension, stress. Facilitate wound healing. Promote restoration of the body. Promote a sense of well-being.	1. Assess client's energy field with a hand scan over the body. 2. Use magnetic passes in client's energy field (hands in motion and/ or hands still) to move congestion and density from the field. 3. Reassess client's energy field with hand scan to determine effects of intervention. 4. Ground the client to the present moment and to feel connection to the earth.
Magnetic clearing	Clear the body's energy field of congestion and emotional debris. Used for: history of drug use, postanesthesia, chronic pain, trauma, systemic disease, after breathing polluted air, history of smoking, environmental sensitivities, emotional clearing and release of unresolved feelings (e.g., anger, fear, worry, tension), chemotherapy or radiation, and kidney dialysis.	1. Assess client's energy field with a hand scan over the body. 2. Place hands 12 to 18 inches above the top of client's head with fingers spread, relaxed and curled, thumbs touching or close together. 3. Move hands very slowly in long continuous raking motions over the body from above the head to off the toes, one to six inches above the body, each sweep taking about 30 seconds (work the middle of the body first, followed by each side). 4. Procedure is repeated 30 times and takes about 15 minutes. 5. Reassess client's energy field with hand scan to determine effects of intervention. 6. Ground the client to the present moment and to feel connection to the earth.

(continued)

Table 17.1 *(continued)*

TECHNIQUES	INDICATIONS	BRIEF DESCRIPTION OF PROCEDURE
Full Body Techniques *(continued)*		
Chakra connection (Joy, 1979)	Connect, open, and balance the energy centers (chakras), enhancing the flow of energy throughout the body.	1. Assess client's energy field with a hand scan over the body. 2. Place hands on or over the minor energy centers (chakras) on the extremities and the major energy centers (chakras) on the trunk in a defined sequential manner, holding each area for at least 1 minute. 3. Reassess client's energy field with hand scan to determine effects of intervention. 4. Ground the client to the present moment and to feel connection to the earth.
Chakra spread	Open the energy centers (chakras) producing a deep clearing of energy blocks. Used for: physical or emotional pain, pre- and post-medical procedures/surgery, severe stress reactions, the terminally ill, stress, and assisting in coping with various life transitions.	1. Assess client's energy field with a hand scan over the body. 2. Hold the client's feet, then hands, one by one in a gentle embrace for at least 1 minute. 3. Place hands (palms up) above each energy center (chakra), moving the hands slowly downward toward the chakra, then spreading the hands outward as far as possible; motion is repeated three times for each energy center, moving from the upper to the lower chakras. 4. Repeat entire sequence two more times. 5. Reassess client's energy field with hand scan to determine effects of intervention. 6. End treatment with holding the client's hand and heart center (procedure is done in silence and takes 10 to 15 minutes; is used very carefully by experienced practitioners for special needs and sacred moments in healing).

(continued)

Table 17.1 *(continued)*

TECHNIQUES	INDICATIONS	BRIEF DESCRIPTION OF PROCEDURE
Localized Techniques		
Energetic ultrasound	Break up congestion, energy patterns, and blockages. Relieve pain. Assist in stopping internal bleeding, sealing lacerations, healing fractures, and joint injuries. Assist in breaking up bronchitis and sinus congestion. Assist in stimulating return of bowel motility after surgery.	1. Hand scan client's localized area to assess energy field. 2. Hold the thumb and first and second fingers together, directing energy from the palm down the fingers. 3. Imagine a beam of light coming from the fingers of one hand into the client's body. 4. Place opposite hand behind the body part being worked on. 5. Move the hand in any direction over the affected part, continuously moving for 3 to 5 minutes. 6. Repeat hand scan to determine effect of intervention.
Energetic laser	Cut, seal, and break up congestion in the energy field. Relieve pain. Help stop bleeding. Assist in wound repair.	1. Hand scan client's localized area to assess energy field. 2. Hold one or more fingers still and pointed toward the problem area. 3. Use for a few seconds to a minute. 4. Repeat hand scan to determine effect of intervention.
Mind clearing	Promote relaxation and focus or quiet the mind.	1. Hold fingertips or palms on designated parts of the neck and head, holding each part 1 to 3 minutes. 2. Gently massage mandibular joint. 3. End with light sweeping touches across the forehead and cheeks three times and a gentle hold around the jaw.

(continued)

Table 17.1 (continued)

TECHNIQUES	INDICATIONS	BRIEF DESCRIPTION OF PROCEDURE
Localized Techniques (continued)		
Pain drain	Ease pain or energy congestion.	1. Place left hand on area of pain or energy congestion and right hand downward away from body. 2. Siphon off congested energy from painful area through left hand and out right hand. 3. Place right hand on painful or congested area and place left hand upward in the air to bring in healing energy from the universal energy field (each position is generally held for 3 to 5 minutes).
Wound sealing	Repair energy field leaks that occur from the physical body experiencing trauma, incisions, or childbirth.	1. Hand scan body above a scar or injury to determine if any leaks of energy are felt coming from the site (may feel like a column of cool air). 2. Move hands over the area, gathering energy. 3. Bring gathered energy down to the client's skin over the injury and hold for a minute with hands. 4. Re-scan the area to determine that the energy field feels evenly symmetrical over the entire body.

Note: Each technique begins with determining the client's specific need for HT and obtaining client permission. Mutual goals are set. This is followed by the practitioner centering, physically and psychologically, and setting the intention for the client's highest good. Assessment of energy field disturbances are determined. Each technique ends with evaluating the energy field and the client's experience and asking for feedback.

Adapted from Hover-Kramer (2002) and Mentgen et al. (2007).

rapid. In the hands-still position, the practitioner holds his or her hands over an area of the client's body for one to several minutes, either lightly touching the skin or just above it. The practitioner uses "intent" to facilitate a transfer of energy to the specific body part of the client from a "universal source" of energy, with the practitioner as the conduit of this energy.

Although several of the HT techniques can be done with the client in a seated position, most are done while the client is lying down in the most relaxed state possible, to promote a more profound effect. The practitioner briefly describes HT and what he or she plans to do, invites the client to ask any questions at any time, and receives permission to do the treatment and to touch the client. HT practitioners practice holistic principles, which encourage openness in communication during the healing process, enhancing the depth of the healing experience (McKivergin, 2009).

Measurement of Outcomes

HT outcomes that have been measured have included patient satisfaction; anxiety and stress reduction; improved mood and reduced fatigue in cancer patients; pain reduction; improved sense of well-being; decrease in depression; positive changes in blood pressure, blood glucose, and salivary immunoglobulin A; decreased length of hospitalization and adverse periprocedural outcomes after cardiac procedures; diminished agitation levels in dementia patients; improved behaviors in Alzheimer's patients; and improved functional status for patients with mobility issues. Studies currently in progress are also examining HT's effects on cellular immune function, radiation-induced tissue damage, peripheral neuropathy and wound healing as cancer treatment side effects; quality-of-life perception with serious inflammatory skin disorders and with chemotherapy patients; cost-effectiveness outcomes; stress recovery in a neonatal intensive care unit; stress responses with veterans suffering from post-traumatic stress disorder symptoms or homelessness; and bariatric surgery recovery. Until a reliable and easily available tool is developed to measure changes in the energy system, objective measurement of changes in the flow of an energy field is not possible. Practitioners do report a change in clients' energy field that they perceive through the use of their senses, most commonly through touch.

Outcomes measured must reflect the specific client need and presenting symptoms, and the particular HT technique used to treat. Tools that have been used to measure client outcomes have included measuring patient satisfaction and well-being using Likert-type scale responses; the Spielberger State/Trait Anxiety Inventory, Profile of Mood States, or an Anxiety Visual Analog Scale; a Pain Visual Analog Scale, the McGill-Melzack Pain Questionnaire, or the Chronic Pain Experience

Instrument; Beck's Depression Inventory; cardiovascular variables (heart rate, systolic/diastolic blood pressure, and mean arterial blood pressure); oxygenation variables (pH, CO_2, PO_2, and HCO_3); Recovery Index; goniometer readings; length of stay; Functional Behavioral Profile; the Cohen-Mansfield Agitation Inventory; Ashworth Scale for grading spasticity; the HELP Strands for Preschooler for assessing gross motor skills; SF-36 to measure health-related quality of life; and immunoglobulin concentrations pre- and post-treatments.

It is difficult to determine whether the outcome of the HT intervention is due solely to the treatment or to other factors as well. The effect of the practitioner's presence has always been considered a confounding variable affecting client outcome, but this is also true in many nursing interventions.

Precautions

Precautions to be aware of when using HT techniques include the following:

- The energy field of infants, children, older people, the extremely ill, and the dying are sensitive to energy work, so treatments should be gentle and time limited.
- Gentle energy treatments are also required for pregnant women because the energy field also includes the fetus.
- Energy work with a cancer patient should be focused on balancing the whole field rather than concentrating on a particular area.
- The effect of medications and chemicals in the body may be enhanced with energy work so one must be alert to the possibility of side effects and sensitivity reactions to these substances.

It is recommended that experienced practitioners work with clients in the above situations. However, to help develop a knowledgeable practice, a student or an apprentice in HT can provide treatments in these situations if supervised by a mentor (Umbreit, 2000). HT is not considered a curative treatment and must always be used in conjunction with conventional medical care. However, practitioners and clients have reported that clients have experienced a sense of healing at a more holistic level of mind, body, and spirit, even if a cure is not possible. Umbreit (2000) reports anecdotal comments from clients that include feeling "wonderful," "relaxed," "peaceful," "in a meditative state," "warm," "soothed," "safe," "reassured," "more balanced," "mellow," "happier with life," "as if all my tension was melting," and a "sense of inner peace." Slater (2009) states, "[a]fter a session, most people experience a sense of relaxation, lessened stress, increased energy, and other signs of increased vitality" (p. 664). Because HT is a noninvasive intervention, these clients' responses have enormous implications for improving quality of life in their striving toward wellness.

USES

HT interventions have been used on all age groups, from the neonate to the elderly. Besides the general curriculum for learning HT, there are also classes available for specifically working with infants (Kluny, 2009). Healing Touch is being utilized within diverse health care facilities: hospitals, long-term care facilities, private practices, hospices, and spas (Healing Touch International, 2008). Models of delivering services range from volunteer to staff-provided programs. There are also well-established community service models that provide support for individuals with cancer while they are receiving conventional medical treatment (Anselme, peronal communication, 2005).

HT interventions have been supported by a limited number of rigorous research studies; the majority of reports are from anecdotal stories in a variety of clinical situations in all age groups and states of illness or wellness (Bulbrook, 2000; Hover-Kramer, 2002; Scandrett-Hibdon et al., 1999; Umbreit, 1997, 2000) and from studies that unfortunately were missing some vital information, which led to problems with both internal and external validity (Wardell & Weymouth, 2004). HT studies have shown positive results in the following clinical situations:

- Reduction of anxiety and stress
- Promotion of relaxation
- Reduction in acute and chronic pain
- Acceleration of postoperative recovery
- Aid in preparation for medical treatments and procedures
- Improvement of cancer treatment side effects
- Reduction in symptoms of depression
- Promotion of a sense of well-being

■ Reduction in agitation levels
■ Improvement in quality of life physically, emotionally, relationally, and spiritually.

Table 17.2 lists several research studies that have supported the use of HT interventions in some of these clinical situations over the past 12 years. Many studies are not published in medical, nursing, or psychology journals, but information can be accessed through Healing Touch International's research department (www.healingtouchinternational.org). The research continues to be controversial because the exact mechanism of action cannot be seen or easily explained in our Western view of what constitutes sound scientific research, and few double-blind studies have been done in this area.

CULTURAL APPLICATIONS

HT is being taught and practiced in 35 countries around the world, including impoverished communities with few economic resources, with more countries continuing to request HT education each year. As of 2008, HT has been taught in Argentina, Australia, Belize, Bermuda, Bolivia, Cambodia, Canada, Colombia, Denmark, Ecuador, El Salvador, England, Finland, France, Germany, Guatemala, Hungary, India, Ireland, Italy, Japan, Korea, Mexico, Nepal, Netherlands, New Zealand, Nicaragua, Peru, Romania, South Africa, Sweden, Thailand, Tibet, Trinidad/Tobago, and the United States (Energy magazine, 2008; Healing Touch International, 2008b). The skills of HT can be communicated across cultures by appropriately adapting teaching styles to the culture and available resources. The HT students are then able to use their skills in their communities, whether it be in a hospital setting, clinic, homes, rural areas, villages, and places where health care may be limited and living conditions very difficult. Even in impoverished places of the world, where strife, abject poverty and hidden hopelessness pervades daily life, learning and practicing HT has helped empower the people to address their serious social and public health issues by decreasing their suffering, especially where women and children are marginalized (Starke, 2008), and offering tools to address difficult situations and ways to work in the absence of medications (Goff, 2007).

Table 17.2

RESEARCH STUDIES USING HEALING TOUCH INTERVENTIONS (1996–2008)

USES	SELECTED SOURCES
Anxiety/stress reduction	Dubrey (2008a); Gehlhaart & Dail (2000); Guevara, Silva, & Menidas (2008); Taylor (2001); Wilkinson et al. (2002)
Promotion of relaxation/ relief of spasticity in pediatric populations	Speel (2008); Verret (2000)
Acute and chronic pain reduction	Cordes, Proffitt, & Roth (2008); Darbonne (2008); Diener (2001); Kiley (2008); Merritt & Randall (2008); Peck (2007); Protzman (2008); Slater (2008); Smith & Jones (2008); Wardell (2000); Wardell et al. (2006); Wardell, Rintala, & Tan (2008); Welcher & Kish (2001); Weymouth & Sandberg-Lewis (2000)
Acceleration of postoperative recovery	Laffey & Neizgoda (2008); MacIntyre et al. (2008); Silva (1996)
Aid in medical procedures/treatments	Seskevich et al. (2004)
Improvement of cancer treatment side effects	Cook et al. (2004); Danhauer et al. (2008); Post-White et al. (2003); Rexilius, Mundt, Megel, & Agrawal (2002)
Mental health	Bradway (1998); Dubrey (2008b); Van Aken (2004)
Elderly	Gehlhaart & Dail (2000); Ostuni & Pietro (2008); Peck (2007); Wang & Hermann (2006)
Personal growth and transformation; spiritual meaning and awareness	Geddes (1999); Wardell (2001); Ziembroski, Gilbert, Bossarte, & Guldbery, (2003)

FUTURE RESEARCH

Research studies and anecdotal cases in HT offer promising, yet certainly not conclusive data on the positive outcomes from this complementary therapy. Qualitative responses from clients have been especially important in helping guide the direction of the research and may provide insight into the phenomenon of energy exchange in the future. Some of the problems encountered in nursing research include insufficient funding to support the work, multiple variables that are hard to control in a clinical setting versus a laboratory setting, and the use of small sample sizes that can be easily affected by highly variable data and sampling error.

There is the additional difficulty of testing the efficacy of an energy-based therapy in which the energy exchange between practitioner and client cannot be seen by most people, but is only observed as subjective responses from clients. The whole conceptual framework of energy fields and energy exchange does not fit the cause–effect model that Western science is focused on. Rogers' theory (1990) speaks about energy changing, exchanging, and patterning, one moment in time never replicating itself. The focus is on nature's restoring universal order and balance, and restoring energy balance is the goal of HT. This is a huge area of research that obviously will require a multidisciplinary effort by Western and Eastern medicine, quantum physics, biology, psychology, philosophy, spirituality, and nursing. Outcome studies, as well as studies of mechanism, will help support the development and understanding of the phenomenon of energy exchange. There are medi-ating factors that may contribute to decreases in pain intensity, anxiety reduction, acceleration of healing, immune system enhancement, dimin-ished depression, and increased sense of well-being. More studies that measure some of these mediating mechanisms are recommended.

The choice of valid instruments for measuring outcomes is critical in HT studies. Results can be skewed in either direction if the instru-ments are not reliable. However, to obtain subject cooperation when working with persons who are ill, measuring instruments must be easy to use and not burdensome to patients who are already facing difficulties.

Other challenges to be controlled in conducting HT research studies include the experience of the HT practitioner, the phenomenon of the caregiver's "presence," the type of HT treatment modality chosen, the length and number of treatments, when the treatment is done, and when measurements are done. There is a wide range of skill levels of HT practitioners from novice to certified practitioner and comparable skill level is important in planning a research study. It is important to note that "the deepest and longest lasting healing will be at the hands of a healer who has the greatest breadth and depth of training, practice, and personal healing" (Slater, 2009, p. 649). The phenomenon of pres-ence of the HT practitioner may also affect the outcome of the research and needs to be controlled in the study design. Because there are many HT interventions that can be used, a research study may need to be consistent in the type of therapy chosen. The challenge with length and number of treatments is that, under normal circumstances, a HT intervention is not used for a prescribed length of time or number of treatments. The practitioner does the work until he or she intuits that it is time to stop or that no more treatments are needed. Research could restrict this professional decision-making process. Choosing when to give a HT treatment and when to measure outcomes and ascertaining how long the outcome may last continue to be challenging. Experienced HT practitioners must have input into determining these time lines by observing patterns they may typically see in their own professional practice.

The next steps for research must build upon the studies already completed. Replication of studies would help strengthen the validity of HT. The following are questions related to specific areas to build upon:

1. Is HT equally effective in acute versus chronic pain? How long and how frequent do treatments need to be for the client to report a decrease in pain? How long does this improvement last?
2. How is postoperative recovery affected by administering HT (pain relief, wound healing, restoring of bowel function, ease of physical activity, length of stay in the hospital)?
3. Does HT have a positive effect on degenerative diseases such as arthritis, multiple sclerosis, fibromyalgia, stroke, immune deficiency disorders, chronic lung conditions, and living with a cancer diagnosis?
4. Does HT assist in managing the side effects of treatments in cancer patients?
5. What are the psychological and spiritual benefits reported by HT recipients?
6. What tools are effective in measuring a change in energy in the recipient before and after HT or an exchange of energy between practitioner and recipient?
7. Does HT reduce medical costs for pharmaceuticals, hospital stays, and clinic time?

In the quest to examine the impact of HT scientifically, we must not be too quick to dismiss the overwhelming positive client feedback from its clinical application. Creativity is necessary in conducting research of this phenomenon that cannot be seen by the naked eye, but is so often felt by the human spirit.

WEB RESOURCES

For more information on Healing Touch:

Healing Touch International: www.healingtouchinternational.org

Healing Touch Program: www.healingtouchprogram.com

American Holistic Nurses Association (AHNA): www.ahna.org

For more information on Therapeutic Touch: www.therapeutictouch.org

REFERENCES

Bailey, A. (1984). *Esoteric healing*. Albany, NY: Lucis Trust.
Bradway, C. (1998). The effects of healing touch on depression. *Healing Touch Newsletter: Research Edition, 8*(3), 2.
Brennan, B. (1986). *Hands of light*. New York: Bantam.
Bruyere, R. L. (1989). *Wheels of light*. New York: Simon & Schuster.
Bulbrook, M. J. (2000). *Healing stories to inspire, teach and heal*. Carrboro, NC: North Carolina Center for Healing Touch.
Carpentito-Moyot, L. (2006). *Nursing diagnosis: Application to clinical practice* (11th ed., pp. 288–291). Philadelphia: Lippincott, Williams, and Wilkins.
Cook, C., Guerrerio, J., & Slater, V. (2004). Healing touch and quality of life in women receiving radiation treatment for cancer: A randomized controlled trial. *Alternative Therapies, 10*(3), 34–41.
Cordes, P., Proffitt, C., & Roth, J. (2008). The effect of healing touch therapy on the pain and joint mobility experienced by patients with total knee replacements. In D. Wardell (Ed.), *Healing touch research survey* (9th ed., pp. 49–50). Lakewood, CO: Healing Touch International.
Danhauer, S., Tooze, J., Holder, P., Miller, C., Jesse, M., Carroll, S., et al. (2008). Healing touch as a supportive intervention for adult acute leukemia patients: A pilot investigation of effects on distress and treatment-related symptoms. In D. Wardell (Ed.), *Healing touch research survey* (9th ed., p. 13). Lakewood, CO: Healing Touch International.
Darbonne, M. (2008). The effects of healing touch modalities on patients with chronic pain. In D. Wardell (Ed.), *Healing touch research survey* (9th ed., p. 57). Lakewood, CO: Healing Touch International.

Diener, D. (2001). A pilot study of the effect of chakra connection and magnetic unruffle on perception of pain in people with fibromyalgia. *Healing Touch Newsletter: Research Edition, 01*(3), 7–8.

Dowd, T., Kolcaba, K., Steiner, R., & Fashinpaur, D. (2007). Comparison of a healing touch, coaching, and a combined intervention on comfort and stress in younger college students. *Holistic Nursing Practice, 21*(4), 194–202.

Dubrey, R. (2008a). Perceived effectiveness of healing touch treatments by healees. In D. Wardell (Ed.), *Healing touch research survey* (9th ed., pp. 63–64). Lakewood, CO: Healing Touch International.

Dubrey, R. (2008b). The effect of healing touch on in-patients going through stage 1 recovery from alcoholism. In D. Wardell (Ed.), *Healing touch research survey* (9th ed., pp. 78–79). Lakewood, CO: Healing Touch International.

Duerden, T. (2004). An aura of confusion. Part 2: The aided eye—"imaging the aura?" *Complementary Therapies in Nurse Midwifery, 10*, 116–123.

Energy Magazine. (2008, July). *Growing Healing Touch worldwide*. Arvada, CO: Healing Touch Program.

Engebretson, J., & Wardell, D. W. (2002). Experience of a reiki session. *Alternative Therapies, 8*(02), 48–53.

Eschiti, V. (2007). Healing touch: A low-tech intervention in high-tech settings. *Dimensions of Critical Care Nursing, 26*(1), 9–14.

Feinstein, D., & Eden, D. (2008). Six pillars of energy medicine: Clinical strengths of a complementary paradigm. *Alternative Therapies, 14*(1), 44–54.

Forbes, M. A., Rust, R., & Becker, G. J. (2004). Surface electromyography (EMG) as a measurement for biofield research: Results from a single case study. *Journal of Alternative & Complementary Medicine, 10*(4), 617–626.

Geddes, N. (1999). The experience of personal transformation in healing touch practitioners: A heuristic inquiry. *Healing Touch Newsletter, 9*(3), 5.

Geddes, N. (2002). Research related to healing touch. In D. Hover-Kramer (Ed.), *Healing touch: A guidebook for practitioners* (2nd ed.; pp. 24–40). Albany, NY: Delmar.

Gehlhaart, C., & Dail, P. (2000). Effectiveness of healing touch and therapeutic touch on elderly residents of long term care facilities on reducing pain and anxiety level. *Healing Touch Newsletter, 0*(3), 8.

Goff, R. (2007). Carrying light into South Africa. *Healing Touch International, Inc. Quarterly Newsletter, 1*, 1, 6–7.

Guevara, E., Silva, C. & Menidas, N., (2008). The effect of healing touch therapy on post traumatic stress disorder (PTSD) symptoms on domestic violence abused Mexican women. In D. Wardell (Ed.), *Healing touch research survey* (9th ed., p. 79). Lakewood, CO: Healing Touch International.

Healing Touch International. (2008). *What is healing touch?* Retrieved October 12, 2008, from www.healingtouchinternational.org

Healing Touch Program. (2008a). *Healing touch history*. Retrieved October 12, 2008, from www.healingtouchprogram.com

Healing Touch Program. (2008b). *Healing touch program information*. Retrieved October 12, 2008, from www.healingtouchprogram.com

Healing Touch Program. (2008c). *What is healing touch?* Retrieved October 12, 2008, from www.healingtouchprogram.com

Hover-Kramer, D. (2002). *Healing touch: A guidebook for practitioners* (2nd ed.). Albany, NY: Delmar.

Hover-Kramer, D., Mentgen, J., & Scandrett-Hibdon, S. (1996). *Healing touch: A resource for health care professionals*. Albany, NY: Delmar.

Hutchison, C. (1999). Healing touch: An energetic approach. *American Journal of Nursing, 99*(4), 43–48.

Jackson, C., & Keegan, L. (2009). Touch. In B. Dossey & L. Keegan (Eds.), *Holistic nursing: A handbook for practice* (5th ed.). Sudbury MA: Jones & Bartlett.

Joy, B. (1979). *Joy's way*. New York: G. P. Putnam's Sons.

Kiley, S. (2008). The evaluation of healing touch for headache pain. In D. Wardell, D. (Ed.), *Healing touch research survey* (9th ed., p. 58). Lakewood, CO: Healing Touch International.

Krieger, D. (1979). *The therapeutic touch: How to use your hands to help or to heal*. New York: Simon & Schuster.

Krieger, D. (1993). *Accepting your power to heal*. Santa Fe, NM: Bear & Co.

Krucoff, M., Crater, S., Gallup, D., Blankenship, J., Cuffe, M., Guarneri, M., et al. (2005). Music, imagery, touch, and prayer as adjuncts to interventional cardiac care: The monitoring and actualization of noetic trainings (MANTRA) II randomized study. *Lancet, 366*(9481), 211–217.

Krucoff, M., Crater, S., Green, C., Massa, A., Seskevich, J., Lane, J., et al. (2001). Integrative noetic therapies as adjuncts to percutaneous intervention during unstable coronary syndromes: Monitoring and actualization of noetic training (MANTRA) feasibility pilot. *American Heart Journal, 142*(5), 760–767.

Laffey, E., & Neizgoda, J. (2008). Wound care and complementary medicine: The impact of healing touch. A case study. In D. Wardell (Ed.), *Healing touch research survey* (9th ed., p. 75). Lakewood, CO: Healing Touch International.

MacIntyre, B., Hamilton, J., Fricke, T., Ma, W., Mehle, S., & Michel, M. (2008). The efficacy of healing touch in coronary artery bypass surgery recovery: A randomized clinical trial. *Alternative Therapies in Healing and Medicine, 14*(4), 24–32.

Maville, J., Bowen, J., & Benham, G. (2008). Effect of healing touch on stress perception and biological correlates. *Holistic Nursing Practice, 22*(2), 103–110.

McCraty, R., Atkinson, M., Tomasino, D., & Tiller, W. (1998). The electricity of touch: Detection and measurement of cardiac energy exchange between people. In K.H. Pribram (Ed.), *Brain and values: Is a biological science of values possible?* (pp. 359–379). Mahwah, NJ: Lawrence Erlbaum.

McKivergin, M. (2009). The nurse as an instrument of healing. In B. Dossey & L. Keegan (Eds.), *Holistic nursing: A handbook for practice* (5th ed.). Sudbury, MA: Jones & Bartlett.

Mentgen, J., Bulbrook, M. J., Hutchison, C., Wardell, D. W., & Komitor, C. (2007). *Healing touch level 1 notebook*. Golden, CO: Healing Touch Program.

Merritt, P., & Randall, D. (2008). The effect of healing touch and other forms of energy work on cancer pain. In D. Wardell (Ed.), *Healing touch research survey* (9th ed, p. 18–19). Lakewood, CO: Healing Touch International.

NCCAM: National Center for Complementary and Alternative Medicine. (2007, March). *Energy medicine: An overview*. Retrieved October 12, 2008, from www.nccam.nih.gov

Oschman, J. L. (2000). *Energy medicine: The scientific basis.* Dover, NH: Churchill Livingston.

Oschman, J. (2008, September). *Validating the heart's work.* Presented at the Healing Touch International Conference, Milwaukee, WI.

Ostuni, E., & Pietro, M. J. (2008). Effects of healing touch on nursing home residents in later stages of Alzheimer's. In D. Wardell (Ed.), *Healing touch research survey* (9th ed., pp. 33–34). Lakewood, CO: Healing Touch International.

Peck, S. (2007). Aftermath of an unexpected, unexplained and abrupt termination of healing touch and extrapolation of related costs. *Complementary Health Review, 12*(144), 144–160.

Post-White, J., Kinney, M. E., Savik, K., Gau, J. B., Wilcox, C., & Lerner, I. (2003). Therapeutic massage and healing touch improve symptoms in cancer. *Integrative Cancer Therapies, 2*(4), 332–344.

Protzman, L. (2008). The effect of healing touch on pain and relaxation. In D. Wardell, D. (Ed.), *Healing touch research survey* (9th ed., p. 58). Lakewood, CO: Healing Touch International.

Rexilius, S., Mundt, C., Megel, M., & Agrawal, S. (2002). Therapeutic effects of healing touch and massage therapy on caregivers of autologous hematopoietic stem cell transplant patients. *Oncology Nursing Forum, 29*(3), 1–14.

Rogers, M. (1990). Nursing: Science of unitary, irreducible, human beings: Update 1990. In E. A. M. Barrett (Ed.), *Vision of Rogers' science-based nursing* (pp. 5–11). New York: National League for Nursing.

Scandrett-Hibdon, S. (1996). Research foundations. In D. Hover-Kramer, J. Mentgen, & S. Scandrett-Hibdon (Eds.), *Healing touch: A resource for health care professionals* (pp. 27–42). Albany, NY: Delmar.

Scandrett-Hibdon, S., Hardy, C., & Mentgen, J. (1999). *Energetic patterns: Healing touch case studies, Vol. 1.* Lakewood, CO: Colorado Center for Healing Touch.

Seskevitz, J., Crater, S., Lane, J., & Krucoff, M. (2004). Beneficial effects of noetic therapies on mood before percutaneous intervention for unstable coronary symptoms. *Nursing Research, 53*(2), 116–121.

Silva, C. (1996). The effects of relaxation touch on the recovery level of postanesthesia abdominal hysterectomy patients. *Alternative Therapies, 2*(4), 94.

Slater, V. (2008). Safety, elements, and effects of healing touch on chronic non-malignant abdominal pain. In D. Wardell (Ed.), *Healing touch research survey* (9th ed., pp. 59–60). Lakewood, CO: Healing Touch International.

Slater, V. (2009). Energy healing. In B. Dossey & L. Keegan (Eds.), *Holistic nursing: A handbook for practice* (5th ed., pp. 647–673). Sudbury, MA: Jones & Bartlett.

Smith, C., & Jones, S. (2008). The effects of healing touch on pain and anxiety with end stage liver disease. In D. Wardell (Ed.), *Healing touch research survey* (9th ed.; p. 59). Lakewood, CO: Healing Touch International.

Speel, L. (2008). A pilot study on the effect of healing touch–mind cleaning and magnetic unruffling on high school students with mental and physical disabilities. In D. Wardell (Ed.), *Healing touch research survey* (9th ed., pp. 70–72). Lakewood, CO: Healing Touch International.

Starke, B.A. (July, 2008). Presence in Nepal. *Energy Magazine, 25,* 11–14.

Stouffer, D., Kaiser, D., Pitman, G., & Rolf, W. (1998, January). *Electrodermal testing to measure the effect of a healing touch treatment.* Paper presented at the Healing Touch Research Symposium, Denver, CO.

Taylor, B. (2001, February). The effect of healing touch on the coping ability, self esteem, and general health of undergraduate nursing students. *Complementary Therapies in Nursing and Midwifery, 7*(1), 34–42.

Therapeutic touch. (2008). *What is therapeutic touch?* Retrieved October 12, 2008, from www.therapeutictouch.org

Umbreit, A. (1997). Therapeutic touch: Energy-based healing. *Creative Nursing, 3,* 6–7.

Umbreit, A. (2000). Healing touch: Applications in the acute care setting. *AACN Clinical Issues, 11*(1), 105–119.

Van Aken, R. (2004). The experiential process of healing touch for people with moderate depression. In D. Wardell (Ed.), *Healing touch research survey* (9th ed., pp. 80–81). Lakewood, CO: Healing Touch International.

Verret, P. (2000). Healing touch as a relaxation intervention in children with spasticity. *Healing Touch Newsletter: Research Edition, 0*(3), 6–7.

Wang, K., & Hermann, C. (2006). Pilot study to test the effectiveness of healing touch on agitation levels in people with dementia. *Geriatric Nursing, 27*(1), 42–40.

Wardell, D. (2000). The trauma release technique: How it is taught and experienced in healing touch. *Alternative and Complementary Therapies, 6*(1), 20–27.

Wardell, D. (2001). Spirituality of healing touch participants. *Journal of Holistic Nursing, 19*(1), 71–86.

Wardell, D. (Ed.). (2008). *Healing touch research survey* (9th ed.). Lakewood, CO: Healing Touch International.

Wardell, D., Rintala, D., Tan, G., & Duan, A. (2006). Pilot study of healing touch and progressive relaxation for chronic neuropathic pain in persons with spinal cord injury. *Journal of Holistic Nursing, 24*(4), 231–240.

Wardell, D., Rintala, D., & Tan, G. (2008). Study descriptions of healing touch with veterans experiencing chronic neuropathic pain from spinal cord injury. *Explore, 4*(3), 187–195.

Wardell, D. W., & Weymouth, K. F. (2004). Review of studies of healing touch. *Journal of Nursing Scholarship, 36*(2), 147–154.

Watson, J. (1985). *Nursing: The philosophy and science of caring.* Boulder: Colorado Associated University Press.

Welcher, B., & Kish, J. (2001). Reducing pain and anxiety through healing touch. *Healing Touch Newsletter, 1*(3), 19.

Weymouth, K., & Sandberg-Lewis, S. (2000). Comparing the efficacy of healing touch and chiropractic adjustment in treating chronic low back pain: A pilot study. *Healing Touch Newsletter, 0*(3), 7–8.

Wilkinson, D., Knox, P., Chatman, J., Johnson, T., Barbour, N., Myles, Y., et al. (2002). The clinical effectiveness of healing touch. *Journal of Alternative and Complementary Medicine, 8*(1), 33–47.

Ziembroski, J., Gilbert, N., Bossarte, R., & Guldbery, G. (2003). Healing touch and hospice care: Examining outcomes at the end of life. *Alternative and Complementary Therapies, 9*(3), 146–151.

18 Reiki

DEBBIE RINGDAHL

Reiki is an energy healing method that can be used as an alternative or complementary therapy for a broad range of acute and chronic health problems. Increasingly, it is gaining acceptance as an adjunct to management of chronic conditions: pain management, hospice and palliative care, and stress reduction. Miles and True (2003) identified hospitals and community-based programs in the United States that utilize Reiki in the areas of general medicine, surgery, treatment of HIV/AIDS and cancer, and elder and hospice care, as well as for staff and family members.

According to the National Center for Complementary and Alternative Medicine (NCCAM) of the National Institutes of Health, Reiki is a biofield therapy. Therapies in this category affect energy fields that both surround and interpenetrate the human body. Bioenergy therapies involve touch or placement of the hands into a biofield, the existence of which has not been scientifically proven (NCCAM, 2007). The NIH has completed trials investigating Reiki use for fibromyalgia, AIDS, and painful neuropathy, and clinical trials of Reiki use for stress and prostate cancer are currently underway (NCCAM, 2006a, 2006b, 2006c, 2008, 2009).

A Reiki practitioner does not need to be prepared as a health care practitioner, but nurses, physical therapists, massage therapists, and doctors who practice Reiki may have greater access and acceptability within the health care system in performing hands-on treatments. The nursing profession is in a unique position to incorporate this healing modality into direct care, because so much of nursing care involves direct contact and hands-on work with patients.

The origins of Reiki are unclear, but Reiki historians generally agree that this therapy may have its roots in hands-on healing techniques that were used in Tibet or India more than 2,000 years ago. Reiki emerged in modern times around 1900 through the work of a Japanese businessman and practitioner of Tendai Buddhism, Mikao Usui (Miles, 2006). According to William Lee Rand (2000), founder of The International Center for Reiki Training, Usui searched many years for knowledge of healing methods until he had a profound, transformative experience and received direct revelation of what became known as Reiki. Following this experience, Usui worked with the poor in Kyoto and Tokyo, teaching classes and giving treatments in what he called "The Usui System of Reiki Healing." One of Dr. Usui's students, Chujiro Hayashi, wrote down the hand positions and suggested ways of using them for various ailments.

Mrs. Hawayo Takata is credited with the spread of Reiki in the Americas and Europe. In 1973, Mrs. Takata began to train Reiki teachers (Miles, 2006). The Reiki Alliance, a professional organization of Reiki masters, grew from 20 to nearly 1,000 members between 1981 and 1999 (Horrigan, 2003). Currently, the International Center for Reiki Training estimates there are more than 50,000 Reiki masters and 1 million Reiki practitioners worldwide ("Federally Funded," 2004).

DEFINITION

The word *Reiki* is composed of two Japanese words—*rei* and *ki*. *Rei* is usually translated as "universal," although some authors suggest that it also has a deeper connotation of all-knowing spiritual consciousness. *Ki* refers to life force energy that flows throughout all living things, known in certain other parts of the world as *Ch'i*, *prana*, or *mana*. When *Ki* energy is unrestricted, there is thought to be less susceptibility to illness or imbalances of mind, body, or spirit (Rand, 2000). In its combined form, the word *Reiki* is taken to mean spiritually guided life force energy or universal life force energy.

The mind–body component to Reiki healing is evidenced in the underlying belief that the deepest level of healing occurs through the spirit. The emphasis is on healing, not cure, which is believed to occur by Reiki energy connecting individuals to their own innate spiritual wisdom. Reiki flows through, but is not directed by, the practitioner, leaving the healing component to the individual receiving the treatment.

Reiki is not only a healing technique, but a philosophy of living that acknowledges mind–body–spirit unity and human connectedness to all things. This philosophy is reflected in the Reiki principles for living: *Just for today do not worry. Just for today do not anger. Honor your teachers, parents, and elders. Earn your living honestly. Show gratitude to all living things* (Mills, 2001).

The ability to practice Reiki is transmitted in stages directly from teacher to student via initiations called attunements. This attunement process differentiates Reiki from other hands-on healing methods. During attunements, teachers open up the students' energy channels by using specific visual symbols that were revealed to Dr. Usui. There are three degrees of attunement preparatory to achieving the status of Master Teacher, at which stage the practitioner is considered fully open to the flow of universal life force energy. By tradition, the Usui Reiki symbols and their Japanese names are confidential. This arises from the sacred nature of the techniques rather than from proprietary motives; the symbols are believed not to convey Reiki energy if used by noninitiates.

Level I Reiki is taught as a hands-on technique that includes basic information about Reiki principles and hand positions. In Level II, students are taught symbols that allow transfer of energy through space and time, also known as absentee or distance healing. The higher vibration of energy available at Level II is considered to work at a deeper level of healing. Level III, or the mastery level, is typically achieved through an apprenticeship with a Reiki Master, and includes more in-depth study of Reiki practice and teaching. At all levels, Reiki skill develops through committed practice.

In recent years, additional branches of Reiki with further degrees of attunement have developed; two of these are Karuna Reiki and Reiki Seichim. There are currently no uniform standards in Reiki education. Because of the noninvasive nature of the treatments, this does not present problems in personal practice. However, this lack of standardization does pose problems when working to integrate Reiki into the conventional health care system (Horrigan, 2003).

SCIENTIFIC BASIS

An emerging body of evidence confirms the existence of energy fields and suggests new ways of measuring energy; these are not specific to Reiki. Traditional electrical measurements such as electrocardiograms and electroencephalograms can now be supplemented by biomagnetic field mapping to obtain more accurate information about the human condition. Superconducting quantum interference devices have been used to show the effect of disease on the magnetic field of the body, and pulsating magnetic fields have been used to improve healing (Oschman, 2002). In a small experimental study of the effects of one type of energy therapy, researchers found consistent, marked decreases in gamma rays measured at several sites within intervention subjects' electromagnetic fields during treatment (Benford, Talnagi, Doss, Boosey, & Arnold, 1999). To a lesser extent, the findings indicated a decrease also during sham treatment, but not among control subjects. The authors hypothesized that the effect among sham treatment recipients resulted from human touch. Brewitt, Vittetoe, and Hartwell (1997) studied electrical skin resistance at selected body points to measure effects of Reiki treatments. Charman's research (2000) suggests that intention to heal transmits measurable wave patterns to recipients. These studies suggest that in the future it may be possible to directly measure subtle elements of the human energy field, to elucidate mechanisms by which Reiki and other energy healing techniques lead to changes in health outcomes.

Methodological problems have been identified in studies of Reiki. It is difficult to demonstrate validity in studies of energy therapies. Although case studies and anecdotal examples have been relatively consistent in reporting positive responses to Reiki treatments, this does not represent the scientific rigor that is demanded within an evidence-based health care system. Mansour, Beuche, Laing, Leis, and Nurse (1999), in an effort to standardize treatments, demonstrated that it is possible to blind subjects to real vs. placebo Reiki, opening the door to placebo-controlled studies in Reiki research.

It has also been speculated that energy healing impacts outcome in a way that is difficult to measure. Engebretson and Wardell (2002) concluded that many research models are not complex enough to capture the experience of a Reiki session. In their qualitative study they found that participants had a diverse and descriptive language that accompanied their experience. They also measured the effects of Reiki on objective measures for stress and anxiety. These measures demonstrated a decrease in perceived anxiety, an increase in signs of relaxation, and an increase in humoral immunological functioning (Wardell & Engebretson, 2001). These two studies demonstrate the potential for increasing the understanding of Reiki energy by utilizing more qualitative research designs.

INTERVENTIONS

Technique

The Reiki practitioner acts as a conduit for this healing-intended energy to self or others. During treatments, a Level I Reiki practitioner employs a series of 12 to 15 hand positions. A Level II Reiki practitioner also uses hand positions, but may use various Reiki symbols to focus the Ki energy or perform distance healings. If touch is contraindicated for any reason, the hands can be held one to four inches above the body. A full Reiki session usually lasts 45 to 90 minutes. Reiki practitioners, especially if they are nurses working in a clinical setting, often do not have the luxury of providing a full session. At such times, shorter and more targeted treatments may be offered for specific purposes. In *The Original Reiki Handbook of Dr. Mikao Usui* (Petter, 1999), the use of particular hand positions is recommended for addressing specific health problems.

Unlike other energy healing modalities, Reiki energy flows through the hands without employing cognitive, emotional, or spiritual skills. The attunement process provides access to the energy without requiring ongoing practice or conscious intention. This makes Reiki particularly easy to learn and simple to use. Potter (2003) compared her experience with therapeutic touch after receiving a Level I attunement. She found that her work became less directive and the effort to stay centered was no longer a concern.

Guidelines for Full Hands-on Reiki Session

The recipient may sit or lie down, but because Reiki tends to be very relaxing it is often preferable to lie down. Patients may remain clothed during a Reiki treatment. A massage table or hospital bed is frequently used, providing comfort for both client and practitioner. After practitioners center themselves and establish an intent to heal with Reiki, the energy flows automatically from their hands without cognitive effort. The hands rest gently on the person's body with the fingers straight and touching so that each hand functions as a unit. The sequence of hand positions may vary, but will generally include all seven major *chakras* and the endocrine glands. The success of a Reiki treatment does not depend on the use of certain hand positions, for the *Ki* energy goes where it is needed.

As more health care institutions offer complementary therapies, policies and guidelines must be developed that provide standards for implementation. Sawyer (1998) chronicles the development of a policy for Reiki use in the operating room at a large medical center. Brill and Kashurba (2001) provide an outline for starting a Reiki Program in a health care facility, including development of program objectives, training health care providers, and tracking and reporting outcomes. This author developed a Reiki protocol for use by nurses providing care to chemotherapy patients.

Measurement of Outcomes

Recipients' subjective feelings during a Reiki session are not considered indications of effectiveness. Patients may feel sensations similar to those of the practitioner, but they may also feel nothing. Sensations may include heat, cold, numbness, involuntary muscle twitching, heaviness, buoyancy, trembling, throbbing, static electricity, tingling, color, and heightened or decreased awareness of sound (Engebretson & Wardell, 2002). It is not uncommon for clients to fall asleep during a treatment with reports of increased relaxation, peacefulness, and reconnecting to their center.

Physiologic outcome measures examined in other healing touch studies are also appropriate for Reiki, such as hematologic tests, blood pressure and heart rate, bioelectric measures, wound healing rate, inhibition of harmful microorganisms, and body temperature changes. Mackay, Hansen, and McFarlane (2004) concluded that Reiki has some effect on the autonomic nervous system by comparing heart rate, cardiac vagal tone, blood pressure, cardiac sensitivity to baroreflex, and breathing activity among three groups of subjects: those resting, receiving

Reiki, or receiving placebo Reiki. Psychological measures are equally important, including perceived pain, cognitive function, memory, and levels of anxiety, depression, or hostility.

Precautions

No serious adverse effects of Reiki treatments have been published. Some patients, however, may experience emotional release that may be uncomfortable or disturbing. Therefore, practitioners must be prepared to provide assistance and appropriate referrals if emotional distress persists. Moreover, some individuals may dislike being touched. Practitioners can avoid this discomfort by assessing the person's level of comfort with touch and taking into account gender and cultural considerations. Few patients who are fully informed object, and even among vulnerable populations such as victims of torture, responses to Reiki have been found to be favorable (Kennedy, 2001).

USES

The range of potential practical applications with patients is broad and depends on the setting. Reiki has been used in hospice and palliative care, among cancer patients, in HIV/AIDS programs, for pre- and postoperative patients, and in stroke rehabilitation. The common theme described in many of these programs is the benefit of Reiki for pain relief, stress and anxiety reduction, and promoting relaxation. Reiki may have particular application for people suffering from chronic physical and mental health conditions, such as fibromyalgia and depression. A study by Shore (2004) provides evidence that Reiki may reduce symptoms of depression that last as long as one year following treatment. This author is currently serving as coinvestigator in a study testing feasibility, acceptability, and safety of Reiki touch for premature infants (Duckett, 2008), a new area of Reiki application.

Achieving institutional approval for Reiki use requires both evidence of safety and effectiveness and the development of policies or clinical guidelines. In a recent Cochrane Database Systematic Review of touch therapies for pain relief in adults (So, Jiang, & Qin, 2008), the authors concluded that, although the studies were inconclusive, the evidence supports the use of touch therapies for pain relief and there were no adverse effects identified. Four systematic reviews on Reiki research have been published from 2007 to 2008 (Herron-Marx, Price-Knol, & Hicks, 2008; Lee, 2008; Lee, Pittler, & Ernst, 2008; Vitale, 2007), suggesting increased interest in developing evidence-based practice guidelines for Reiki use. Of the 23 studies (nine randomized controlled trials) included in the systematic reviews, four studies showed evidence that Reiki reduced pain (Dressen & Singh, 2000; Olson, Hanson, & Michaud, 2003; Vitale & O'Connor, 2006; Wirth, Brenlan, Levine, & Rodriguez, 1993), one study showed Reiki decreased depression and anxiety symptoms (Shore, 2004), and one study demonstrated decreased fatigue and increased quality of life among cancer patients who received Reiki (Tsang, Carlson, & Olson, 2007). The variation in populations and outcomes measured serves to reinforce the notion that Reiki may have application among populations with diverse health needs.

Nurses are increasingly engaging in Reiki practice and research, leading to greater awareness of the potential for integrating Reiki into nursing practice. Several authors have documented effective use of Reiki in the direct provision of nursing care (Brathovde, 2006; Brill & Kashurba, 2001; Engebretson, 2002; Gallob, 2003; Lipinski, 2006; Pierce, 2007; Vitale, 2006). Reiki as a nursing intervention has the potential for reducing pain and stress for people experiencing a variety of chronic health problems, including cancer. Robb (2006) studied the lived experience of registered nurse Reiki practitioners to contribute to the knowledge about Reiki as a nursing intervention.

Exhibit 18.1 provides a list of populations/settings in which Reiki has been used. In a biomedical treatment setting Reiki is best seen as a complementary healing modality, whereas in other circumstances it can either be used alone or along with other approaches.

Self-Treatment and Practitioner Benefits

One of the more unique features of Reiki therapy is its capacity to self-treat. A Reiki practitioner can self-treat by using hand positions on the head, abdomen, chest, or other areas of the body, reducing pain and/or increasing a sense of relaxation. The concepts of empowerment and self-treatment have particular value when considering chronic health problems. For some Reiki practitioners, teaching their clients Level I Reiki provides the client with a greater sense of control over some of

Exhibit 18.1

Applications for Reiki in Clinical Settings

Application	Reference
Promoting relaxation in labor and delivery	Mills, 2003
HIV/AIDs	Schmehr, 2003; Vanderbilt, 2004
Supporting pre- and postoperative surgical patients	Potter, 2007; Sawyer, 1998; Vitale & O'Connor, 2006
Hospice and palliative care	Hemming & Maher, 2005; Mramor, 2004
Supporting oncology patients	Ameling & Potter, 2000; Bossi, Ott, & DeCristofaro, 2007; Pierce, 2007; Tsang, Carlson, & Olson, 2007
Pain management	Gillipsie, Gillipsie, & Stevens, 2007; Olson, Hanson, & Michaud, 2003; Wirth, Brenlan, Levine, & Rodriguez, 1993
Decreasing depression and/or anxiety and stress levels	Dressen & Singg, 1998; Shore, 2004
Trauma, posttraumatic stress disorder	Dey & Emmanuel, 2008; Kennedy, 2001
Enhancing immune function	Wardell & Engebretson, 2001
Promoting wound healing	Papantonio, 1998
Rehabilitation	DiNucci, 2005; Hall, 2004; Pocotte & Salvador, 2008
Support for nursing home residents	Silva, 2002; Thomas, 2005
Improving hematologic measures	Wirth, Chang, Eidelman, & Paxton, 1996

their health problems, including pain management and stress reduction (Miles & True, 2003; Mills, 2001). This author teaches Levels I and II to clients with a variety of health problems, including fibromyalgia, mood disorders, cancer, and neurological problems, such as advanced amyotrophic lateral sclerosis (ALS). Clients with physical limitations may gain particular benefits from learning Level II, or distance healing.

Reiki energy, by moving through the practitioner's crown and out through the hands, also has positive effects on the practitioner. A Reiki practitioner is simultaneously giving and receiving Reiki energy while giving a Reiki treatment. Reiki practitioners report feeling energized, relaxed, and/or more centered after performing a Reiki treatment. Research on Reiki use by nurses has demonstrated positive effects on the practitioner, including greater job satisfaction and increase in caring behaviors (Brathovde, 2006; Fortune & Price, 2003; Whelan & Wishnia, 2003). The increased sense of well-being that occurs when giving and receiving Reiki may influence the patient/nurse relationship and create a less stressful work environment. Reiki may also be used for health care provider self-care, with the potential for reducing stress (Ameling & Potter, 2000; Raingruber & Robinson, 2007). Fortune and Price have identified Reiki as an energy therapy that can be used to prevent and treat burnout among nurses.

CULTURAL ASPECTS

Energy and touch therapies are found in the health traditions of most cultures. Like Reiki, *Johrei,* originated in Japan. It is a spirituality-based energy modality that aims to release negativity from the individual's spiritual self (Brooks, Schwartz, Reece, & Nangle, 2006). Anagami healing practices include massage, bonesetting, and curing sprains (Joshi, 2004). The healing practices of Siberian shamans include touching the sore place of a person with a bundle of twigs or blowing the disease out of the dwelling, shaking off the illness, or banishing the illness by ringing a bell (Sem, 2009). Shamanic healing practices can also include the shaman sucking directly on the skin over the area where the harmful spiritual intrusion is thought to reside or seeking to remove this harmful spirit by cupping the hands over the area (Shamanic Healing, 2009).

Although health care workers may find that some of the energy and healing practices used in non-Western cultures differ greatly from Western health practices, and even from the more frequently used complementary therapies, respecting the person's belief in these practices is important in the person's healing process. The patient's strong belief in the unity of body and spirit warrant the nursing staff to find ways to include these therapies in the care regimen unless these interfere with needed medical therapies.

FUTURE RESEARCH

Most published research on Reiki has been conducted with small, non-random, convenience samples, raising questions about the validity and generalizability of findings. Overall, few studies on Reiki have used randomized control trials, and measuring Reiki outcomes has proved challenging. Outcomes for touch therapies such as Reiki are typically not disease-specific and establishing an appropriate time frame to detect effect is variable (Engebretson & Wardell, 2007). New models of research that enlarge our definition of outcomes need to be explored (Schiller, 2003). Clinical evaluation of Reiki represents a challenge using our current standards of assessment. Combining subjective and physiologic measures in such research studies will allow broader assessment of the effects of Reiki (Liverani, Minelli, & Ricciuti, 2000). Because the goals of Reiki may be broader than symptom relief and include concepts of physiologic and psychological balance, qualitative studies that can address values and meaning are also important, as evidenced in the research by Wardell and Engebretson (2001).

Vitale (2007) identified limitations in research design and the use of linear research methods as problematic in conducting Reiki research. Current outcome measures may not accurately reflect or measure all aspects of a Reiki treatment. Lack of standardization in Reiki practice also impacts reliability and validity. Some research studies do not identify all components of the Reiki intervention used, including length of treatment, type of treatment, or level/training of the Reiki practitioner.

Although both hands-on and distance healing are forms of energy healing, the presence of touch has the capacity to confound the research results, as all touch may have some healing properties. A review of studies of the efficacy of distance healing (Astin, Harkness, & Ernest, 2000) identified both methodological limitations and positive outcomes meriting further study. Shore (2004) compared outcomes between hands-on and distant Reiki healing, and found a greater reduction in depression symptoms with distance healing.

There is a need to develop research designs that consider more subtle and longer lasting outcomes than those that have typically been

Exhibit 18.2

Reiki Web Sites

IARP—International Association of Reiki Professionals: www.iarp.org

The International Center for Reiki Training: www.reiki.org

The Reiki Alliance: www.Reikialliance.com

The Reiki Page: www.reiki7gen.com

Usui Reiki: www.usuireiki.com

Reiki Module through the University of Minnesota Center for Spirituality and Healing: http://takingcharge.csh.umn.edu/therapies/reiki/what

---

used. If energy treatment works on a different level than the conventional medical model, the results may not be as dramatic and may require larger groups and a longer treatment period to show a positive outcome (Nield-Anderson & Ameling, 2000). Additional information about Reiki can be obtained on the Web sites found in Exhibit 18.2.

Suggested questions for future research include:

1. What are the physiologic and/or psychological effects of Reiki treatments for specific conditions when used alone or in conjunction with other therapies?
2. What is the relative effectiveness of noncontact Reiki (distance healing) and hands-on Reiki?
3. What is the best way to use Reiki in providing stress reduction for health care providers?
4. What are the differences in selected outcome measures between Reiki and other energy therapies?

REFERENCES

Ameling, A., & Potter, P. (2000). Reiki: Caring for self, caring for others. *Innovations in Breast Cancer Care, 5*(2), 44–48.

Astin, J., Harkness, E., & Ernst, E. (2000). The efficacy of 'distant healing': A systematic review of randomized trials. *Annals of Internal Medicine, 132*(11), 903–910.

Benford, M. S., Talnagi, J., Doss, D. B., Boosey, S., & Arnold, L. E. (1999). Gamma radiation fluctuations during alternative healing therapy. *Alternative Therapies, 5*(4), 51–56

Bossi, L. M., Ott, M. J., & DeCristofaro, S. (2007). Reiki as a clinical intervention in oncology nursing practice. *Clinical Journal of Oncology Nursing, 12*(3), 489–494.

Brathovde, A. (2006). A pilot study: Reiki for self-care and healthcare providers. *Holistic Nursing Practice, 20*(2), 95–101.

Brewitt, B., Vittetoe, T., & Hartwell, B. (1997). The efficacy of Reiki hands-on healing: Improvements in spleen and nervous system function as quantified by electrodermal screening. *Alternative Therapies, 5*(4), 51–56.

Brill, C., & Kashurba, M. (2001). Each moment of touch. *Nursing Administration Quarterly, 25*(3), 8–14.

Brooks, A. J., Schwartz, G., Reece, K., & Nangle, G. (2006). The effect of *Johrei* healing on substance abuse recovery: A pilot study. *Journal of Alternative and Complementary Medicine, 12,* 625–631.

Charman, R. A. (2000). Placing healers, healees, and healing into a wider research context. *Journal of Alternative and Complementary Medicine, 6*(2). 177–180.

Dey, M., & Emanuel, M. (2008). Reiki for veterans. *Reiki News Magazine, 7*(4), 41–43.

DiNucci, E. (2005). Energy healing: A complementary treatment for orthopaedic and other conditions. *Orthopaedic Nursing, 24*(4), 259–269.

Dressen, L. J., & Singh, S. (2000). Effects of Reiki on pain and selected affective and personality variables of chronically ill patients. *Subtle Energies and Energy Medicine, 9*(1), 51–82.

Duckett, L. (2008). *Testing feasibility, acceptability, and safety of Reiki touch for premature infants.* University of Minnesota IRB application.

Engebretson, J. (2002). Hands on: The persistent metaphor in nursing. *Holistic Nursing Practice, 16*(4), 20–35.

Engebretson, J., & Wardell, D. (2002). Experience of a reiki session. *Alternative Therapies, 8*(2), 48–53.

Engebretson, J., & Wardell, D. (2007). Energy-based modalities. *Nursing Clinics of North America, 42,* 243–259.

Federally funded Reiki study underway in Washington. (2004). *Acupuncture Today, 5*(3), 1, 8.

Fortune, M., & Price, M. (2003, Spring/Summer). The spirit of healing: How to develop a spirituality based personal and professional practice. *Journal of New York State Nurses Association,* 32–38.

Gallob, R. (2003). Reiki: A supportive in nursing practice and self-care for nurses. *Journal of the New York State Nurses Association, 34*(1), 9–13.

Gillipsie, E., Gillipsie, B., & Stevens, M. (2007). Painful diabetic neuropathy: Impact of an alternative approach. *Diabetes Care, 30,* 999–1001.

Hall, M. (2004) Treating stroke and other neurological disorders. *Reiki News Magazine, 3*(2), 38–42.

Hemming, L., & Maher, D. (2005). Complementary therapies in palliative care: A summary of current evidence. *British Journal of Community Nursing, 10*(10), 448–452.

Herron-Marx, S., Price-Knol, F., & Hicks, C. (2008). A systematic review of the use of Reiki in health care. *Alternative and Complementary Therapies, 14*(1), 37–42.

Horrigan, B. (2003). Pamela Miles: Reiki vibrational healing. *Alternative Therapies, 9*(4). 75–83.

Joshi, V. (2004). Human spiritual agency in Angami healing. Part 1. Divinational healers. *Anthropology and Medicine, 11,* 269–291.

Kennedy, P. (2001). Working with survivors of torture in Sarajevo with Reiki. *Complementary Therapies in Nursing and Midwifery, 7*(1), 4–7.

Lee, M. S. (2008). Is Reiki beneficial for pain management? *Focus on Alternative and Complementary Therapies, 12*(2), 78–81.

Lee, M. S., Pittler, M. H., & Ernst, E. (2008). Effects of Reiki in clinical practice: A systematic review of randomized control trials. *International Journal of Clinical Practice, 62*(6), 947–954.

Lipinski, K. (2006). Finding Reiki: Applications for your nursing practice. *Beginnings, 26*(1), 6–7.

Liverani, A., Minelli, E., & Ricciuti, A. (2000). Subjective scales for the evaluation of therapeutic effects and their use in complementary medicine. *Journal of Alternative and Complementary Medicine, 6*(3), 257–264.

Mackay, N., Hansen, S., & McFarlane, X. O. (2004). Autonomic nervous system changes during Reiki treatment: A preliminary study. *Journal of Alternative and Complementary Medicine, 10*(6), 1077–1081.

Mansour, A. A., Beuche, M., Laing, G., Leis, A., & Nurse, J. (1999). A study to test the effectiveness of placebo Reiki standardization procedures developed for a planned Reiki efficacy study. *Journal of Alternative and Complementary Medicine, 5*(2), 153–164.

Miles, P. (2006). *Reiki: A comprehensive guide.* New York: Jeremy P. Tarcher/Penguin.

Miles, P., & True, G. (2003). Reiki—review of a biofield therapy: History, theory, practice, and research. *Alternative Therapies, 9*(2), 62–72.

Mills, J. (2001). *Tapestry of healing: Where Reiki and medicine intertwine.* Green Valley, AZ: White Sage Press. www.TapestryofHealing.Com

Mills, J. (2003). How I introduced Reiki treatments into my obstetrics and gynecologic practice. *Reiki News, 2*(2), 16–21.

Mramor, J. (2004, February/March). Reiki in hospice care: Miranda's story. *Massage and Bodywork,* 51–59.

NCCAM. (2006a). *Effects of Reiki on painful neuropathy and cardiovascular risk factors.* Study begun: February 2, 2001; last updated: August 17, 2006. ClinicalTroals.gov Identifier: NCT00010751. Retrieved February 28, 2009, from http://clinicaltrials.gov/ct2/show/NCT00010751?term=%28NCCAM%29+%5BSPONSOR%5D+%28reiki%29+%5BTREATMENT%5D&rank=5

NCCAM. (2006b). *The efficacy of Reiki in the treatment of fibromyalgia.* Study begun: January 9, 2003; last updated: August 16, 2006. ClinicalTroals.gov Identifier: NCT00051428. Retrieved February 28, 2009, from http://clinicaltrials.gov/ct2/show/NCT00051428?term=%28NCCAM%29+%5BSPONSOR%5D+%28reiki%29+%5BTREATMENT%5D&rank=3

NCCAM. (2006c). *The use of Reiki for patients with aqdvanced AIDS.* Study begun: March 29, 2002; last updated: August 17, 2006. ClinicalTroals.gov Identifier: NCT00032721. Retrieved February 28, 2009, from http://clinicaltrials.gov/ct2/show/NCT00032721?term=%28NCCAM%29+%5BSPONSOR%5D+%28reiki%29+%5BTREATMENT%5D&rank=2

NCCAM. (2007, February). *What is CAM?* Retrieved February 28, 2009, from http:// nccam.nih.gov/health/whatiscam/overview.htm#types

NCCAM. (2008). *Effects of Reiki on stress.* Study begun: June 29, 2006; last updated: October 7, 2008. ClinicalTroals.gov Identifier: NCT00346671. Retrieved February 28, 2009, from http://clinicaltrials.gov/ct2/show/NCT00346671?term=%28NCCAM %29+% 5BSPONSOR%5D+%28reiki%29+%5BTREATMENT%5D&rank=1

NCCAM. (2009). Study begun: July 18, 2003; last updated: February 9, 2009. ClinicalTroals.gov Identifier: NCT00065208. Retrieved February 28, 2009, from http:// clinicaltrials.gov/ct2/show/NCT00065208?term=%28NCCAM%29+% 5BSPONSOR%5D+%28reiki%29+%5BTREATMENT%5D&rank=4

Nield-Anderson, L., & Ameling, A. (2000). The empowering nature of Reiki as a complementary therapy. *Holistic Nursing Practice, 14*(3), 21–29.

Olson, K., Hanson, J., & Michaud, M. (2003). A Phase II trial of reiki for the management of pain in advanced cancer patients. *Journal of Pain and Symptom Management, 26*(5), 990–997.

Oschman, J. (2002). Clinical aspects of biological fields: An introduction for health care professionals. *Journal of Bodywork and Movement Therapies, 6*(2), 117–125.

Papantonio, C. (1998). Alternative medicine and wound healing. *Ostomy/Wound Management, 44*(4), 44–55.

Petter, F. (1999). *The original Reiki handbook of Dr. Mikao Usui.* Twin Lakes, WI: Lotus Press.

Pierce, B. (2007). The use of biofield therapies in cancer care. *Clinical Journal of Oncology Nursing, 11*(2), 253–258, 269–273.

Pocotte, S., & Salvador, D. (2008). Reiki as a rehabilitative nursing intervention for pain management: A case study. *Rehabilitation Nursing, 33*(6), 231–232.

Potter, P. (2003). What are the distinctions between Reiki and therapeutic touch? *Clinical Journal of Oncology Nursing, 7*(1), 89–91.

Potter, P. (2007). Breast biopsy and distress: Feasibility of testing a Reiki intervention. *Journal of Holistic Nursing, 25,* 238–248.

Raingruber, B., & Robinson, C. (2007). The effectiveness of Tai Chi, Yoga, meditation, and Reiki healing sessions in promoting problem solving abilities of registered nurses. *Issues in Mental Health Nursing, 28,* 1141–1155.

Rand, W. (2000). *Reiki, the healing touch: First and second degree manual.* Southfield, MI: Vision Publications.

Robb, W. (2006). *The lived experience of registered nurse Reiki practitioners: A phenomenologic study using computer mediated communication.* Doctoral dissertation, Widener University.

Sawyer, J. (1998). The first Reiki practitioner in our OR. *AORN Journal, 67*(3), 674–676.

Schiller, R. (2003). Reiki: A starting point for integrative medicine. *Alternative Therapies in Health and Medicine, 9*(2), 20–21.

Schmehr, R. (2003). Enhancing the treatment of HIV/AIDS with Reiki training and treatment. *Alternative Therapies, 9*(2), 120–121.

Sem, T. (2009). Shamanic healing rituals. *Messages from the Museum Directors, Illinois State Museum.* Retrieved March 12, 2009, from http://www.museum.state.il.us/exhib its/changing/journey/healing.html

Shamanic healing. (2009). *Earth Shamans*. Retrieved March 12, 2009, from http://www.geocities.com/athens/troy/7922?SHAMANHEALER.html?200911

Shore, A.G. (2004). Long-term effects of energetic healing on symptoms of psychological depression and self-perceived stress. *Alternative Therapies, 10*(3), 42–48.

Silva, T. (2002). Treating Alzheimer's disease with Reiki. *Reiki News Magazine, 1*(2), 37–39.

So, P., Jiange, Y., & Qin, Y. (2008). Touch therapies for pain relief in adults. *Cochrane Database of Systematic Reviews*, Issue 3.

Thomas, T. (2005). Reiki adds a new dimension to the term "quality of life" in the nursing home community. *American Journal of Recreation Therapy*, 43–48.

Tsang, K. L., Carlson, L. E., & Olson, K. (2007). Pilot crossover of Reiki versus rest for treating cancer-related fatigue. *Integrative Cancer Therapies, 6*(1), 25–35.

Vanderbilt, S. (2004). Somatic research: Moving energy forward in the scientific realm. *Massage and Bodywork, 19*(1), 136–139.

Vitale, A. (2006). The use of selected energy touch modalities as supportive nursing interventions: Are we there yet? *Holistic Nursing Practice, 20*(4), 191–196.

Vitale, A. T. (2007). An integrative review of Reiki touch therapy research. *Holistic Nursing Practice, 21*(4), 167–179.

Vitale, A. T. & O'Connor, P. C. (2006). The effect of Reiki on pain and anxiety in women with abdominal hysterectomies: A quasi-experimental pilot study. *Holistic Nursing Practice, 20*(6), 263–274.

Wardell, D., & Engebretson, J. (2001). Biological correlates of Reiki touch healing. *Journal of Advanced Nursing, 33*(4), 439–445.

Whelan, K. M., & Wishnia, G. S. (2003). Reiki therapy: The benefits to a nurse-Reiki practitioner. *Nursing Practice, 17*(4), 209–217.

Wirth, D. P., Brenlan, D. R., Levine, R. J., & Rodriguez, X, C. M. (1993). The effect of complementary healing therapy on postoperative pain after surgical removal of impacted third molar teeth. *Complementary and Alternative Medicine, 1*, 133–138.

Wirth, D. P., Chang, R. J., Eidelman, W. S., & Paxton, J. B. (1996). Hematological indicators of complementary healing intervention. *Complementary Therapies in Medicine, 4*, 4–20.

19 Acupressure

PAMELA WEISS-FARNAN

Touch has been central to the practice of nursing since its inception. This chapter will discuss a form of touch known in traditional Chinese medicine as acupressure and its application in nursing care. This method of treatment is common in many cultures. As Dossey, Keegan, and Guzzetta (2000) note, "[a]ll cultures have demonstrated that some form of rubbing, pressing, massaging or holding are [sic] natural manifestations of the desire to heal and care for one another" (p. 615). Acupressure is also integral to the practice of *shiatsu, tui na, tsubo*, and *jin si ju jitsyu*.

DEFINITIONS

Acupressure is defined by Gach (1990) as "an ancient healing art that uses the fingers to press certain points on the body to stimulate the body's self-curative abilities" (p. 3). To assist the reader, the following definitions are also provided:

- *Acupuncture*—"[a] procedure used in or adapted from Chinese medical practice in which specific body areas are pierced with fine needles for therapeutic purposes or to relieve pain or produce regional anesthesia" (Freedictionary, 2009).

- *Auriculotherapy*—"also called ear acupuncture, applies the principles of acupuncture to specific points on the ear" (Firsthealth, 2009).
- *Jin Shin Jyutsu*—"a non-massage form of shiatsu—using pressure points to 'harmonize' the flow of 'energy' through the body" (Heall, 2006).
- *Meridians*—"specific interconnected channels through which Qi circulates" (Answers.com, 2006).
- *Moxibustion*—"[t]he burning of moxa or other substances on the skin, to treat diseases or to produce analgesia" (Freedictionary, 2009).
- *Qi* (pronounced *chee*)—"[t]he vital force believed in Taoism and other Chinese thought to be inherent in all things. The unimpeded circulation of chi and a balance of its negative and positive forms in the body are held to be essential to good health in traditional Chinese medicine" (Freedictionary, 2009).
- *Shiatsu*—"A form of therapeutic massage in which pressure is applied with the thumb and palms to those areas of the body used in acupuncture. Also called acupressure" (Freedictionary, 2009).

TRADITIONAL CHINESE MEDICINE

Traditional Chinese medicine (TCM) is an ancient system of health developed more than 3,000 years ago in Asia. This system is based on the concept that *qi* flows throughout the body and that balance of *yin* and *yang* forces represents health and well-being. As Kaptchuk (1983) describes it:

> This system of care is based on ancient texts and is the result of a continuous process of critical thinking, as well as extensive clinical observation and testing. It represents a thorough formulation and reformulation of material by respected clinicians and theoreticians. It is also, however, rooted in the philosophy, logic and sensibility, and habits of a civilization entirely foreign to our own. It has therefore developed its own perception of the body and health and disease. (p. 2)

The focus of care within this system is to restore balance in the body. To do so, *yin* and *yang* must be balanced. *Yin* aspects are associated with cold, passivity, interiority, and decreases. *Yang* aspects are associated with warmth, activity, external forces, and increases. *Yin* and *yang* are always in relation to each other (Kaptchuk, 1983). According to this conceptualization, they are in continuous flux and there is always *yin* within *yang* and *yang* within *yin*.

Unschuld (1999) reflects that TCM theory is a mixture of beliefs that pathogenic influences from the outside combine with the lack of balance or harmony within the person and result in illness. TCM is also concerned with the concept of *qi*. *Qi* flows in the body through specific pathways identified as meridians or channels. If the *qi* is blocked or diminished, a person experiences pain or illness.

There are 12 bilateral meridians and 8 extra meridians. All meridians have an exterior and an interior pathway and are named according to the organ system. Located on the meridians are specific points. In the 12 major meridians, the points are bilateral and in the West are called acupuncture points. This nomenclature implies that the points are designated for needle insertion and does not fully reflect the TCM concept of the point.

Acupuncture points are also used for acupressure. The points do not have a corresponding anatomic structure but are described by their location relative to other anatomical landmarks. This contributes to the skepticism of many Western-trained scientists about their existence. In Chinese, the name of the point usually is descriptive of its function or location. Mistranslation over the years has often limited the substantial amount of anatomical basis for the nomenclature of points and the apparent knowledge of anatomy of Chinese scholars (Schnorrenberger, 1996).

There are 365 (Kaptchuk, 1983) to 700 (Jwing-Ming, 1992) major points on the meridians. Jwing-Ming stated that 108 could be stimulated using the fingers. In a traditionally formulated TCM treatment plan, whether the modality is needles or pressure, the points are combined to achieve maximum benefit for the patient. Rarely is only one point used. There are also points that should not be stimulated, especially during pregnancy, which are referred to as "forbidden points."

SCIENTIFIC BASIS

Western medicine is the dominant system of health care in the United States. It is characterized by hospitals; clinics; pharmaceutical resources;

and a workforce of physicians, nurses, specialized therapists, and various support service personnel. There are many differences between Western medicine and TCM, which become more evident as nurses seek to add TCM modalities to their practice. Western medicine emphasizes disease, causal agents, and treatments that are designed to control or destroy the cause of disease (Kaptchuk, 1983). Once a causal agent or mechanism is identified, treatment plans are developed that focus on the agent or mechanism as a consistent factor in all human manifestations of the disease. In Western journals, almost all studies using the modality of acupuncture and acupressure emphasize the specific effects of needling one point known to address a specific symptom. Medical researchers are eager to find the mechanism by which acupuncture alleviates the symptoms. Some of the mechanisms have been suggested in Western medical research (National Center for Complementary/Alternative Medicines [NCCAM], 2000; National Institutes of Health [NIH], 1997). The therapeutic effect that seems to be produced by stimulation of the points with needles or with pressure may be due to the following:

Conduction of electromagnetic signals that may start the flow of pain-killing biochemicals, such as endorphins, and of immune system cells to specific sites in the body that are injured or vulnerable to disease (Dale, 1997; Takeshige, 1989).

Activation of opioid systems, which also reduces pain (Han, 1997).

Changes in brain chemistry, sensation, and involuntary responses by changing the release of neurotransmitters and neurohormones in a health-promoting way (Wu, 1995; Wu, Zhou, & Zhou, 1994).

The scientific research into an underlying mechanism demonstrates one of the differences between Western medicine and the TCM system. The focus in TCM is the imbalance in the patient, and the causality is always multifactorial. The function of the points is described in terms of TCM diagnosis. For example, Western medicine research has focused on pericardium 6, or *nei guan*, for the treatment of nausea. In English its name means "inner border gate." Lade (1986) describes the point:

The name refers to the point's role as the gateway or connecting point of the triple burner channel and the yin-linking vessel. Inner refers to the palmar aspect of the forearm and to the point's location on the yin channel. The actions of this point are: to regulate and tonify the heart, transform heart phlegm, facilitate qi flow, regulate the yin-linking vessel and clear heart fire, redirect rebellious qi downward, expand and relax the chest and benefit the diaphragm. The indications for use of the point are: asthma, bronchitis, pertussis, hiccups, vomiting, diaphragmatic spasms, intercostal neuralgia, chest fullness, and pain and dyspnea. (pp. 196, 197)

Whereas Western medicine focuses on the treatment of nausea for this point, the TCM paradigm suggests multiple uses. In TCM theory, nausea is considered rebellious *qi* (*qi* that flows in the wrong direction). Nausea and vomiting are examples of this. *Nei guan* (pericardium 6) is used as one of the points in the treatment of a patient who presents with nausea. In TCM theory, nausea is considered one of the external manifestations of the imbalance, but in an authentic TCM treatment, a practitioner would evaluate the imbalances that set up the manifestation and treat the underlying condition. Therefore, a combination of points to treat nausea would be used, possibly including other primary points for antiemesis (Hoo, 1997): Stomach 36 on the stomach meridian located on the knee, Ren 12 on the ren/conception meridian located on the upper abdomen, or the Spleen 4 on the spleen meridian located on the foot. Application of multiple acupoints may be more effective for the treatment of nausea; however, in Western medicine, the focus on finding the single active point or the mechanism creates an almost insurmountable challenge to the fullest application of the therapy.

In 1997, the National Institutes of Health held the first consensus conference on acupuncture. The conference concluded that:

Acupuncture is effective in the treatment of adult nausea and vomiting in chemotherapy and probably pregnancy and in postoperative dental pain. The conference members stated there is an indication that acupuncture may be helpful in the treatment of addiction, stroke rehabilitation, headache, menstrual cramps, tennis elbow, fibromyalgia, myofascial pain, osteoarthritis, low back pain, carpal tunnel syndrome, and asthma, in which acupuncture may be useful as an adjunct treatment or an acceptable alternative or be included in a comprehensive management program. (NIH, 1997)

Research evidence underlying the use of the point called *nei guan* (pericardium 6) for nausea is reviewed in the text that follows. This

NIH statement was the springboard for increasing the number of studies completed for the treatment of nausea and vomiting that include the use of devices to apply pressure or stimulation to pericardium 6. These devices included an elastic bracelet with a pressure button called Sea-Bands® or an electrical stimulation device called a Reliefband®.

In recent years, the research focusing on the effectiveness of pericardium 6 for the treatment of nausea and vomiting have increased. Table 19.1 demonstrates that studies continue to find conflicting results about the effectiveness of using pericardium 6 for the treatment of nausea and vomiting from any condition. However, in addition to the research focusing on these symptoms, several studies have been completed showing the efficacy of using Pericardium 6 for many conditions. Although, again, the studies are limited in size, generally the outcomes are highly suggestive of the effectiveness of acupressure on Pericardium 6.

Table 19.2 presents a brief overview of recent studies examining the use of acupressure in a variety of patients. The conditions treated include wandering in Alzheimer's disease, dyspnea, sleep in elderly patients, pain of labor, dysmenorrhea, and stress of patients transported by emergency vehicles. Many of the studies are done outside of the United States, where the cultural barriers about the use of this ancient type of medicine are lower because the use of acupressure is an accepted part of the cultural health practices.

Pediatric patients have not been studied extensively using acupuncture as an intervention, but, in the framework of TCM, children are considered sensitive to any type of energy and may enjoy the same benefits that are found in adult populations.

The number of studies continues to increase, and yet scarce funding has yielded studies with small sample sizes, thus limiting their generalizability. However, these limited studies do provide the incentive for nurses to consider incorporating acupressure techniques into their practices, as it is a noninvasive treatment that may have an impact on patient outcomes.

INTERVENTION

A diagnostic process is used to choose the correct points to stimulate. In TCM, the process includes an extensive history, observing the patient's appearance and demeanor, noticing the patient's odor, checking the

Table 19.1

SAMPLE OF STUDIES USING P6 FOR NAUSEA

NAUSEA	MODALITY	AUTHOR/DATE	CONCLUSION
Nausea of chemotherapy	Acupressure on P6 and Stomach 36	Dibble, Chapman Mack, & Shih (2000)	During the first 10 days of the chemotherapy cycle, women with breast cancer who were taught and practiced acupressure of P6 experienced a decreased intensity and frequency of nausea.
Nausea of chemotherapy	Acupressure	Klein & Griffiths (2004)	Acupressure may decrease nausea among patients undergoing chemotherapy, but further study is required.
Nausea of chemotherapy	Acupressure	Shin, Kim, Shin, & Juan (2004)	Acupressure on P6 point appears to be an effective adjunct treatment.
Nausea of chemotherapy	Acupressure	Lee, Dodd, Dibble, & Abrams (2008)	A review of ten acupressure studies concluded that acupressure should be strongly recommended as an effective intervention when supported by further studies.
Nausea of chemotherapy	Acupressure	Collins & Thomas (2004)	Acupressure in addition to antiemetics provides better control of the nausea of chemotherapy.
Nausea of chemotherapy	Use of acupressure wrist bands	Molassiotis, Helen, Dabbour, & Hummerston (2007)	Nausea and retching experience and nausea and vomiting/retching events were reduced at statistically significant level.
Nausea of pregnancy	Acupressure and acu-stimulation bands	Roscoe et al. (2003)	This review article concludes that stimulation of the point is positive, but many of the studies have limitations that leave questions about effectiveness.
Nausea of early pregnancy	Compared pressure on P6 to a sham point	Werntoft & Dykes (2001)	The treatment group had a significant reduction of nausea.

(continued)

Table 19.1 *(continued)*

NAUSEA	MODALITY	AUTHOR/DATE	CONCLUSION
Nausea of HIV/ AIDS	Acupressure	Capili (2002)	Symptoms of nausea were decreased; however, reports of the quality of life did not improve.
Postoperative nausea and vomiting	Acupressure	Ming, Kuo, Lin, & Lin (2002)	In view of the absence of side effects, acupressure is a safe alternative to treatment of nausea and vomiting.
Postoperative vomiting in children after strabismus surgery	Use of Korean hand acupuncture pressure on the P6 point on the hand 30 minutes before induction anesthesia	Schlager, Boehler, & Puhringer (2000)	Vomiting was significantly reduced.
Postoperative nausea and vomiting after gyneconlogy surgery	Group that received acupressure on Pericardium 6 point compared to group who received sham and no treatment	Alkaissi, Evertson, Johnsson, Ofenbartl, & Kalman (2002)	P6 is a method to reduce emesis during gynecological surgery.
Nausea and vomiting with myocardial infarction	Acupressure using continuous pressure (wrist bands)	Dent (2003)	Continuous pressure on P6 reduced need for antiemetic meds and is feasible and well tolerated by patients.

tongue, palpating the abdomen and points on the body, and palpating the pulses at the radial location on the wrists. A diagnosis is formulated and a treatment plan, which may use a variety of techniques, is implemented. Nurses will not follow this process and will therefore be using a Western, symptom-based system of determining the correct treatment plan.

Guidelines for Use

Nurses can incorporate acupressure into the care of patients by using some common points that have specific actions to relieve common

Table 19.2

SAMPLE OF STUDIES OF EFFECTIVE USES OF ACUPUNCTURE/ ACUPRESSURE

CONDITION	MODALITY	AUTHOR/DATE	CONCLUSION
Wandering behaviors in Alzheimer's disease	Foot acupressure	Sutherland, Reakes, & Bridges (1999)	Foot acupressure may produce a decrease in wandering and an increase in quiet time.
Agitated behaviors in dementia	Used five acupoints based on the effect of reducing agitation	Yang, Wu, Lin, & Lin (2007)	On all measures, agitation behaviors were reduced and the authors recommend acupressure as a noninvasive effective therapy.
Dyspnea of COPD	Acupressure	Wu, Wu, Lin, & Lin (2004)	Pulmonary function, dyspnea scores, and other physiological measures were improved with the use of acupressure of appropriate points.
Quality of life of patients with obstructive asthma	Eight weeks of self administered acupressure with standard care	Maa et al. (2003)	Patients experience improved qualify of life when acupressure supplements standard care.
Sleep of elderly	Magnetic auricular beads	Suen, Wong, & Leung (2002)	Three-week treatment of placing magnetic beads in the ear significantly increased sleep time in the elderly.
Dysmenorrhea	Relief Brief® (a brief that puts pressure on acupuncture points)	Taylor, Miaskowski, & Kohn (2002)	Wearing of the acupressure brief relieved pain symptoms and reduced the need for medication in subjects.
Low-back pain	Acupressure	Hsieh, Kuo, Yen, & Chen (2004)	Acupressure is another effective alternative medicine for reducing low back pain. However, careful assessment should be made in future studies.

(continued)

Table 19.2 *(continued)*

CONDITION	MODALITY	AUTHOR/DATE	CONCLUSION
Primary dysmenorrhoea	Acupressure at Spleen 6	Chen & Chen (2004)	Acupressure reduced both pain and anxiety typical of dysmenorrhoea.
Pain of labor	Ice massage at the Large Intestine 4 (LI 4) point	Waters & Raisler (2003)	Ice massage assisted women in reducing their pain perception on a scale from distressing to uncomfortable.
Pain of labor	Acupressure using Large Intestine 4 (LI 4) and Bladder 67 (BL 67) points	Chung, Hung, Kuo, & Huang (2003)	Acupressure reduced the pain of labor while not diminishing the quality of contractions in first stage labor.
Pain and duration of labor	Use of Spleen 6 with continuous pressure	Lee, Change, & Kange (2004)	Pain and duration of labor were reduced in the treatment group.
Stress experienced during transport in EMS vehicle	Auricular acupressure	Kober et al. (2003)	Auricular acupressure reduced anxiety, decreased pain, and resulted in more positive attitudes about potential outcomes.
Alertness of students in the classroom	Acupressure was self-administered by the subject to improve alertness.	Harris et al. (2005)	Evidence suggests that there is an effect on Sleepiness Scale indicating efficacy.
Preoperative parental anxiety	Acupressure at *yintang* point compared to a sham point.	Wang, Gaal, Maranets, Caldwell-Andrews, & Kain, 2005	Parents in the treatment group reported significantly less anxiety at 20 minutes postinterventions.
Fatigue in patients with end stage renal disease.	Acupressure group had less fatigue and less depression than the treatment group.	Tsay (2003)	Treatment group reported reduction in fatigue in the postdialysis period.

symptoms. The nurse can treat the patient with acupressure or teach the patient or family members how to use acupressure as part of a care plan.

Prior to touching any patient, the nurse must assess the readiness of the client. Shames and Keegan recommend the following assessment of clients:

- Perception of mind–body situation
- Pathophysiological problems that may require referral
- History of psychological disorders
- Cultural beliefs about touch
- Previous experience with body therapies (2000, p. 264).

Each point is located using an anatomical marker. There are many books describing point location. The standard measure is the *cun*, which is different for each individual. One *cun* for a particular patient is defined as the "width of the interphalangeal joint of the patient's thumb" or as "the distance between the two radial ends of the flexor creases of a flexed middle finger of the patient. Two cun is the width of the index finger, the middle finger and the ring finger" (Hoo, 1997).

Stimulating the Point

There are several different types of techniques to stimulate the points, according to Gach:

- *Firm stationary pressure*—using the thumbs, fingers, palms, the sides of hands, or knuckles
- *Slow motion kneading*—using the thumbs and fingers along with the heels of the hands to squeeze large muscle groups
- *Brisk rubbing*—using friction to stimulate the blood and lymph
- *Quick tapping*—with the fingertips, to stimulate muscles on unprotected areas of the body such as the face (1990, p. 9).

Evaluating Acupressure's Effect

Gach has developed guidelines for assessing results. The elements of the assessment include:

- Identifying the problems being addressed with acupressure
- Identifying the points being used for the treatment
- The length of time for the acupressure
- Identifying what makes the condition worse (e.g., standing, cold weather, menstruation, constipation, lack of exercise, stress, traveling, and other variables)
- Describing the changes experienced by the patient after 3 days and after 1 week of treatment
- Describing the changes in the condition and overall feeling of well-being (Gach, 1990, p. 13).

USES

There are many uses for acupressure. Some conditions for which it has been used are shown in Table 19.2. The use of acupuncture for nausea, pain, and gastrointestinal disorders is described below.

Nausea

Point: Pericardium 6 (nei guan, "Inner Gate")

Location: Pericardium 6 is located on the inner aspect of the wrist 2 *cun* (units) proximal to the transvese crease of the wrist between the tendons of the palmaris longus and flexor carpi radialis muscles (Lade, 1986). Have the patient place the middle three fingers (index, middle, and ring fingers) on the opposite hand that is palm upward. The point under the ring finger between the two tendons is pericardium 6 (see Figure 19.1).

Functions: Its functions were outlined previously in the discussion on the research on this point.

Method of Stimulation: The point can be stimulated using firm pressure either with a rotating pattern with the thumb or the static pressure of a SeaBand®.

Indications in Nursing: This point can be used for the treatment of nausea in many situations, but research, as cited previously, has focused on postoperative nausea, the nausea of pregnancy, and the nausea accompanying chemotherapy.

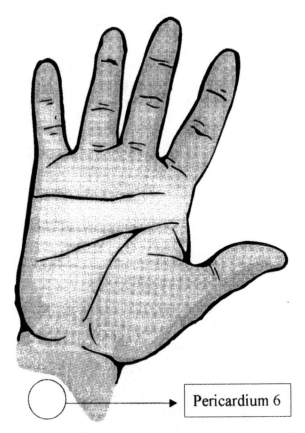

Pericardium 6

Figure 19.1 Pressure point pericardium 6. This point has multiple functions and is one of the most important points.

Pain and Gastrointestinal Disorders

Point: Large Intestine 4 (LI 4) (Hoku, "Joining the Valley")

Location: This point is on the back of the hand halfway between the junction of the first and second metacarpal bones, which form a depression or valley when the thumb is abducted (Lade, 1986). There are two ways to locate this point easily. Have the patient hold the hand with the thumb touching the index finger; hold the hand at eye level and the highest mound at the base of the thumb and index finger is the location of LI 4. Or instruct the patient to place the thumb of one hand in the web between the thumb and index finger of the opposite hand. The patient should match the first crease on the thumb of one hand to the web of the other and then rotate the thumb to touch the fleshy area between the index finger and thumb. The point is where the tip of the thumb touches the area between the thumb and the index finger.

Functions: This point has multiple functions and is one of the most important points of the body. It alleviates pain, tones *qi*, and generates protective *qi* (in Western medicine this would be considered an immune system–building function); moistens the large intestine and in so doing relieves diarrhea or constipation; clears the nose; regulates the lungs in asthma, bronchitis, or the common cold; and expedites labor. This point is contraindicated in pregnancy because of the latter function (Lade, 1986, pp. 40–41).

Method of Stimulation: Firm pressure can be applied on this point with a rotating thumb massage technique. This point is often sensitive and the patient will report a feeling of discomfort. This is normal and not indicative of a problem.

Indications in Nursing: This point will relieve any pain in the body. In addition, persons with diarrhea or constipation may feel relief because stimulating the point balances the gastrointestinal functions. This point can be used to induce labor and, coupled with its pain-relieving effect, may be helpful.

Precautions

There are overall guidelines and precautions carefully outlined by Michael Reed Gach (1990) in his book, *Acupressure Potent Points*:

- Never press any area in an abrupt, forceful, or jarring way. Apply finger pressure in a slow, rhythmic manner to enable layers of tissues and the internal organs to respond (p. 11).
- Use abdominal points cautiously, especially if the patient is ill. Avoid the abdominal area altogether if the patient has a life-threatening disease, especially intestinal cancer, tuberculosis, or

leukemia. Avoid the abdominal area during pregnancy (pp. 11–12).

■ During pregnancy, strong stimulation of certain points should be avoided: LI 4 (fourth point on the large intestine meridian), K 3 (third point on the kidney meridian), and SP 6 (sixth point on the spleen meridian). Each of these points may have an effect on the pregnancy (p. 192).

■ Lymph areas such as the groin, the area of the throat just below the ears, and the outer breast near the armpits are very sensitive. Touch these areas lightly (p. 12).

■ Do not work directly on a serious burn, ulcer, or area of infection.

■ Do not work directly on a newly formed scar. New surgical or other wounds should not be touched directly. Continuous holding on the periphery of the injury will stimulate the injury to heal (p. 12).

■ After an acupressure treatment, tolerance to cold is lowered and the energy of the body is focused on healing, so advise the patient to wear warm clothes and keep out of drafts (p. 12).

■ Use acupressure cautiously in persons with a new acute or serious illness (p. 12).

■ Acupressure is not a sole treatment for cancer, contagious skin disease, or sexually transmitted disease (pp. 11–12).

■ Brisk rubbing, deep pressure, or kneading should not be used for persons with heart disease, cancer, or high blood pressure (Gach, 1990, p. 9).

CULTURAL CONSIDERATIONS

Nurses work with patients from differing cultural backgrounds. Multiple cultures throughout the world use manual therapies to either promote or maintain health or to treat illness. Although the therapies are part of the indigenous healing methods used by different groups of people, currently they are classified as complementary and alternative medicine (CAM) in the United States (Wing, 1998). However, within many cultures, individuals and families treat manual therapies as mainstream and integral to their health practices.

Folk and indigenous healing practices are common not only for the people of Asian origin (Chinese, Thai, Cambodian, Vietnamese, and Japanese), but also almost every other culture. The practices include massage: pressure, rubbing, stretching and pulling the skin, with and without herbal preparations, oils, or poultices. For example, many indigenous practices are focused on preparing for childbirth. To illustrate, in Oaxaca (a Mexican state), a practice called *sobada* massage is used as a diagnostic tool for gestational age, and to relieve the aches and pain of pregnancy and delivery, and then stimulating the baby immediately after birth. In India, infant massage with various oils is a regular practice and recent research has confirmed that massage with coconut oil enhances the baby's weight gain. (Sankaranarayanan et al., 2005).

Although Western-trained nurses may not understand how different cultural groups incorporate skin massage and rubbing and may misinterpret what they may observe, it is important for the nurse to allow the family to express the types of practices they use as part of their routine caring for each other and their children (Davis, 2000). Struthers (2008) emphasizes there is a "need for nurses and other health care providers to become knowledgeable regarding traditional indigenous health that their clients may be receiving—to foster open communication" (p.74). What the practices are called will vary from one cultural group to another, but each uses skin stimulation as part of health routines and family bonding.

FUTURE RESEARCH

There are many areas of research in which the methods of traditional Chinese medicine and the underlying theory can be tested using Western medical research techniques. Research questions about the usefulness of acupressure techniques can be posed in many areas of nursing, including their use for palliative care, rehabilitation nursing, support of women in labor, and health promotion and disease prevention. Gach (2004) has expanded his self-care manuals to include trauma, stress, and common emotional imbalances.

Acupressure is used by millions of persons around the world. Incorporating this technique into nursing care plans will unite us in the commonality we share—the desire to relieve human suffering (Serizawa, 1976).

Klein, J., & Griffiths, P. (2004). Acupressure for nausea and vomiting in cancer patients receiving chemotherapy. *British Journal of Community Nursing, 9*(9), 383–386, 388.

Kober, A., Scheck, T., Schubert, B., Strasser, H., Gustorff, B., Bertalanffy, P., et al. (2003). Auricular acupressure as a treatment for anxiety in prehospital transport settings. *Anesthesiology, 98*(6), 1328–1332.

Lade, A. (1986). *Images and functions.* Seattle, WA: Eastland.

Lee, J., Dodd, M., Dibble, S., & Abrams, D. (2008). Review of acupressure studies for chemotherapy-induced nausea and vomiting. *Journal of Pain and Symptom Management, 36*(5), 529–544.

Lee, M. K., Chang, S. B., & Kange, D. H. (2004). Effects of P6 on labor pain and length of delivery time in women during labor. *Journal of Alternative and Complementary Medicine, 10*(6), 959–965.

Maa, S. H., Sun, M. F., Hsu, K. H., Hung, T. J., Chen, H. C., Yu, C. T., et al. (2003). Effect of acupuncture or acupressure on qualify of life patients with chronic obstructive asthma: a pilot study. *Journal of Alternative and Complementary Medicine, 9*(5), 659–670.

Ming, J., Kuo, B. I., Lin, J., & Lin, L. (2002). The efficacy of acupressure to prevent nausea and vomiting in post-operative patients. *Journal of Advanced Nursing, 39*(4), 343–351.

Molassiotis, A., Helen, A. B., Dabbour, R., & Hummerston, S. (2007). The effects of P6 acupressure in the prophylaxis of chemotherapy-related nausea and vomiting in breast cancer. *Complementary Therapies in Medicine, 15*(1), 3–12.

National Center for Complementary/Alternative Medicines. (2000). *Acupuncture information and resources.* Retrieved July 31, 2009, from http://nccam.nih.gov/health/acupuncture/

National Institutes of Health. (1997). *NIH Consensus Development Conference Statement. Acupuncture.* Retrieved April 30, 2004, from http://consensus.nih.gov/1997/1997Acupuncture107html.htm

Roscoe, J. A., Morrow, G. R., Hickok, J. T., Bushunow, P., Pierce, H. I., Flynn, P. J., et al. (2003). The efficacy of acupressure and acustimulation wrist bands for the relief of chemotherapy-induced nausea and vomiting: A University of Rochester Cancer Center Community Clinical Oncology Program multicenter study. *Journal of Pain and Symptom Management, 26*(2), 731–742.

Sankaranarayanan, K., Mondkar, J. A., Chauhan, M. M., Mascarenhas, B. M., Mainkar, A. R., & Salvi, R. Y. (2005). Oil massage in neonates: An open randomized controlled study of coconut versus mineral oil. *Indian Pediatric, 42*(9), 877–84.

Schlager, A., Boehler, M., & Puhringer, F. (2000). Korean hand acupressure reduced postoperative vomiting in children after strabismus surgery. *British Journal of Anaesthesia, 85*(2), 267–70.

Schnorrenberger, C. C. (1996). Morphological foundations of acupuncture: An anatomical nomenclature of acupuncture structures. *Acupuncture in Medicine, 14*(2), 89–103.

Serizawa, K. (1976). *Tsubo.* Tokyo: Japan Publications.

Shames, K. H., & Keegan, L. (2000). Touch: Connecting with the healing power in 2000. In B. Dossey, L. Keegan, & C. E. Guzzetta (Eds.), *Holistic nursing* (3rd ed., pp. 613–635). Gaithersberg, MD: Aspen.

Shin, Y. H., Kim, T. I., Shin, M. S., & Juan, H. (2004). Effect of acupressure on nausea and vomiting during chemotherapy cycle for Korean postoperative stomach cancer patients. *Cancer Nursing, 27*(4), 267–274.

Struthers, R. (2008). The experience of being an Anishinabe man healer: Ancient healing in the modern world. *Journal of Cultural Diversity, 15*(2). 70–75.

Suen, L. K., Wong, T. K., & Leung, A. W. (2002). Effectiveness of auricular therapy on sleep promotion in the elderly. *American Journal of Chinese Medicine, 30*(4), 429–449.

Sutherland, J. A., Reakes, J., & Bridges, C. (1999). Foot acupressure and massage for patients with Alzheimer's disease and related dementias. *Image: The Journal of Nursing Scholarship, 31*(4), 347–348.

Takeshige, C. (1989). *Mechanism of acupuncture analgesia based on animal experiments: Scientific bases of acupuncture.* Berlin: Springer-Verlag.

Taylor, D., Miaskowski, C., & Kohn, J. (2002). A randomized clinical trial of the effectiveness of an acupressure device (Relief Brief) for managing symptoms of dysmenorrhea. *Journal of Alternative and Complementary Medicine, 8*(3), 357–370.

Tsay, S. (2004). Acupressure and fatigue in patients with end-stage renal disease—A randomized controlled trial. *International Journal of Nursing Studies, 41*(1), 99–106.

Unschuld, P. (1999). The past 1,000 years of Chinese medicine. *Lancet, 354*(Suppl.), SIV9.

Waters, B. L., & Raisler, J. (2003). Ice massage for the reduction of labor pain. *Journal of Midwifery & Women's Health, 48*(5), 317–321.

Wang, S. M., Gaal, D., Maranets, I., Caldwell-Andrews, A., & Kain, Z. N. (2005). Acupressure and preoperative parental anxiety: A pilot study. *Anesthesia Analgesia, 101*, 666–669.

Werntoft, E., & Dykes, A. K. (2001). Effect of acupressure on nausea and vomiting during pregnancy. A randomized, placebo controlled study. *Journal of Reproductive Medicine, 46*(9), 835–839.

Wing, D. M. (1998). A comparison of traditional folk healing concepts with contemporary healing concepts. *Journal of Community Health Nursing, 15*(3), 143–154.

Wu, B. (1995). Effect of acupuncture on the regulation of cell-mediated immunity in patients with malignant tumors. *Chen Tzu Yen Chiu Acupuncture Research, 20*(3), 67–71.

Wu, B., Zhou, R. X., & Zhou, M. S. (1994). Effect of acupuncture on interleukin-2 level and NK cell immunoactivity of peripheral blood of malignant tumor patients. *Chung Kuo Chung Hsi I Chieh Ho Tsa Chich, 14*(9), 537–539.

Wu, H., Wu, S., Lin, J., & Lin, L. (2004). Effectiveness of acupressure in improving dyspnoea in chronic obstructive pulmonary disease. *Journal of Advanced Nursing, 45*(3), 252–259.

Yang, M. H., Wu, S. C., Lin, J. G., & Lin, L. C. (2007). The efficacy of acupressure for decreasing agitated behaviour in dementia: A pilot study. *Journal of Clinical Nursing, 16*, 308–315.

20 Reflexology

THORA JENNY GUNNARSDOTTIR

Reflexology, although ancient, is one of a number of complementary therapies that has gained popularity in recent years. In reflexology, the whole body has been mapped out in the hands and in the feet and can be manipulated directly using specific massage techniques. The corresponding areas on the feet are easier to locate because they cover a larger area and are more specific, rendering them easier to work on than the hands. Therefore reflexology of the feet will be the main focus of this chapter. Reflexology shares the philosophical base of holism congruent with nursing. As such, it provides the nurse an opportunity to show caring and presence with the aim of helping the patient to become more whole in a fragmented health care system. This gentle intervention has been shown to affect symptoms, but the scientific basis behind reflexology needs to be further established.

DEFINITION

Reflexology is defined as a holistic healing technique aimed at treating the individual as an entity, incorporating the body, mind, and spirit. It is a specific pressure technique that works on precise reflex points of the feet that correspond to other body parts as depicted in Figure 20.1. Because the feet represent a microcosm of the body, all organs,

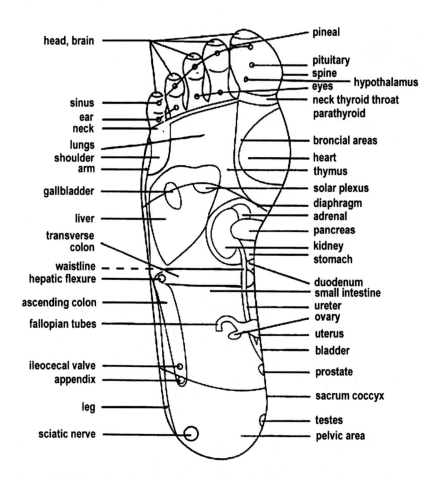

Figure 20.1 Relationship of body parts with reflexology points on the foot (Retrieved May 25, 2005, from http://www.ivy-rose.co.uk)

glands, and other body parts are laid out in a similar arrangement on the feet (Dougans, 1999). Different definitions have been put forth, but they all express the basic principle behind reflexology, which is that the soles of the feet and the palms of the hands are connected to all parts of the human body, including its internal organs, and that by applying specific pressure techniques to the soles of the feet, healing effects can be wrought over the entire body.

The International Institute of Reflexology defines reflexology as a manual technique based on the theory that there are reflex areas in the feet and hands that correspond to all glands, organs, and all body parts as laid out in Figure 20.1 (Byers, 1983). Kunz and Kunz (2003) state that the pressure techniques stimulate specific reflex areas on the feet and hands with the intention of invoking a beneficial response in other parts of the body. Vennells (2001) uses the word "reflex" to mean a stimulus or reaction in the form of an increase, decrease, or rebalance of a particular physical, mental, or emotional function in the body. The literature also suggests that reflexology is useful for achieving and maintaining health, enhancing well-being, relieving the symptoms of illness and disease (Tiran, 2002), aiding relaxation, and triggering the body's own innate self-healing (Lett, 2000).

Other various definitions of reflexology have been offered, but they all convey the basic principle behind reflexology, which is that the extremities are connected to all other parts and internal organs of the human body, and that there is a relationship between organs, systems, and processes. By using specific pressure techniques on the foot or hand, healing the whole body is possible. The left foot/hand represents the left side of the body and the right foot/hand represents the right side of the body. Numerous schools of reflexology have been established throughout the world.

SCIENTIFIC BASIS

The foundations of reflexology can be traced to two different theories or schools of thought documented in the reflexology literature. The first theory originated in traditional Chinese medicine (TCM) and the second one in a Western technique known as *zone therapy*.

Traditional Chinese Medicine

The Chinese first began using reflexology roughly 5,000 years ago; however, its reputation has since declined. Its decline is believed to have been due to a rise in the popularity of acupuncture, which emerged from similar roots (Kunz & Kunz, 2003). Reflexology is thought to be Eastern in origin (Dougans, 1999), and it is congruent with the principle of organ representation from TCM: *the whole represents itself in the parts* (Kaptchuk, 2000). This statement means that the feet are seen as a microcosm of the body, as a kind of holographic image in which all organs, glands, and other body parts are mirrored on the soles of the feet. The idea that the whole body can be represented in its parts is not new. For example, tongue diagnosis has been documented in China for at least 2000 years. It is also evident in the iris of the eye, the face, and the ear (Omura, 1994).

TCM posits that there are a number of invisible energy pathways, or meridians, within the body, that carry an energy called *Qi*, which is the vital energy behind all processes. All organs are interconnected with each other by a meridian network system and, to maintain health, energy needs to be flowing in balance. Factors impeding the free circulation of *Qi* are divided into categories of "excess" and "deficiency." Excess refers to the presence of something that is "too much" for the individual to handle—too much food to digest, too much waste to eliminate, and so forth. Deficiency refers to the absence or relative insufficiency of one or more aspects of the life energies necessary for sustaining health and well-being. A deficiency or excess of life energy can allow outside factors to overwhelm the individual, thus inducing pathology, and leading to pain and illness (Ehling, 2001; Kaptchuk, 2000).

In a healthy person with energy in balance, the feet feel soft when palpated and should have the same texture in every area. When an area is felt to be "empty" or is lacking in texture when palpated, it is an indication of deficiency in the energy of that particular organ or area in the body. If an area feels stiff and hard in texture when palpated, it indicates an excess of energy. If a lack of energy is found in one area that means that some other area has too much energy, because the energy must be in balance. On empty areas, it is necessary to slowly build aggressive pressure to increase the energy flow, and more vigorous, light but firm pressure is applied on the area that has too much energy to direct the flow out and away from this area. In that way, reflexology redirects excess energy from one area into another where there is an apparent deficiency, so as to supplement a deficiency or to "sedate" an excess pattern. This process guides the client back to balancing the whole.

Zone Therapy

The second theory, often referred to as zone therapy, originated in the West. At the beginning of the twentieth century, Dr. William Fitzgerald found that pressure applied to some parts of the feet induced anesthesia in specific parts of a client's body. He than determined that the entire body and all its organs were "laid out" in a certain configuration on the soles of the feet. He divided the body into ten longitudinal zones, running from the top of the head to the toes, and proposed that parts of the body within a certain zone were linked with one another; hence the name "zone" therapy.

An American therapist, Eunice Ingham, is credited with establishing reflexology in its present form. She used the zones as a guiding map, but began to chart the feet according to where pressure would produce distinct effects in the body. She developed a map of the entire body on the feet and called the areas "reflexes." Her proposition was that when the bloodstream becomes blocked with waste materials or excess acid, calcium deposits start to form in the nerve endings, impeding the normal circulation of the blood and creating an imbalance in the various parts of the body, depending on where the blockage is. She believed that by using the specific pressure of reflexology, the calcium deposits on the feet can be detected as "gritty areas," which may feel painful when touched. Ingham describes these as "particles of frost" or "crystal blocks" when examined under a microscope. The pressure and massage techniques taught in reflexology are designed to dissipate these formations and break down their crystalline structures. By doing so, the corresponding area connected with this particular nerve ending will receive an added supply of blood. In this way, the circulatory and lymphatic systems are stimulated, thus encouraging the release and removal of toxins, and the body starts to heal itself (Ingham, 1984). Other theories have been considered in the literature, but will not be detailed in this chapter.

None of these theories has been directly proven, which may partially explain why there is not universal agreement on how to classify reflexology. The National Center for Complementary and Alternative Medicine classifies reflexology as a manipulative and body-based method (NCCAM, 2008). However, many reflexologists see reflexology as energy therapy (Dougans, 1999; Vennells, 2001).

INTERVENTION

The patient will be lying comfortably, covered in a blanket, somewhat higher than the chair in which the reflexologist sits, and will have pillows under the knees and the head to induce relaxation. In addition, the patient will be barefoot and in a comfortable position, with any tight clothes loosened so as to not hinder circulation. Then the patient will be assessed continuously for tolerance of the amount of pressure applied. The pressure needs to be firm enough to activate the body's healing potentials, but must also be tolerable to the patient. Sensitivity varies in each individual, and the feet usually become more sensitive with subsequent treatments. Each area is worked, finishing the toe area on the one foot and then treating the toe area on the other, and so on, going from one foot to the other.

Although it is emphasized that reflexology is to be applied to the feet as a whole, it is important to work specifically on several systems of the body. These specific systems are, for example: the digestive system to increase proper elimination, the lymphatic system, to increase the clearance of waste materials, the bladder and kidneys, to increase urine and energy flow (the kidneys are one source of *Qi*); the solar plexus (where feelings and emotions are stored), to increase relaxation; all internal glands, to stimulate their respective functions; and the lungs, to increase oxygen consumption. By using reflexology on these body systems, the reflexologist is both increasing circulation and elimination and affecting the flow of *Qi*, because all organs are interconnected with each other by meridians.

Techniques

There are several techniques used, depending on what area of the feet is worked on. One hand is used to support the foot while the fingers and the thumb of the other are used to massage the skin. A period of 45 minutes to one hour is estimated to be enough time to perform the reflexology on both feet and will allow for extra time to work on specific areas that need further care. At the end of each session the client is encouraged to relax for several minutes. There are some standard pressure techniques for working on the reflexes of the feet. The two techniques described here are: *thumb walking* and *hook and back up* (Kunz & Kunz, 2003). Other grips are used depending on which area one is working on. It is important to not forget any area and to finish one area before starting the next one (see Exhibit 20.1).

Exhibit 20.1

Techniques

THUMB WALKING

The goal of the thumb-walking technique is to apply a constant, steady pressure to the surface of the foot or the hand:

1. With the other hand (holding hand) stretch the sole of the foot. Rest your working thumb on the sole and your fingers on the top of the foot. Drop your wrist to create leverage, which exerts pressure with the thumb.
2. Bend and unbend the thumb's first joint, moving it forward a little bit at a time. When your working hand feels stretched, reposition it and continue walking it forward. Take a little step forward with each unbend. The goal is to work with a small area in each step to create a feeling of constant, steady pressure. Always walk in a forward direction, not backward. Keep your thumb slightly cocked as you work to prevent overextending it.

HOOK AND BACK UP

The hook-and-back-up technique is used to work a specific point rather than to cover a large area. It is a relatively stationary technique, with only small movements of the working thumb involved. To avoid digging your fingernail into the flesh, apply pressure using more of the flat of the thumb:

1. Support and protect the area to be worked with holding hand. The hand wraps around the area while the thumb and fingers hold it in place. Place the fingers of the working hand over those of the holding hand.
2. Place the working thumb in the center of the area to be worked. Hook and back up, using the edge of the thumb.

Note: Adapted from Kunz and Kunz (2003).

Measurement of Outcomes

The philosophy behind reflexology states that it affects the body as whole, but, based on the literature (which will be discussed in detail later), more studies have measured physiological or psychological outcomes of reflexology than its overall effects. It is important to measure the effect of reflexology over a number of sessions to gain insight into its overall benefits.

Precautions

It must be emphasized that many people do not like to have their feet touched and approval from the patient is needed before starting. Before massage, the condition of the feet must be examined for swelling, color, ulcerations, toe deformities, and odor (Kunz & Kunz, 2003). The physical condition of the patient is also very important; hence, the health history of the patient is reviewed. If there is a problem regarding the blood flow to the limbs because of diabetes, neurological diseases (Dougans, 1999; Ingham, 1984), or arteriosclerosis, the therapist must be careful about the pressure of the massage and the patient should also be more alert to pain. The elderly may need special precautions, due to such concerns as restricted movement, incontinence, arthritis, and aching joints. When dealing with such conditions, it may be better to consider the patient's comfort and feel of the touch as the primary goals.

It must also be emphasized that no adverse reactions to reflexology have been documented in the literature, and reports from patients have indicated reflexology to be a largely pleasant experience, leaving the client both calm and relaxed. Nevertheless, certain reactions have been described. Reflexology is thought to activate the body's own healing power (Dougans, 1999). Consequently, some form of reaction is inevitable as the body rids itself of toxins. This phenomenon, known as a *healing crisis*, is a cleansing process manifested in the eliminating systems—the kidneys, bowels, skin, and lungs. Dougans (1999) has described the general reactions to be: increased urination, flatulence, more frequent bowel movements, aggravated skin conditions, increased perspiration, increased secretions of the mucous membranes, disrupted sleep patterns (either deeper or more disturbed sleep), fatigue, feverishness, headaches, dizziness, depression, or an overwhelming desire to weep. These reactions have been reported in the early stages of treatment and tend to last for relatively short periods of time, such as a few hours (Gunnarsdottir, 2007).

USES

Research testing the effects of reflexology is limited and includes studies of many approaches to and practices of reflexology. Some conditions for which it has been used are listed in Exhibit 20.2.

Reflexology has been found to significantly reduce the anxiety and pain of patients with lung and breast cancer after one session (Stephenson, Weinrich & Tavakoli, 2000). In another study, the duration of the effects of reflexology on pain was tested on patients with various

Exhibit 20.2

Uses of Reflexology

Decrease pain (Gunnarsdottir, 2007; Hodgson & Andersen, 2008; Launsö et al., 1999; Stephenson et al., 2003; Stephenson et al., 2007; Stephenson et al., 2000)

Decrease anxiety (Gambles et al., 2002; Stephenson et al., 2000; Stephenson et al., 2007)

Reduce physiologic distress (Hodgson & Andersen, 2008)

Improve the quality of life (Gambles et al., 2002; Hodgson, 2000; Milligan et al., 2002)

Reduce the symptoms of multiple sclerosis (Joyce & Richardson, 1997; Siev-Ner et al., 2003)

Promote relaxation (Gambles et al., 2002; Hodgson, 2000; Joyce & Richardson, 1997; Launsö et al., 1999; Milligan et al., 2002; Ross, et al., 2002)

Improve sleep (Gambles et al., 2002; Joyce & Richardson, 1997; Milligan et al., 2002)

types of cancer. The immediate effects on pain were supported, but the pain-relieving effects were not significant at 3 hours and 24 hours after the reflexology session (Stephenson, Dalton & Carlson, 2003). In a study by Ross and colleagues (2002), the effects of reflexology on anxiety and depression were compared with those of simple foot massage on two groups of cancer patients. These cancer patients received six sessions of intervention, and depression and anxiety were measured at baseline and within 24 hours after each session. No significant differences were found between the groups with respect to anxiety and depression, but both groups indicated experiencing relaxing effects from the treatment.

In a study by Hodgson and Andersen (2008), 21 nursing home residents with dementia were given four reflexology treatments over four weeks. The primary efficacy endpoint that was obtained was a significant reduction of physiologic distress as measured by salivary á-amylase. Furthermore, the residents demonstrated significant reduction in observed pain during the study period.

Quality of life (QoL) has been found to be enhanced in cancer patients after reflexology. To examine whether reflexology had any impact on QoL, Hodgson (2000) studied 12 cancer patients. They were randomized in two groups to receive either reflexology or placebo for 40 minutes. All of the participants in the reflexology group reported an increase in QoL, compared with 33% in the placebo group. To investigate patient satisfaction with reflexology therapy and its impact on QoL, an audit was undertaken in a Scottish hospice (Milligan, Fanning, Hunter, Tadjali, & Stevens, 2002). Twenty cancer patients completed self-report questionnaires after receiving from three to more than five reflexology sessions from a nurse trained in the therapy. The patients reported that reflexology reduced pain, improved sleep, enhanced relaxation, and reduced stress. In England, a similar study took place in which 34 cancer patients under palliative care were asked to comment about the reflexology therapy they had received (Gambles, Crooke, & Wilkinson, 2002). The patients received from four to six individually tailored reflexology interventions. They commented on reflexology as being emotionally beneficial in reducing anxiety and tension, improving sleep, and coping with the side effects of medications.

Patients with multiple sclerosis (MS) tend to suffer from a variety of chronic muscular symptoms, and two studies have reported improvements in symptoms after sessions of reflexology. In a study by Joyce and Richardson (1997), improvements were found in sleep, balance, pain, and spasms; however, these findings were based only on subjective responses. Siev-Ner, Gamus, Lerner-Geva, and Achiron (2003) conducted a randomized, controlled clinical trial to determine the effects of reflexology on the symptoms of multiple sclerosis (MS). Statistically significant positive differences in the scores for paresthesia, urinary symptoms, and spasticity were found in the group receiving reflexology compared with the control group.

Reflexology has been found to have an impact on migraine headaches (Launsö, Brendstrup, & Arnberg, 1999). Two-hundred-and-twenty migraine headache patients receiving reflexology sessions for 6 months reported a decrease in their medication consumption, but by the final treatment, 23% of the patients reported being cured, and 55% were completely relieved of their symptoms.

A case study design was used to test the effects of reflexology on six cases of women with fibromyalgia (Gunnarsdottir, 2007). Each case had 10 sessions of reflexology over a period of 10 weeks. Data were collected by observation, interviews, and diaries and then analyzed within each case and across cases. The findings showed that symptoms of pain in multiple areas started to localize and decrease in severity. The areas that responded best were the head, shoulders, neck and arms.

Domestic partners can be taught by qualified professionals to perform foot reflexology on patients with metastases from cancer. Stephenson, Swanson, Dalton, Keefe, and Engelke (2007) showed that partner-delivered foot reflexology had significant effects, resulting in a decrease of pain and anxiety as compared with a control group that received reading sessions from their partners. Social benefits of such use of reflexology were reported by some participants.

CULTURAL APPLICATIONS

The roots of reflexology are embedded in ancient history, when pressure therapies were recognized as preventive and therapeutic. Evidence indicates that therapeutic foot massage has been practiced throughout history by a variety of cultures. The oldest documentation depicting the practice of reflexology was unearthed in Egypt, dating around 2500–2330 B.C. The use of reflex pressure applied to the feet as a healing therapy has been practiced by the North American native peoples for generations.

As discussed earlier in the chapter, there are different perspectives on the effects of reflexology in eastern and western cultures. The TCM energy channels are one of the main concepts in both reflexology and acupuncture, as in both therapies energy is channeled throughout the body. Energy is channeled through the meridians and through the zones in reflexology. Both practices assert that diseases are caused by blockages in energy channels. In acupuncture/acupressure, energy is stimulated or sedated with needles/finger pressure. Six meridians are present in the feet, where they either end or begin. The other ends of the meridians going from or to the feet start or end in the fingers. Therefore, the meridians in the upper and lower parts of the body are connected.

Reflexology on the whole foot is also done on the acupuncture points there, and thus can help clear congestions in the meridians. It can also be used purposively, as it may be very helpful to push, press, or massage these points to increase energy in the meridians. Such stimulation is helpful in increasing energy movement along the meridians and in the organs to which they are connected. In this way the use of reflexology is based more on energy and assessment and movement of energy through out the body. Zone therapy as developed by Eunice Ingham is mostly practiced in Europe and the United States.

Reflexology, reflex zone therapy, and reflexotherapy are all terms that refer to the current use of the treatment, with distinctions apparently being due to scientific, philosophical, and political differences of opinion between authorities. Reflexology has become one of the most common therapies practiced by nurses and midwives in the United Kingdom (Mackereth & O'hara, 2002). In fact, the practice of reflexology is on the rise. In the UK, there are an estimated 12,500 registered reflexologists, with approximately 4.33 million visits per year (Poole, 2002).

FUTURE RESEARCH

In the pursuit of greater integration of complementary therapies into conventional health care, it is inevitable that reflexology will evolve and will need to be adapted to meet the needs of the system in which it finds itself. Practitioners need to be critical and acknowledge the value of research and inquiry in this process. The scientific basis for reflexology is growing, and promising results of its use for some symptoms are beginning to emerge, but more rigorous research is needed if it is to be used effectively by nurses in health care settings.

A recent systematic review of reflexology concluded that there is no evidence for any specific effect of reflexology in any conditions, with the exception of urinary symptoms associated with MS (Wang, Tsaai, Lee, Chang, & Wang, 2008). However another critical review on studies of reflexology (Gunnarsdottir, 2007) suggests that the reasons for limited scientific evidence of reflexology's effects are several. The methods used in the studies differ and are often not adequately explained. The amount of time and frequency of sessions are different and the principle behind reflexology states that it can affect the body as a whole. However, the latter phenomenon has not been captured in the studies reviewed. Nurses are in a primary position to conduct research on reflexology because their holistic background is in tune with the philosophies behind reflexology. Some questions for future research are:

1. What are the specifics of reflexology among other complementary therapies and how can the specifics of reflexology be captured in research?

2. What is the mechanism behind reflexology?

It is important to continue researching the effectiveness of reflexology to know how patients can be best served. Collaboration between therapists in private practice and those researching complementary and alternative therapies would enable a broad range of possibilities for future study.

REFLEXOLOGY-SPECIFIC WEB SITES

The International Council of Reflexologists was established in Toronto and holds an international conference on reflexology every other year. The Council's Web site is www.icr-reflexology.org.

Kevin and Barbara Kunz have developed and maintain two Web sites offering the basics on reflexology theory and practice, and information on developments in reflexology research: www.reflexology-re search.com and www.foot-reflexologist.com.

Other selected Web sites offer more information, including lists of worldwide reflexology organizations, as well as interactive information on reflexology products and practice: www.reflexology-usa.net; www.reflexology.org; www.myreflexologist.com; and www.aor.org.uk.

REFERENCES

Byers, D. C. (1983). *Better health with foot reflexology*. St. Petersburg, FL: Ingham.

Dougans, I. (1999). *The complete illustrated guide to reflexology*. Boston: Element Books.

Ehling, D. (2001). Oriental medicine: An introduction. *Alternative Therapies in Health and Medicine, 7*(4), 71–82.

Gambles, M., Crooke, M., & Wilkinson, S. (2002). Evaluation of a hospice based reflexology service: A qualitative audit of patient perceptions. *European Journal of Oncology Nursing, 6*(1), 37–44.

Gunnarsdottir, T. J. (2007). *Reflexology for fibromyalgia syndrome: A case study*. Unpublished doctoral dissertation, University of Minnesota, Minneapolis, MN.

Hodgson, H. (2000). Does reflexology impact on cancer patients' quality of life? *Nursing Standard, 14*(31), 33–38.

Hodgson, N. A., & Andersen, S. (2008). The clinical efficacy of reflexology in nursing home residents with dementia. *Journal of Alternative and Complementary Medicine, 14*(3), 269–275.

Ingham, E. D. (1984). *Stories the feet can tell thru reflexology/Stories the feet have told thru reflexology*. Saint Petersburg, FL: Ingham Publishing.

Joyce, M., & Richardson, R. (1997). Reflexology can help MS. *International Journal of Alternative and Complementary Medicine, 15*(7), 10–12.

Kaptchuck, T. J. (2000). *The web that has no weaver: Understanding Chinese medicine.* Chicago: Contemporary Books.

Kunz, K., & Kunz, B. (2003). *Reflexology: Health at your fingertips.* New York: DK Publishing.

Launsö, L., Brendstrup, E., & Arnberg, S. (1999). An exploratory study of reflexological treatment for headache. *Alternative Therapies in Health and Medicine, 5*(3), 57–65.

Lett, A. (2000). *Reflex zone therapy for health professionals.* London: Churchill Livingstone.

Mackereth, P. A., Dryden, S. L., & Frankel, B. (2000). Reflexology: recent research approaches. *Complementary Therapies in Nursing and Midwifery, 6,* 66–71.

Mackereth, P. A., & O'Hara, C. S. (2002). Appreciating preparatory and continuing education. In R. A. Mackereth & D. Tiran (Eds.), *Clinical reflexology* (pp. 17–32). Edinburg, Scotland: Churchill Livingstone.

Milligan, M., Fanning, M., Hunter, S., Tadjali, M., & Stevens, E. (2002). Reflexology audit: Patient satisfaction, impact on quality of life and availability in Scottish hospices. *International Journal of Palliative Nursing, 8,* 489–496.

National Center for Complementary and Alternative Medicine [NCCAM]. *About NCCAM.* Retrieved November 3, 2008, from http://nccam.nih.gov/health/whatiscam/

Omura, Y. (1994). Accurate localization of organ representation areas on the feet & hands using the bi-digital O-ring test resonance: Its clinical implication in diagnosis & treatment-part II. *Acupuncture & Electro-Therapeutics Research, International Journal, 19,* 153–190.

Poole, H. (2002). Appreciating preparatory and continuing education. In R. A. Mackereth & D. Tiran (Eds.), *Clinical reflexology* (pp. 61–71). Edinburg, Scotland: Churchill Livingstone.

Ross, C. S. K., Hamilton, J., Macrae, G., Docherty, C., Gould, A., & Cornbleet, M. A. (2002). A pilot study to evaluate the effect of reflexology on mood and symptom rating of advanced cancer patients. *Palliative Medicine, 16,* 544–545.

Siev-Ner, I., Gamus, D., Lerner-Geva, L., & Achiron, A. (2003). Reflexology treatment relieves symptoms of multiple sclerosis: A randomized controlled study. *Multiple Sclerosis, 9,* 356–361.

Stephenson, L. N., Dalton, J. A., & Carlson, J. (2003). The effect of foot reflexology on pain in patients with metastatic cancer. *Applied Nursing Research, 16*(4), 284–286.

Stephenson, L. N., Swanson, M., Dalton, J., Keefe, F. J., & Engelke, M. (2007). Partner-delivered reflexology: Effects on cancer pain and anxiety. *Oncology Nursing Forum, 34*(1), 127–132.

Stephenson, L. N., Weinrich, S. P., & Tavakoli, A. S. (2000). The effects of foot reflexology on anxiety and pain in patients with breast and lung cancer. *Oncology Nursing Forum, 27*(1), 67–72.

Tiran, D. (2002). Reviewing theories and origins. In R. A. Mackereth & D. Tiran. (Eds.), *Clinical reflexology* (pp. 5–15). Edinburg, Scotland: Churchill Livingstone.

Vennells, D. F. (2001). *Reflexology for beginners: Healing through foot massage of pressure points.* St. Paul, MN: Llewellyn.

Wang, M., Tsai, P., Lee, P., Chang, W., & Yang, C. (2008). The efficacy of reflexology: A systematic review. *Journal of Advanced Nursing, 62*(5), 512–520.

21 Creating Optimal Healing Environments

MARY JO KREITZER
TERRI ZBOROWSKY

INTRODUCTION

Nurses have long been leaders in creating optimal healing environments (OHEs). Florence Nightingale, the founder of modern nursing, described the role of the nurse as helping the patient attain the best possible condition so that nature can act and self-healing occur (Dossey, 2000). Nightingale recognized the nurse's role in both caring for the patient and managing the physical environment. She wrote about the importance of natural light, fresh air, noise reduction, and infection control as well as spirituality, presence, and caring. Her philosophy embodied the notion that, as nurses, we don't heal our patients, rather, we recognize that healing occurs within a person and our work is to help people tap into their innate capacities.

Increasingly, a base of evidence about the creation of optimal healing environments is emerging from many disciplines, including nursing, interior design, architecture, neuroscience, psychoneuroimmunology, and environmental psychology, among others. Just as evidence-based practice informs clinical decision making, evidence-based design impacts the planning and construction of health care facilities. Nurses need to be informed about the ways in which the physical environment affects health outcomes, firstly, so that they can contribute to the design of patient care units and clinical facilities that will optimize the health and well-being of patients, their families, and the staff who work in health care environments. Secondly, nurses are in a unique position to carry on needed research on the impact of specific design interventions on intended outcomes.

DEFINITIONS

The word "healing" comes from the Anglo-Saxon word *haelen*, which means "to make whole." Healing environments are designed to promote harmony or balance of mind, body, and spirit; to reduce anxiety and stress; to be restorative. The Samueli Institute, a research center focused on the science of healing, defines an optimal healing environment as a place where all aspects of patient care—physical, emotional, spiritual, behavioral, and environmental—are optimized to support and stimulate healing (see Table 21.1).

As illustrated in Table 21.1, within an optimal healing environment, the attitudes and intentions of all health care providers, and of the patients themselves, are recognized as being important. There are opportunities for personal growth and self-care practices that promote wholeness. Healing relationships are cultivated as patients and their families interact with caring and compassionate health care providers and staff. Healthy lifestyles are promoted and patients have options to choose conventional care and/or complementary therapies and healing practices. A culture is created that supports healing through alignment of the organizational vision, mission, resources, and leadership. This culture is supported by a physical environment that embodies design characteristics known to promote healing, such as nature, light, and color.

The primary emphasis of the present volume, *Complementary & Alternative Therapies in Nursing*, is on the evidence and clinical applications of complementary and alternative therapies that nurses can use to enhance their practice. The present chapter focuses on the dimension of place or space—the physical environment in which care is provided and the ways in which evidence can be used to create environments that contribute to positive health outcomes.

Table 21.1

OPTIMAL HEALTH ENVIRONMENTS

INNER ENVIRONMENT → → OUTER ENVIRONMENT

ENHANCE:

AWARENESS	INTEGRATION	CARING	HEALTH HABITS	HEALTH CARE	PROCESS & STRUCTURE	SENSORY INPUT
Expectation	Self-care	Compassion	Diet	Conventional medicine	Leadership	Nature
Hope	Mind	Empathy	Exercise	Complementary practices	Mission	Color
Understanding	Body	Social support	Relaxation	Entho-cultural traditions	Workforce	Light
Intention	Spirit	Communication	Balance		Technology	Positive distraction
	Energy	Family involvement			Evaluation	Architecture
					Service	Aroma Music
						Green

SCIENTIFIC BASIS

There is a growing body of evidence that links the physical environment to health outcomes. According to a review of the research literature on evidence-based health care design (Ulrich et al., 2008), there have been over 1,000 rigorous empirical studies published that link the design of a hospital's physical environment with health care outcomes. The studies cover a broad scope, with evidence linking:

- *single-bed rooms* with reduced hospital-acquired infections, reduced medical errors, reduced patient falls, improved patient sleep, and increased patient satisfaction;
- *decentralized supplies* with increased staff effectiveness;
- *appropriate lighting* with decreased medical errors and decreased staff stress; and
- *ceiling lifts* with decreased staff injuries.

Although many of the studies focus on such topics as infection control, patient falls, staff productivity, and staff injuries, a growing number of studies focus on other aspects of the environment that contribute to healing.

As described by Malkin (2008), design strategies that focus on creating healing environments have in common the goal of reducing stress and include:

- Connections to nature (e.g., artwork with a nature theme, views to the outside, interior gardens, plants)
- Options that give patients choices and control (e.g., room-service menu, choice of music and art, ability to control lighting and temperature)
- Spaces that provide access to social support (e.g., family zones within patient rooms that offer sleeping space, storage, and adequate seating)
- Positive distractions (e.g., music, water features, aviaries, videos of nature, aquariums, and sculpture)
- Reductions of environmental stressors such as noise and glare from direct light sources (e.g., carpet, indirect lighting, elimination of overhead paging).

Theories Related to Healing Environments and Clinical Applications

Biophilia is the inherent human inclination to "affiliate" with natural systems and processes. The concept, originally proposed by eminent biologist Edward O. Wilson (1984), has grown into a broader framework that increasingly is shaping the design of the man-made environment, including hospitals and other health care facilities. Biophilic design emphasizes the necessity of maintaining, enhancing, and restoring the beneficial experience of nature, and describes attempts to do so through the use of environmental features that embody such characteristics of the natural world as color, water, sunlight, plants, natural materials, and exterior views and vistas (Kellert, 2008).

The theory of biophilia has been empirically tested in clinical settings. Outcomes measured most often include stress and pain reduction. For example:

- A study of elderly residents in an urban long-term care facility revealed that residents attach considerable importance to having access to window views of outdoor spaces with prominent features such as plants, gardens, and birds (Kearney & Winterbottom, 2005).
- Patients in a dental clinic reported less stress on days when a large nature mural was hung in the waiting room compared to days when there was no nature scene (Heerwagen, 1990).
- In a prospective randomized trial of blood donors, it was found that donors who viewed a wall-mounted television playing a nature videotape had lower blood pressure and pulse rates than subjects who were viewing a television playing either a videotape of urban scenes or game or talk shows (Ulrich, Simons, & Miles, 2003).
- Ulrich, Lunden, and Eltinge (1993) found that patients following heart surgery who viewed photos of trees and water required fewer doses of strong pain medication and reported less anxiety than patients who viewed abstract images or were assigned to a control group with no picture.

There is some evidence that the more engrossing a "nature distraction," the greater the potential for pain alleviation. Miller et al. (1992), in a study of burn patients, found that distracting patients during burn dressings by having them view nature scenes on a bedside TV accompanied by music lessened both pain and anxiety. In a randomized prospective trial of patients undergoing bronchoscopy, patients who viewed a ceiling-mounted nature scene and listened to nature sounds reported less pain than patients in the control group who looked at a blank ceiling. Following a review of the literature on the use of virtual reality as adjunct analgesic technique, Wismeijer and Vingerhoets (2005) concluded that "nature exposures" may tend to be more diverting, and hence pain–reducing, if they involve sound as well as visual stimulation and maximize realism and immersion.

A number of studies have examined patient preferences for art and the effect of art on stress, recovery, and pain, among other outcomes. Consistently, studies have documented that patients prefer nature over other subject matter and that they overwhelmingly prefer realistic art and strongly dislike abstract images (Winston & Cupchik, 1992). Findings such as these, consistent with the theory of biophilia, have led to the use of evidence-based design guidelines in health care facilities to guide the selection of art. According to Ulrich and Gilpin (2003), visual art should be unambiguously positive. Recommended subject matter includes waterscapes with calm or nonturbulent water, landscapes with visual depth or openness, nature settings depicted during warmer seasons when vegetation is verdant and flowers are visible, garden scenes, outdoor scenes in sunny conditions, and avoidance of overcast or foreboding weather.

Chronobiology

Chronobiology is an interdisciplinary field of inquiry that focuses on biological rhythms. Discoveries in "chronotherapeutics" have documented that time patterning of medications in synchrony with body rhythms can enhance effectiveness and safety. Other studies have focused on the impact of environmental factors such as light and temperature on body rhythms. There is a significant body of literature focused on the impact of light on depression. In a study of psychiatric patients, Beauchemin and Hays (1996) found that patients in sunnier rooms stayed an average of 2.6 fewer days than those in sunless rooms. A meta-analysis of 20 randomized controlled trials by Golden et al. (2005)

on the impact of light treatment on nonseasonal and seasonal depression quantified the effect of light treatment as equivalent to that of antidepressant pharmacotherapy trials. Light has also been found to be related to patients' perception of pain. In a study (Walch et al., 2005) of postspinal surgery experiences, patients who were admitted to rooms with greater sunlight intensity reported less pain and stress and took 22% fewer analgesic medications. Results such as these support careful site planning to assure adequate access to daylight and provide justification for larger windows in patient rooms or the use of bright (but diffused) artificial light in areas where sufficient daylight is inaccessible.

INTERVENTION

Case Study Applications of Optimal Healing Environment

North Hawaii Community Hospital

North Hawaii Community Hospital embodies the culture of the community in the way in which it has operationalized the concept of optimal healing environment. The footprint of the hospital was aligned so that the front is oriented to the Kohala Mountain, and the back to the mountain Mauna Kea. Earl Bakken, one of the founders of the hospital, had the vision that the hospital itself would be an "instrument of healing," rather than a "warehouse for sick bodies" (E. Bakken, personal communication, January 2008). All patient rooms are private and have access to views of nature and fresh air through sliding doors that open to the outside. Art in patient's rooms is culturally meaningful and can be changed. Hallways are carpeted and there is minimal overhead paging. Soft music is playing in public spaces. Familiar cultural patterns, textures, and colors are used in wallpapers, carpeting, and furniture coverings. Ti plants at all entrances and corners of the building are believed to filter out bad spiritual energy. An interior bamboo garden also offers spiritual protection and represents strength and resilience. All patient rooms have sleep chairs or extra beds for guests to stay over and there are no limits on the number of visitors or visiting hours. An ohama (Hawaiian for "family") room includes a kitchen so that families can prepare special meals. Skylights in halls and windows in the operating rooms were incorporated into the design to enable staff to stay attuned to day/night cycles. In addition to these and many other mechanical, architectural, and engineering adaptations, the hospital embraced a philosophy of blended medicine that encourages the integration of complementary therapies and culturally based healing practices. The vision of North Hawaii Community Hospital is to become the most healing hospital in the world.

Abbott Northwestern Hospital

The design of the Neuroscience/Orthopaedic/Spine Patient Care Center at Abbott Northwestern's new Heart Hospital in Minneapolis, Minnesota, integrates the elements of Abbott Northwestern's Healing Environment Aesthetic Standards, including the principles of *feng shui* and patient-centered care, while acknowledging the needs of staff. This 128–inpatient bed unit located on two floors of the Heart Hospital was designed to incorporate the latest technology to aid in meeting patient and safety requirements as well as implement the organization's holistic approach to healing. To accomplish these goals, patient rooms were "zoned" so that the needs of each user of the space would be addressed:

- The *patient zone* provides a view to the outside from every bed; a flower/card shelf; private safes for valuables; art work and care provider information on the footwall; and a small refrigerator for favorite foods.
- The *family zone* incorporates an upholstered bench seat/sleeper, a reading light with private switch, and a data outlet for internet access.
- The *caregiver zone* includes a bedside work area with a sink, computer, and, in each patient room, a ceiling-mounted patient lift system with a custom track to assist with turning, moving, or toileting a patient.

Other family and patient amenities on the unit include access to a two-story atrium with soothing water walls and a waiting room with a panoramic view of the city, kitchenette, and fireplace (see Figure 21.1). In addition to the bedside computer in each patient room, staff amenities

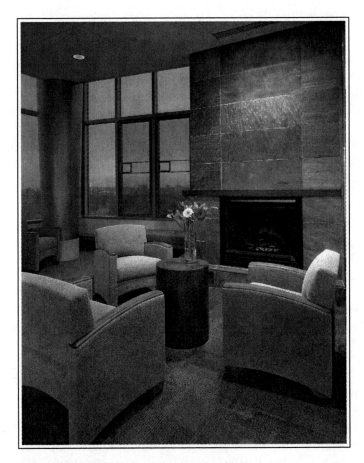

Figure 21.1 The Neuroscience/Orthopaedic/Spine Patient Care Center at Abbott Northwestern's (ANW) Heart Hospital in Minneapolis, MN.

include decentralized support rooms such as clean utility, soiled utility, nutrition, and medication rooms. A staff-respite area, a private room for staff to use, includes a lounge chair, ottoman, a phone, and an outside view. Beyond the clinical outcomes, this design provides balance for the psychological, social, and spiritual needs of the staff, the patients, and their families. Ultimately, the new patient care center design aspired to create a unique health care environment for this center of excellence at Abbott Northwestern Hospital.

Regions Hospital

A primary objective of a recent building project at Regions Hospital, a large tertiary care facility located in St. Paul, Minnesota, was to replace shared patient rooms with private patient rooms. To do this, the hospital undertook the largest construction project ever to occur in the city. The new hospital bed tower includes an expansion of the emergency department, replacement of the operating suite, and the addition of 144 private patient rooms. Design principles included an overarching goal to enhance patient safety.

To accomplish this goal in the bed tower, many new features were built into the design:

- **Standardization of patient rooms.** First, staff realized that standardization of all the patient rooms was imperative. While each floor will have a different service line, even different acuity levels that range from intensive care to orthopedics, all patient rooms are laid out in the same way.
- **Unique staff access and visibility.** Each patient room has a separate doorway for patients and families as well as one for staff. Staff work areas directly adjacent to the patient room include a view window with an integral blind. Staff will share this alcove between two rooms, a design feature particularly important for intensive care unit staff. Patient visibility and ease of access to the patient should enhance patient safety by increasing staff presence.
- **Enhanced family zones.** In addition, family zones in the rooms are generous with the intent to encourage family-centered patient care. Families will have the ability to stay overnight in most rooms.
- **Inclusion of acuity-adaptable patient rooms.** Patient rooms on the cardiac unit were designed to be "acuity adaptable," i.e., allowing patients to stay in the same room as their acuity level varies. The concept is based on data that suggest that decreased transferring of patients decreases medical incidents and errors (Hendrich, Fay, & Sorrels, 2004).
- **Patient access to the toilet.** Finally, as the patient rooms are mirrored, at least half of the patient rooms will have direct access to the patient toilet. No studies to date have been able to document that this is a safer layout for patients, but with a growing number of patient rooms being designed this way, Regions will provide the perfect setting to study the impact of this layout on patient safety.

CULTURAL APPLICATIONS AND PRECAUTIONS

The increased diversity of the U.S. population has added a level of complexity to the design of health care environments. As noted by Kopec and Han (2008), entering a health care environment can be frightening and disempowering, particularly when a patient's traditional and spiritual beliefs differ from that of the dominant culture. Thus, it is becoming increasingly important to carefully weigh all design decisions that impact the physical environment, including the use of color and cultural symbols as well as other visual, auditory, and tactile design elements.

To Asians, for example, the color red symbolizes good luck whereas the color white is associated with mourning and death. The color green has positive associations within the Islamic tradition, as it is associated with vegetation and life and is believed to have been the prophet Mohammed's favorite color. Kopec and Han (2008) have identified a number of ways in which the needs of Muslim patients might be accommodated. A curtain inside the door, for instance, could help patients maintain visual privacy and modesty, while allowing health care providers on rounds to announce their presence, giving patients time to prepare themselves to be seen. Understanding that followers of Islam face the northeast when they pray could be taken into consideration when orienting the bed and furnishings in the room.

Given the diversity of spiritual, religious, and cultural beliefs and practices, however, it would be nearly impossible, from a design perspective (as well as practically and financially), to accommodate all of the specifics and nuances of every tradition. Thus, the goal of design can only be to strive to express core, universal values while seeking to devise design elements that can be flexible.

FUTURE RESEARCH

More research is needed to understand the impact of design interventions on the environment of care. Future studies need to rigorously examine the many factors that contribute to healing environments and should include a focus on staff as well as patient outcomes. Health care outcomes for patients may include the reduction of stress, reduced length of stay, decreased incidence of nosocomial infections, reduced pain, improved sleep, increased patient satisfaction, and reduced patient falls. Outcomes for nursing staff may include decreased staff injuries, decreased staff stress, reduced sick days and increased staff effectiveness, productivity, and satisfaction.

As the United States enters an era of hospital construction that is unprecedented in size and scope and is projected to exceed $70 billion a year by 2011 (Jones, 2007), nurses need to be actively engaged in contributing to the design and evaluation of healing environments that will optimize the health and well-being of patients, family members and staff.

WEB SITES

The Center for Health Design: www.healthdesign.org

Center for Spirituality and Healing, University of Minnesota: http://takingcharge.csh.umn.edu/therapies/environment/what

REFERENCES

Beauchemin, K. M., & Hays, P. (1996). Sunny hospital rooms expedite recovery from severe and refractory depressions. *Journal of Affective Disorders, 40*(1–2), 49–51.
Dossey, B. M. (2000). *Florence Nightingale: Mystic, visionary, healer.* Springhouse, PA: Springhouse.
Golden, R. N., Gaynes, B. N., Ekstrom, R. D., Hamer, R. M., Jacobsen, F. M., Suppes, T., et al. (2005). The efficacy of light therapy in the treatment of mood disorders: A review and meta-analysis of the evidence. *American Journal of Psychiatry, 162*(4), 656–662.
Heerwagen, J. H. (1990). The psychological aspects of windows and window design. In K. H. Anthony, J. Choi, & B. Orland (Eds.), *Proceedings of 21st Annual Conference of the Environmental Design Research Association* (pp. 269–280). Oklahoma City, OK: Environmental Design Research Association.
Hendrich, A., Fay, J., & Sorrells, A. (2004). Effects of acuity-adaptable rooms on flow of patients and delivery of care. *American Journal of Critical Care, 113*(1), 35–45.
Jones, H. (2007). *FMI's construction outlook fourth quarter 2007 report.* Raleigh, NC: FMI.
Kearney, A. R., & Winterbottom, D. (2005). Nearby nature and long-term care facility residents: Benefits and design recommendations. *Journal of Housing for the Elderly, 1*(3/4), 7–28.
Kellert, S. R. (2008). Dimensions, elements and attributes of biophilic design. In S. R. Kellert, J. H. Heerwagen, & M. L. Mador (Eds.), *Biophilic design* (pp. 3–20). Hoboken, NJ: John Wiley.

Kopec, D., & Han, L. (2008). Islam and the healthcare environment: Designing patient rooms. *Health Environments Research and Design Journal, 1*(4), 111–121.

Malkin, J. (2008). *A visual reference for evidence-based design.* Concord, CA: The Center for Health Design.

Miller, A. C., Hickman, L. C., & Lemasters, G. K. (1992). A distraction technique for control of burn pain. *Journal of Burn Care and Rehabilitation, 13*(5), 576–580.

Ulrich, R. S., & Gilpin, L. (2003). Healing arts. In S. B. Frampton, L. Gilpin, & P. Charmel (Eds.), *Putting patients first: Designing and practicing patient-centered care* (pp. 117–146). San Francisco: Jossey-Bass.

Ulrich, R. S., Lunden, O. L., & Eltinge, J. L. (1993). Effects of exposure to nature and abstract pictures on patients recovering from heart surgery. [Paper presented at the Thirty-Third Meeting of the Society for Psychophysiological Research.] *Psychophysiology, 30* (Suppl. 1), 7.

Ulrich, R. S., Simons, R. F., & Miles, M. A. (2003). Effects of environmental simulations and television on blood donor stress. *Journal of Architectural & Planning Research, 20*(1), 38–47.

Ulrich, R. S., Zimring, C., Zhu, X., Dubose, J., Seo, H., Choi, Y., et al. (2008). A review of the research literature on evidence-based healthcare design. *Health Environments Research & Design Journal, 1*(3), 61–125.

Walch, J. M., Rabin, B. S., Day, R., Williams, J. N., Choi, K., & Kang, J. D. (2005). The effect of sunlight on post-operative analgesic medication usage: a prospective study of patients undergoing spinal surgery. *Psychosomatic Medicine, 67,* 156–163.

Wilson, E. O. (1984). *Biophilia: The human bond with other species.* Cambridge, MA: Harvard University Press.

Winston, A. S., & Cupchik, G. C. (1992). The evaluation of high art and popular art by naive and experienced viewers. *Visual Arts Research, 18,* 1–14.

Wismeijer, A. J., & Vingerhoets, J. J. (2005). The use of virtual reality and audiovisual eyeglass systems as adjunct analgesic techniques: A review of the literature. *Annals of Behavioral Medicine, 30*(3), 268–278.

Manipulative and Body-Based Therapies

OVERVIEW

This NCCAM category includes therapies that involve the manipulation and movement of body parts. Three large groups of therapies comprise this category—chiropractic, osteopathic, and massage. But a myriad of relaxation therapies, such as progressive muscle relaxation and breathing modalities, have been relegated to this category. Exercise, a key element of health-promotion programs, is an important body-based therapy. Other manipulative and body-based therapies include Trager bodywork, Bowen technique, rolfing, Tui Na, Alexander technique, and the Feldenkrais method.

Massage, in the form of back rubs, is a basic skill that has been included in nursing curricula since the beginning of modern nursing. In recent years, back rubs have been largely abandoned by nurses, citing "too busy" as the reason for this decline in use. However, a number of nurses have pursued education to become massage therapists; the practice of massage therapy is often separate from their practice of nursing, although some nurses who are massage therapists use this modality in nursing homes and in independent practice as advanced practice nurses.

Although many of the therapies in this group are routinely administered by other therapists, such as chiropractors and massage therapists, a number of therapies in this group are employed by nurses. Back rubs or massage has been part of nursing for centuries. Within other systems of care such as TCM, heat and cold are part of the assessment of the patient and used in determining the types of therapies to use in treating the patient.

Tai Chi, a therapy originating in China, is receiving increasing attention in the Western world. Tai Chi classes in community settings, in long-term care facilities, and in workplaces are common. In addition to relaxation, outcomes of Tai Chi include increased agility and flexibility and improvement in other body functions.

A myriad of relaxation therapies exist. Nurses continue to use these therapies in working with many patient populations, including those with cardiac and pulmonary conditions. Many of these therapies (for example, stress reduction) can be taught to the patient and family and do not require ongoing nursing supervision.

Research on therapies in this category varies according to the specific therapy. Numerous studies exist to support the use of massage, Tai Chi, exercise, and relaxation therapies. Fewer studies have been conducted on therapies such as Trager and hydrotherapy. Nurses can select and use many therapies in this category in their practice.

22 Massage

MARIAH SNYDER
SHIZUKO TANIGUKI

Massage is an ancient therapy. There is evidence that it was used in China more than 5,000 years ago (McRee Noble, & Pasvogel, 2003). It is one of the most widely used complementary therapies and has been a part of the nurse's armamentarium for centuries. At a time when the public use of massage is increasing, the nursing profession is decreasing its use of this traditional intervention. To compensate for this, some health institutions have massage therapists on staff; patients or family, in most instances, pay for this service.

Massage is often combined with other therapies, such as music, aromatherapy, acupressure, or light touch. Thus, it is difficult to differentiate the specific effects of massage from those of the other therapies used. Study findings point to the positive effects of massage with or without other therapies in producing relaxation, improving sleep, and reducing pain.

DEFINITION

The term *massage* is derived from the Arabic word *mass'h*, meaning "to press gently" (Furlan, Brosseau, Imamura, & Irvin, 2004). Massage, as defined by the American Massage Therapy Association, is "the application of manual techniques and adjunctive therapies with the intention of positively affecting the health and well-being of the client" (2004—http://www.amtamassage.org/about/definition/html). Various strokes are used to produce friction and pressure on cutaneous and subcutaneous tissues. The types of stroke and the amount of pressure chosen depend on the desired outcomes and the body part being massaged.

There are a number of types of massage: *Swedish* (a massage using long, flowing strokes); *Esalen* (a meditative massage using light touch); *deep tissue or neuromuscular* (an intense kneading of the body); *sports massage* (a vigorous massage to loosen and ease sore muscles); *Shiatsu* (a Japanese pressure-point technique to relieve stress); and *reflexology* (a deep foot massage that relates to parts of the body). The different types of massage incorporate a variety of strokes, varying levels of pressure, and a multitude of procedures. Massage strokes can be administered to the entire body or to specific areas of the body, such as the back, feet, or hands.

SCIENTIFIC BASIS

The use of massage is a natural healing process that helps to connect the body, mind, and spirit. Massage produces therapeutic effects on multiple body systems: integumentary, musculoskeletal, cardiovascular, lymph, and nervous. Manipulating the skin and underlying muscle makes the skin supple. Massage increases or enhances movement in the musculoskeletal system by reducing swelling, loosening and stretching contracted tendons, and aiding in the reduction of soft-tissue adhesions. Friction to the cutaneous and subcutaneous tissues releases histamines that in turn produce vasodilation of vessels and enhance venous return.

Massage has been found to produce a relaxation response (Hattan, King, & Griffiths, 2002; Holland & Pokorny, 2001; McNamara, Burnham, Smith, & Carroll, 2003). Investigators report that massage has produced a decrease in certain physiological parameters (systolic and diastolic blood pressure, heart rate, and skin temperature), indicative of the relaxation response (Mok & Woo, 2004).

Reduction of pain, a frequent desired outcome of massage, is closely related to the production of the relaxation response. Studies have validated that patients were more comfortable after the administration of massage (Frey Law et al., 2008; Simmons, Chabal, Griffith, Rausch, & Steele, 2004; Wang & Keck, 2004). The positive impact of massage on pain reduction is often posited on the gate control theory, with massage stimulating the large-diameter nerve fibers that have an inhibitory input on T-cells (Furlan et al., 2004). According to Wang and Keck, "massaging the hands and feet stimulates the mechanorecptors that activate the nonpainful nerve fibers, preventing pain transmission from reaching consciousness" (p. 59).

Results from some studies on the use of massage have shown that massage does not always produce relaxation. One factor that may contribute to these findings is that massage of short duration may initially cause stimulation of the sympathetic nervous system and thus cause an increase in blood pressure and heart rate. Few studies have included information about subjects' comfort with touch and massage. For some persons, massage may increase anxiety.

The impact of massage on the psychoneuroimmunological functions of the body and mind is beginning to be explored. Billhult, Lindholm, Gunnarsson, and Stener-Victoria (2008) explored the effect of massage on CD4+ and CD8+ T cells in women with cancer. Findings revealed that massage had no effect on these indices. Anecdotal reports, however, suggest that massage produces positive results in persons with HIV infection.

Massage is a holistic therapy and, as such, promotes overall health. Improvement in well-being has been shown in the following studies: emotional discomfort (Currin & Meister, 2008); psychological well-being (Chang, Wang, & Chen, 2002); and quality of life (Williams et al., 2005).

INTERVENTION

As noted earlier, numerous types of massage exist. The techniques for hand and shoulder massage will be presented.

The environment in which massage is administered is important. The room must be warm enough for the person to be comfortable, as shivering could negate the effects of the massage. In addition, privacy needs to be ensured. Adding music and aromatherapy to massage session has been thought to increase the effectiveness of massage. Fellowes, Barnes, and Wilkinson (2004), however, did not find any convincing evidence that aromatherapy contributed to additional improvement in outcomes. Chapter 6 details intervention with music; aromatherapy is described in chapter 26.

Massage Strokes

Commonly used strokes in administering massage include effluerage, friction, pressure, petrissage, vibration, and percussion.

Effluerage

Effluerage is a slow, rhythmic stroking, with light skin contact. Effleurage may be applied with varying degrees of pressure, depending on the part of the body being massaged and the outcome desired. The palmar surface of the hands is used for larger surfaces, the thumbs and fingers for smaller areas. On large surfaces, long, gliding strokes about 10 to 20 inches in length are applied.

Friction Movements

In *friction movements*, moderate, constant pressure to one area is made with the thumbs or fingers. The fingers may be held in one place or moved in a small circumscribed area.

Pressure Stroke

The *pressure stroke* is similar to the friction stroke, except pressure strokes are made with the whole hand.

Petrissage

Petrissage, or kneading, involves lifting a large fold of skin and the underlying muscle and holding the tissue between the thumb and fingers. The tissues are pushed against the bone, then raised and squeezed in circular movements. The grasp on the tissues is alternately loosened and tightened. Tissues are supported by one hand while being kneaded with the other. Variations include pinching, rolling, wringing, and kneading with fists or fingers. Petrissage is limited to tissues having a significant muscle mass.

Vibration Strokes

Vibration strokes can be administered with either the entire hand or with the fingers. Rapid, continuous strokes are used. Because administering vibration strokes requires much energy, mechanical vibrators are sometimes used.

Percussion Strokes

For percussion strokes, the wrist acts as a fulcrum for the hand, with the hand hitting the tissue. Strokes are made with a rapid tempo over a large body area. Tapping and clapping are variants of percussion strokes.

Shoulder Massage

Shoulder massage can be easily performed by nurses and other persons. The person receiving the massage sits so that the back is accessible to the person administering the massage. The massage can be administered with the person's shoulders uncovered or clothed. If clothed, no oil or lotion is used.

The massage begins with some gentle pressure applied on the shoulders using the palm of the hand. Next, attention is given to stretching the trapezius muscles, moving from the center of the back to the muscle's insertion in the scapula at the shoulder joint. Fingers can be used to massage the fibers in the muscles of the shoulder. Petrissage strokes are used to lift the skin and muscle fibers so as to massage these tissues between the fingers. Attention is given to the attachment of the muscles at the base of the skull by massaging up the neck and stretching the muscles. If a person is unable to hold his or her head upright, a hand can be placed on the forehead to support the head. The massage is concluded with lighter percussion strokes across the top of the shoulders (M. O. Martin, March 2005, personal communication).

Hand Massage

A technique for performing hand massage is outlined in Exhibit 22.1. The technique is easy to use with many populations, including older adults (Kolcaba, Schirm, & Steiner, 2006; Snyder, Eagan, & Burns, 1995) as well as infants and children (Field, 2002). A suggested period

Exhibit 22.1

Techiques for Hand Massage

Each hand is massaged for $2^1/2$ minutes. Do not massage if hand is injured, reddened, or swollen.

1. **Back of hand**
   - Short, medium-length, straight strokes are done from the wrist to the finger-tips; moderate pressure is used (effluerage).
   - Large, half-circle, stretching strokes are made from the center to the side of the hand, using moderate pressure.
   - Small, circular strokes are made over the entire hand, using light pressure (make small O's with the thumb).
   - Featherlike, straight strokes are made from the wrist to the fingertips, using very light pressure.

2. **Palm of hand**
   - Short, medium–length, straight strokes are made from the wrist to the finger-tips, using moderate pressure (effluerage).
   - Gentle milking and lifting of the tissue of the entire palm of the hand is done using moderate pressure.
   - Small circular strokes are made over the entire palm, using moderate pressure (making little O's with index finger).
   - Large, half-circle, stretching strokes are used, from the center of the palm to the sides, using moderate pressure.

3. **Fingers**
   - Gently squeeze each finger from the base to the tip on both sides and the front and back, using light pressure.
   - Gentle range-of-motion of finger.
   - Gentle pressure on nail bed.

4. **Completion**
   - Place client's hand on yours and cover it with your other hand. Gently draw your top hand toward you several times. Turn the client's hand over and gently draw your other hand toward you several times.

for administering massage is $2^1/2$ minutes per hand. The length of time is individualized for each patient, based on his/her response.

Measurement of Outcomes

Both physiological and psychological outcomes have been used to measure the effectiveness of massage. Indices of relaxation (heart rate, blood pressure, respiration rate, skin temperature, cortisol level, and muscle tension) have been measured in many studies. Anxiety inventories and scales to determine pain level and quality of sleep as well as quality-of-life indices have been used to determine the efficacy of massage. It is important that both short- and long-term effects of massage be measured.

Precautions

Ernst (2003) reviewed the literature to determine adverse reactions to massage. Although a number of negative reactions were noted, the majority of these were associated with exotic types of massage and not with the Swedish massage technique.

Before administering massage, the nurse explains the intervention, obtains a history, and secures the permission of the patient. The history provides the nurse with information about past use of massage and any adverse responses. It is also important to find out the person's overall response to touch. Some people may be averse to being touched because of past negative experiences. Others may be hypersensitive to touch. One method for overcoming this sensitivity is beginning with light touch and slowly increasing the pressure. The area to be massaged is assessed for redness, bruises, edema, or rashes.

Massage therapists and nurses have been reluctant to use massage with cancer patients (Gecsedi, 2002) because of the belief that the therapy may initiate or accelerate metastases. Guidelines are being developed to govern the use of massage with persons with cancer. Some therapists request a physician's order about the body region and technique to be used. Factors considered are the location of the tumor, the stage of the cancer, and the location of any metastatic lesions. Pressure in the immediate area of the cancer is to be avoided.

Because blood pressure may be lowered during massage, monitoring for light-headedness is suggested following the initial massage sessions, particularly in older adults. If light-headedness does occur, allowing the person to remain recumbent for several minutes at the conclusion of the massage may help to decrease the likelihood of hypotension and falls. Monitoring of blood pressure and pulse rate are required in persons with cardiac conditions, to determine whether adverse effects are being experienced.

Exhibit 22.2

Uses of Massage

Promote relaxation

Cataract surgery (Simmons et al., 2004)

Decrease aggressive behaviors (Garner et al., 2008)

Promote sleep (Richards, 1998)

Lessen fatigue (Currin & Meister, 2008)

Facilitate communication (Kolcaba et al., 2006)

Lessen pain (Chang et al., 2002; Ernst, 2004; Wang & Keck, 2004)

Improve mobility (Smith, Stallings, Mariner, & Burrall, 1999)

Increase weight in preterm infants (Field, 2002)

Increase psychological well-being (Hattan et al., 2002)

Lessen anxiety (Currin & Meister, 2008; Fellowes et al., 2004)

USES

For a list of conditions for which massage has been used, see Exhibit 22.2. Use of massage to produce relaxation and reduce pain will now be described.

Relaxation

Many people use a massage therapist to ameliorate their stress. Mok and Woo (2004) reported a positive response to a slow-stroke back massage in elders who had had a stroke. In a review of 22 studies in which massage had been used, Richards, Gibson, and Overton-McCoy (2000) found that the most commonly reported outcome was a reduction in anxiety. Using foot massage with cardiac patients, Hattan et al. (2002) found that subjects receiving this therapy reported feeling much calmer.

In addition to using massage with patients, massage can also be used with a patient's family members who are experiencing high levels of stress. A short hand massage may help to relax a family member so they can rest or sleep.

Pain

Reduction of pain is another condition for which massage is often used. Numerous studies have found that massage resulted in a reduction of pain. Ernst (2004), in a meta-analysis of seven studies, found that use of Swedish massage may be effective in lessening pain. However, the author also noted that many methodological concerns about the studies existed. In a review of research on the use of massage and aromatherapy in persons with cancer, Fellowes et al. (2004) found a reduction in pain in 3 of the 10 studies reviewed in which massage and aromatherapy had been used with cancer patients. Wang and Keck (2004) reported a lessening of pain in postoperative patients, and Mok and Woo (2004) found that massage lessened pain in patients with strokes.

CULTURAL ASPECTS

Nurses may encounter patients who have a reddened area that does not appear to be from pressure. Cupping is a therapy, used in Asian countries, that originated in traditional Chinese medicine. A cup (often a plastic cup) is placed over the area and either heat or suction is used to create a partial vacuum which lifts up the underlying tissue. Stasis of the blood occurs, hence the reddened skin. The intended purpose of cupping is to "activate" the underlying tissue or organ. For example, the therapy may be used to release toxins or open up blockages in the colon. Minimal research has been done on the effectiveness of cupping. Ahmadi, Schwebel, and Rezaei (2008) tested the efficacy of wet-cupping to treat tension and migraine headaches. A 66% decrease in severity of pain was reported, and subjects reported 12.6 fewer days of headache per month.

Shiatsu, a pressure-point type of massage, is popular in Japan and other Asian countries. Its underlying purpose is to rebalance the energy system in the body through pressure on specific points. Although Shiatsu may not be "comforting" during administration, relaxation is often felt at the conclusion. Shiatsu may be used to help alleviate other conditions. Tanigaki (2008) found Shiatsu therapy to be highly efficacious in managing constipation in 6 elderly patients (from 81 to 93 years of age) who were on bedrest and receiving home care.

FUTURE RESEARCH

Reviews of the studies that have been conducted using massage have identified a number of methodological issues. One challenge posed in conducting research on massage is having a comparable control group. McNamara et al. (2003) compared massage and standard care in patients undergoing a diagnostic test. Some have compared the effects of massage with those of other therapies such as imagery (Hattan et al., 2002). The following are suggestions for research that is needed so that practitioners may have more direction in using massage in clinical settings:

1. Few investigators have explored the impact massage has on pyschoneuroimmunologcial indices. Studies on the use of massage with patients having HIV infection and cancer would guide nurses in its use with these groups.
2. The period of time for administering massage and the number of sessions that produce the best results need to be established. There is great variation in these two parameters in published studies. Because of time constraints in practice settings, this information would be very helpful to busy practitioners.
3. What, if any, is the effect of the sex of the therapist administering massage on the outcomes obtained? Few studies have reported on the significance of the sex of the therapist in relation to that of the patient.

REFERENCES

Ahmadi, A., Schwebel, D. C., & Rezaei, M. (2008). The efficacy of wet-cupping in the treatment of tension and migraine headaches. *American Journal of Chinese Medicine, 36*, 37–44.

American Massage Therapy Association. Retrieved January 5, 2005, from http://www.amtamassage.org/about/definition.html

Bilhult, A., Lindhom, C., Gunnarsson, R., & Stener-Victoria, E. (2008) The effect of massage on cellular immunity, endocrine and psychological factors in women with breast cancer—a randomized controlled clinical trial. *Autonomic Neuroscience—Basic and Clinical, 140*, 88–95.

Chang, M. Y., Wang, S. Y., & Chen, C. H. (2002). Effects of massage on pain and anxiety during labour: A randomized controlled trial in Taiwan. *Journal of Advanced Nursing, 38*, 68–73.

Currin, J., & Meister, E. A. (2008). A hospital-based intervention using massage to reduce distress among oncology patients. *Cancer Nursing, 3*, 214–221.

Ernst, E. (2004). Manual therapies for pain control: Chiropractic and massage. *Clinical Journal of Pain, 20,* 8–12.

Ernst, E. (2003). The safety of massage therapy. *Rheumatology, 42,* 1101–1106.

Fellowes, D., Barnes, K., & Wilkinson, S. (2004). Aromatherapy and massage for symptom relief in patients with cancer. *Cochrane Database for Systematic Reviews, 2.*

Field, T. (2002). Preterm infant massage therapy studies: An American approach. *Seminars in Neonatology, 7,* 487–494.

Frey Law, L. A., Evans, S., Kundston, J., Nus, S., Scholl, K., & Sluka, K.A. (2004). Massage reduces pain perception and hyperalgesia in experimental muscle pain: A randomized, controlled trial. *Journal of Pain, 9,* 714–721.

Furlan, A. D., Brosseau, L., Imamura, M., & Irvin, E. (2004). Massage for low-back pain. *Cochrane Database of Systematic Reviews, 2.*

Garner, B., Phillips, L. J., Schmidt, H. M., Markulev, C., O'Connor, J., Wood, S.J., et al. (2008). Pilot study evaluating the effect of massage therapy on stress, anxiety, and aggression in a young adult psychiatric inpatient unit. *Australian & New Zealand Journal of Psychiatry, 45,* 414–422.

Gecsedi, R. A. (2002). Massage therapy for patients with cancer. *Clinical Journal of Oncology Nursing, 6,* 52–54.

Hattan, J., King, L., & Griffiths, P. (2002). The impact of foot massage and guided relaxation following cardiac surgery: A randomized controlled trial. *Journal of Advanced Nursing, 37,* 199–207.

Holland, B., & Pokorny, M. W. (2001). Slow stroke back massage on patients in a rehabilitation setting. *Rehabilitation Nursing, 26,* 182–186.

Kolcaba, K., Schirm, V., & Steiner, R. (2006). Effects of hand massage on comfort of nursing home residents. *Geriatric Nursing, 27,* 85–91.

McNamara, M. E., Burnham, D. C., Smith, C., & Carroll, D. L. (2003). The effects of back massage before diagnostic cardiac catheterization. *Alternative Therapies in Health and Medicine, 9*(1), 50–57.

McRee, L. S., Noble, S., & Pasvogel, A. (2003). Using massage and music therapy to improve postoperative outcomes. *AORN, 78,* 433–440, 445–447.

Mok, E., & Woo, C. P. (2004). The effects of slow-stroke massage on anxiety and shoulder pain in elderly stroke patients. *Complementary Therapies in Nursing & Midwifery, 10,* 209–216.

Richards, K. C. (1998). Effect of a back massage and relaxation intervention on sleep in critically ill patients. *American Journal of Critical Care, 7,* 288–299.

Richards, K. C., Gibson, R., & Overton-McCoy, A. L. (2000). Effects of massage in acute and critical care. *AACN Clinical Issues, 11,* 77–96.

Simmons, D., Chabal, C., Griffith, J., Rausch, M., & Steele, B. (2004). A clinical trial of distraction techniques for pain and anxiety control during cataract surgery. *Insight (American Society of Ophthalmic Registered Nurses), 29*(4), 13–16.

Smith, M. C., Stallings, M. A., Mariner, S., & Burrall, M. (1999). Benefits of massage therapy for hospitalized patients: A descriptive and qualitative evaluation. *Alternative Therapies in Health and Medicine, 5*(4), 64–71.

Snyder, M., Egan, E. C., & Burns, K. R. (1995). Efficacy of hand massage in decreasing agitation behaviors associated with care activities in persons with dementia. *Geriatric Nursing, 16*(2), 60–63.

Tanigaki, S. (2008). Use of Shiatsu with home care patients. Unpublished manuscript.

Wang, H. L., & Keck, J. F. (2004). Foot and hand massage as an intervention for postoperative pain. *Pain Management Nursing, 5,* 59–65.

Williams, A., Selwyn, P., Liberti, L., Molde, S., Njike, V. Y., McCorkle, R., et al. (2005). A randomized controlled trial of meditation and massage effects on quality of life in people with late-stage disease: A pilot study. *Journal of Palliative Medicine, 8,* 939–952.

23 Exercise

DIANE TREAT-JACOBSON
ULF G. BRONÄS
DANIEL L. MARK

Exercise is recognized as a lifelong endeavor essential for energetic, active, and healthy living. Mortality and morbidity are reduced in physically fit individuals, compared with sedentary individuals (Kujala, Kapiro, Sarna, & Koskenvuo, 1998; Paffenbarger et al., 1993; Sherman, D'Agostino, Cobb, & Kannel, 1994). Although the research supporting the benefits of exercise is substantial, it is often overlooked in the conventional practice of Western medicine.

Exercise, either alone or as an alternative or complementary therapy, has been linked to many positive physiological and psychological responses, from reduction in the stress response to an increased sense of well-being (Crews & Landers, 1987; Pender, 1996). Surprisingly, despite the tremendous benefits of exercise, it is an activity largely ignored by the general population. Indeed, the U.S. Surgeon General (1996) issued a report identifying millions of inactive Americans as being at risk for a wide range of chronic diseases and ailments, including coronary heart disease (CHD), adult-onset diabetes, colon cancer, hip fractures, hypertension, and obesity. The U.S. Department of Health and Human Services (USDHHS) publication *Healthy People 2010* (USDHHS, 2000) specified several objectives for improving health, including physical activity and exercise. These include reducing the percentage of adults who do not participate in any physical activity, increasing the percentage of adults who engage in moderate physical activity on most days of the week, and increasing the percentage of adults participating in vigorous exercise, as well as exercises to improve strength and flexibility. There are additional objectives related to physical activity and exercise habits of children and adolescents, including goals to increase participation in daily school physical education classes. The alarmingly low percentage of children participating in physical activity in school and outside of school (<27%) is reportedly contributing to the nation's growing childhood obesity problem (Andersen, Crespo, Bartlett, Cheskin, & Pratt, 1998; McKenzie et al., 1996).

In 2007 the American Heart Association (AHA) and the American College of Sports Medicine (ACSM) issued several updates (Haskell et al., 2007; Nelson et al., 2007; Williams et al., 2007) to the Surgeon General's 1996 guidelines. This was followed in 2008 by a report and revised guidelines from the USDHHS Physical Activity Advisory Committee (DHHS-PAAC, 2008). These updated guidelines are based on new data from several large-scale trials completed since the 1996 report.

It is important to recognize the role of exercise as a component of good health. Exercise *must* be an integral part of one's personal lifestyle if it is to have optimum effects. During the past few decades, there has been an increase in the popularity of non-Western styles of exercise and physical activity, such as *qigong* and the related movements in yoga and *Tai Chi*. These forms of exercise and physical activity also build on meditative moments and, as such, may provide a more enjoyable form of physical activity for older adults than walking exercise.

Maintaining physical fitness should be enjoyable and rewarding for persons of all ages and can contribute significantly to extending longevity and improving quality of life. Nurses' knowledge of exercise and its application in multiple populations will assist in the delivery of expert nursing care. This chapter discusses the definition, physiological basis, and application of exercise as a nursing intervention.

DEFINITION

Physical activity is defined as "any bodily movement produced by skeletal muscles that results in caloric expenditure" (Pender, 1996, p. 185). Definitions of exercise are complex and vary according to scientific discipline; however, they all incorporate physical activity into their descriptions. Exercise is commonly considered to be a planned, recurring subset of physical activity that results in physical fitness, a term used to describe cardiorespiratory fitness, muscle strength, body composition, and flexibility related to the ability of a person to perform physical activity (Thompson et al., 2003).

Exercise is commonly classified according to the rate of energy expenditure, which is expressed in either absolute terms as metabolic equivalents (MET) or in relative terms according to what percentage of maximal heart rate or maximal oxygen consumption is achieved (Astrand, Rodahl, Dahl, & Stromme, 2004; Thompson et al., 2003). Exercise is aerobic when the energy demand by the working muscles is supplied by aerobic ATP (adenosine triphosphate) production as allowed by inspired oxygen and mitochondrial enzymatic capacity (Astrand et al.). In general, aerobic exercise increases demand on the respiratory, cardiovascular, and musculoskeletal systems. Sustained periods of work require aerobic metabolism of energy at a level compatible with the body's oxygen supply capabilities (i.e., oxygen uptake equals oxygen requirements of the tissues). Anaerobic exercise is exercise during which the energy demand exceeds what the body is able to produce through the aerobic process or when the body is performing short bursts of high intensity exercise (Astrand et al.; Kisner & Colby, 1996).

SCIENTIFIC BASIS

Better understanding of exercise physiology and the body's response to various stages of physical activity will assist in the development of exercise programs appropriate for the individual and the goal of the exercise. The response of the body to exercise occurs in stages. The initial response to acute exercise is a withdrawal of parasympathetic stimulation of the heart through the vagal nerve. This results in a rapid increase in heart rate (HR) and cardiac output. The sympathetic stimulation occurs more slowly and becomes a dominant factor once HR is above approximately 100 beats per minute. Sympathetic stimulation is fully completed after approximately 10 to 20 seconds, during which time a large sympathetic outburst occurs and the heart overshoots the rate needed, but then returns to the rate required for increased activity

(Rowell, 1993). The brain stimulates the initial cardiovascular response together with impulses from muscles being exercised, which impulses are sent to the brain; an increase in HR is initiated and the blood flow is shunted toward the exercising muscles (Astrand et al., 2004; Fletcher, 1982; Rowell, 1993). During this phase, there is a sluggish adjustment of respiration and circulation, resulting in an O_2 deficit; the initial energy needed by the exercising tissue is mainly fueled by the anaerobic metabolism of creatine phosphate and anaerobic glycolysis (glucose) (Kisner & Colby, 1996).

As exercise continues, oxygen consumption (VO_2) increases in a linear fashion in relation to the intensity of exercise. The increase in VO_2 is caused by an increase in oxygen extraction by the working muscles and an increase in cardiac output. Oxygen extraction by the working muscle tissues is approximately 80 to 85%, or a three-fold increase from rest, in sedentary and moderately active individuals. This is caused by an increase in the number of open capillaries, thereby reducing diffusion distances and increasing capillary blood volume (Fletcher et al., 2001; Rowell, 1993). Cardiac output is increased to meet the increased O_2 demands of the working muscle. The increase in cardiac output is caused by increased stroke volume, which is due to an increase in ventricular filling pressure brought on by increased venous return and decreased peripheral resistance offered by the exercising muscles. Together with the withdrawal of parasympathetic stimulation and increases in sympathetic stimulation, the increase in HR further accentuates the increase in cardiac output as well as increased myocardial contractibility (from positive inotropic sympathetic impulses to the heart) (Astrand et al., 2004; Fletcher, 1982). In normal individuals, cardiac output can increase 4 to 5 times, allowing for increased delivery of O_2 to exercising muscle beds and facilitating removal of lactate, CO_2, and heat. Respiration increases to deliver O_2 and to allow for elimination of CO_2. Blood pressure increases as a result of increased cardiac output and the sympathetic vasoconstriction of vessels in the nonexercising muscles, viscera, and skin. During this "steady state" exercise phase, O_2 uptake equals O_2 tissue requirement, aerobic metabolism of glucose and fatty acids occurs, and there is no accumulation of lactic acid.

As exercise becomes more strenuous, there is a shift toward anaerobic metabolism of glucose, resulting in increased production of lactic acid (Balady & Weiner, 1992). The anaerobic threshold is a point during exercise at which ventilation abruptly increases despite linear increases in work rate. As exercise goes beyond steady state, the O_2 supply does not meet the oxygen requirement, and energy is provided through anaerobic glycolysis and creatine phosphate breakdown. This increases proton release and phosphate accumulation, increasing acidosis (Robergs, Ghiasvand, & Parker, 2004; Westerblad, Allen, & Lannergren, 2002). Shortly beyond the anaerobic threshold, fatigue and dyspnea ensue and work ceases. This usually coincides with a significant drop in blood glucose levels (Hargraves, 1995). Exercise at a level that allows for aerobic metabolism and reduces the need for anaerobic metabolism and reliance on glucose metabolism as the primary fuel may delay onset of these symptoms.

Following cessation of exercise, there is a period of rapid decline in oxygen uptake followed by a slow decline toward resting levels. This slow phase of oxygen uptake return is termed excess postexercise oxygen consumption. During this period, the body attempts to resynthesize used creatine phosphate, remove lactate, restore muscle and blood oxygen stores, decrease body temperature, return to resting levels of HR and BP, and lower circulating catecholamines (Astrand et al., 2004; Fleg & Lakatta, 1986). It is important to facilitate this phase of exercise by performing a 5- to 10-minute cool-down, as will be discussed below.

INTERVENTION

Healthy People 2010 is a set of objectives for the nation to try to achieve by the year 2010 (www.healthypeople.gov). One of these objectives is to improve health, fitness, and quality of life through daily physical activity. The updated guidelines from the AHA/ACSM and DHHS-PAAC affirm the Surgeon General's 1996 report, specifically stating that exercise is considered to be beneficial to health with a class 1A (highest) evidence base and that physical activity: (a) decreases the risk of premature death; (b) decreases risk of premature death from heart disease; (c) decreases risk of acquiring type 2 diabetes; (d) decreases risk of incurring high blood pressure; (e) decreases high blood pressure in hypertensive individuals; (f) decreases risk of acquiring colon cancer; and (g) decreases feelings of uneasiness and despair. The updated report further confirms that exercise also (h) aids in weight control; (i) helps in the strengthening and maintenance of muscles, joints, and bones; (j) assists older adults with balance and mobility; and (k) fosters feelings of psychological well-being. In addition to these benefits, the AHA/ACSM (Haskell et al., 2007) and the DHHS-PAAC (DHHS-PAAC, 2008) have published scientific statements summarizing evidence confirming physical activity as a significant factor in both primary and secondary prevention of cardiovascular disease. There is a relationship between lack of physical activity and development of coronary artery disease and increased cardiovascular mortality (Haskell et al., 2007; DHHS-PAAC, 2008). Further, there is evidence that persons who engage in regular exercise as part of their recovery postmyocardial infarction have improved rates of survival (Fletcher et al., 1996).

Given that the benefits apply to all age groups across a broad spectrum of health and disease, it is important for nurses to recognize opportunities to promote exercise as a nursing intervention. There are countless activities included under the umbrella of exercise. Finding the activity that fits an individual's capabilities and that meets the purposes for which exercise is prescribed is key to the success of the intervention (Gavin, 1988). When prescribing an intervention, it is important to take into account the recommended exercise intensity for the patient population being served.

Evidence suggests that exercise is more likely to be initiated if the individual: (a) recognizes the need to exercise; (b) perceives the exercise to be beneficial and enjoyable; (c) perceives that the exercise has minimal negative aspects, such as expense, time burden, or negative peer pressure; (d) feels capable and safe engaging in the exercise; and (e) has ready access to the activity and can easily fit it into the daily schedule (DHSS-PAAC, 2008).

Technique

An aerobic exercise session should involve three phases: warming up, aerobic exercise, and cooling down. These phases are designed to allow the body an opportunity to sustain internal equilibrium by gradually adjusting its physiological processes to the stress of exercise and thus maintaining homeostasis. It should be noted that the new guidelines have explicitly stated that, to achieve optimal health benefits, the exercise should be in addition to activities of daily living that are not of moderate intensity or lasting 10 minutes or longer. Further, although resistance training will not be discussed in depth in here, the new guidelines recommend that resistance training should be performed on at least 2 nonconsecutive days per week, and should involve 8 to 10 of the major muscle groups and one set of 8 to 12 repetitions at a resistance that causes significant fatigue (Haskell et al. 2007; DHHS-PAAC, 2008).

Warm-Up Phase

The goal of the warm-up is to allow the body time to adapt to the rigors of aerobic exercise. Warming up results in an increase in muscle temperature, a higher need for oxygen to meet the increased demands of the exercising muscles, dilatation of capillaries resulting in increased circulation, adjustments within the neural respiratory center to the demands of exercise, and a shifting of blood flow centrally from the periphery, resulting in increased venous return (Kisner & Colby, 1996). In addition, a good warm-up increases flexibility and decreases or prevents arrhythmias and ischemic electrocardiographic changes (Kisner & Colby).

Warming-up exercises should be done for 10 minutes, involve all major body parts, and achieve a heart rate within 20 beats per minute of the target HR for the subsequent aerobic exercise (Kisner & Colby). In addition, a good warm-up should incorporate stretching exercises. Stretching exercises are done at a slow, steady pace and help maintain a full range of motion in body joints while strengthening tendons, ligaments, and muscles.

Aerobic Exercise Phase

The aerobic phase of exercise is also known as the stimulus phase. It consists of four essential components: intensity (which is usually measured as the relative percentage of maximal aerobic capacity), frequency, duration, and mode of exercise. The combination of these components determines the effectiveness of the exercise and is known as the activity dose. The mode of exercise should involve rhythmic, continuous movement of large muscle groups, such as walking, jogging, cycling, swimming, or cross-country skiing. The frequency should be 5 days per week, with a duration of at least 30 minutes for health benefits, 60 minutes for prevention of weight gain, and 60 to 90 minutes for aiding in weight loss and preventing weight regain following weight loss. The new guidelines explicitly state that achieving weight loss by exercise alone is difficult and therefore recommends that weight loss regimen should be a combination of calorie restriction and increased physical activity.

The updated guidelines further reaffirm that the duration of exercise is cumulative and can be achieved by exercising 3 times for a minimum of 10 minutes. The intensity can be either moderate or vigorous. If the exercise performed is vigorous, the duration can be shortened to 20 minutes. Moreover, the 2007–2008 guidelines clarify that the moderate and vigorous exercise can be combined to achieve the recommended activity dose per week (for more information, see DHSS-PAAC, 2008). To simplify this concept, the new guidelines recommend using the activity dose of MET x minutes to meet the minimum physical activity recommendations of approximately 500 MET-min per week (450–750 MET-min per week). To find the specific MET that each activity requires, the reader is encouraged to visit the University of South Carolina's Prevention Research Center Web site (http://prevention.sph.sc.edu/tools/compendium.htm). For individual determination of intensity, the HR range can be used. For most individuals, physical fitness improvements may be gained with an intensity of exercise sufficient to achieve 55 to 75% of maximal HR. However, the updated guidelines recommend using the MET-min method for determination of activity dose (Haskell et al. 2007; DHHS-PAAC, 2008).

As physical fitness improves, it may be necessary to increase one of the components to gain additional benefits (Institute of Medicine [IOM] Report, 2005; Haskell et al. 2007; DHHS-PAAC, 2008). It should be emphasized that it is the accumulated amount of daily moderate physical activity and exercise that is important. Although individuals who perform 30 minutes of accumulated moderate physical activity show significant health benefits compared to sedentary individuals, those who perform more than 60 minutes show additional health benefits, including prevention of weight gain. A balance needs to be achieved to obtain maximal benefit with the least risk and discomfort. Adjustment of intensity is important not only for safety reasons, but also for comfort and enjoyment of the activity (Foster & Tamboli, 1992). If exercise can be kept at a comfortable level, the individual is more likely to continue to perform the activity. As tolerance develops, any or all of the exercise components can be increased to meet the individual's aerobic capacity. For example, if an individual is comfortable with the intensity of the exercise, the duration and frequency can be increased to further improve training effect.

Cool-Down

Immediately following the endurance exercises, the person should engage in a cooling-down period. The cool-down allows the body to return to its normal resting state. This allows the HR and BP to return to resting levels and attenuates any postexercise hypotension by improving venous return. The cool-down also improves heat dissipation and elimination of blood lactate and provides a means to combat any potential postexercise rise in catecholamines (Fleg & Lakatta, 1986). Five to 10 minutes are needed for the body to adjust to a slower pace. Cooling-down exercises may include walking slowly, deep breathing, and stretching.

Maintenance

The maintenance phase begins after 6 months of regular training, with the goal of maintaining achieved improvements in physical fitness (DHHS-PAAC, 2008). Maintaining the exercise program is the key to the effectiveness of the intervention. Setting both short- and long-term goals helps improve adherence. The individual can experience a sense of accomplishment upon meeting short-term goals while still striving for overall goals. Keeping a record or graph supplies a visual demonstration of progress and may provide insight into adjustments to the exercise program that may assist in achievement of goals.

Reversibility and Detraining

Once participation in exercise has ceased, there is a rapid return to pre-exercise levels of physical fitness. Most of the rapid decline occurs during the first 5 weeks following cessation of exercise and is usually complete within 12 weeks (Coyle et al., 1984; Saltin et al., 1968). With disuse, the muscle tissues atrophy. Additionally, the decreased caloric expenditure leads to a positive energy balance, which can result in increased accumulation of adipose tissue.

Specific Technique: Walking

One of the strategies identified by *Healthy People 2010* to improve health and quality of life through daily physical activity is an increase in "trips made by walking." Walking has declined rapidly in the United States and has reached the point at which 75% of all trips of 1 mile or less are made by car (U.S. Department of Transportation [DOT], 1994). Walking is an easy and enjoyable activity that has significant health benefits. Moreover, it is an exercise in which persons of all age groups and varying levels of ability can engage to improve endurance. A major advantage is that walking requires no special equipment, facilities, or new skills. It is also safer and easier to maintain than many other forms of exercise. Intensity, duration, and frequency are easily regulated and adjusted to accommodate a wide range of physical capabilities and limitations. The initial intensity should be outlined at the start of the program and is dependent on baseline level of conditioning, physical or disease-related limitations or precautions, and outcome goals.

A walking program can be approached in two ways. The exercise can be completed in one or more daily sessions. For example, a previously sedentary individual may wish to begin an exercise program consisting of 10-minute walks and progressively increase the time or intensity as physical fitness increases. The more traditional alternative is to engage in one longer session at least five times per week; the recommended frequency for optimal benefits is 60 to 90 minutes of enjoyable moderate physical activity five days of the week (Haskell et al. 2007; DHHS-PAAC, 2008). These sessions would include a warm-up session of 5 to 10 minutes, an aerobic period that could start at 10 to 15 minutes and be gradually increased to 30 to 60 to 90 minutes, and a cool-down period of 5 to 10 minutes (Haskell et al.; DHHS-PAAC). Tips for fitness walking are presented in Exhibit 23.1.

Exercising individuals should monitor their body's response to the activity, to ensure that the intensity is appropriate. This can be done in several ways.

Monitor Target Heart Rate

The target HR for a previously sedentary individual should be between 50 and 75% of the maximal HR, which is calculated by subtracting one's age from 220 (AHA, 1995), to gain improvements in physical

Exhibit 23.1

Tips for Fitness Walking

- Warm up by performing a few stretches.
- Think tall as you walk. Stand straight with your head level and your shoulders relaxed.
- Your heel will hit the surface first. Use smooth movements rolling from heel to toe.
- Keep your hands free and let your arms swing naturally in opposition to your legs.
- When you're ready to pick up the pace, quicken your step and lengthen your stride, but don't compromise your upright posture or smooth, comfortable movements.
- To increase your intensity, burn more calories, and tone your upper body, bend your arms at the elbows and pump your arms. Keep your elbows close to your body.
- Breathe in and out naturally, rhythmically, and deeply.
- Use the "Talk Test" to check your intensity, or take your pulse to see if you are within your target heart rate.
- Cool down during the last 3 to 5 minutes by gradually slowing your pace to a stroll.

Source: American Heart Association (1995).

fitness. The HR should be assessed one-third to halfway through the exercise session and immediately after stopping exercise. Exercise intensity can be increased or decreased based on this measurement.

The Talk Test

The talk test can replace target HR monitoring when an individual is exercising at a moderate intensity. If the exercise prevents the individual from talking comfortably, the intensity should be decreased. A variation of this technique is to whistle; if the individual is unable to whistle, the intensity is too great and should be decreased.

Rating of Perceived Exertion

This is a scale that describes the sense of effort during the exercise. This scale can be ranked from 1 to 10, with 1 being no effort and 10 being maximal effort (AHA, 1995).

CONDITIONS/POPULATIONS IN WHICH THE INTERVENTION HAS BEEN USED

Several populations for whom exercise is particularly beneficial include children, the elderly, those with affective disorders, individuals with heart disease, and those with peripheral arterial disease. The application and demonstrated effects of exercise intervention in each of these populations are discussed below.

Overweight Children and Adolescents

The number of overweight children and adolescents is rapidly increasing. Of particular concern are the increasing rates of type 2 diabetes mellitus and metabolic syndrome diagnosed in overweight children and adolescents, problems that used to be primarily limited to adults. Lack of physical activity and excess caloric intake cause central obesity, which, in turn, is believed to promote development of these conditions. Treatment includes dietary modification and initiation of physical activity. Increased physical activity has been shown to improve insulin sensitivity, BP, cholesterol, and vascular function, and prevent further weight gain. The current recommendations are essentially the same as for healthy adults: 60 to 90 minutes of enjoyable, moderate physical activity 5 days a week. An additional goal is to achieve less than 2 hours per day of consecutive sedentary activity, and at least 90 minutes of physical activity to achieve weight loss and prevent weight regain (DHHS-PAAC, 2008).

The Elderly

The fastest growing segment of the population in the United States is individuals over the age of 65. The benefit of exercise as a therapy to prevent or delay functional decline and disease and improve quality of life is demonstrated by the numerous favorable changes occurring in response to exercise. Improvements in cardiovascular function have been shown to help lower risk factors for disease and reduce the need for assisted living (Mazzeo et al., 1998). The elderly are especially prone to the "hazards of immobility" that affect many of the body's systems. Exercise results in increased bone strength (Smith & Reddan, 1976) and increased total body calcium (Dalsky et al., 1988), as well as improved coordination, which may result in a reduction in falls (Bassett, McClam-rock, & Schmelzer, 1982). Exercise has also been shown to improve body functioning and overall well-being. Blumenthal, Schocken, Nee-dles, and Hindle (1982) reported in their study that 40% of the elderly who exercised felt healthier, were more satisfied with life, and had more self-confidence and improved mood.

It is particularly important to "tailor" or customize exercise pro-grams for the elderly, who may have specific limitations. Exercise needs to be initiated at lower levels and increased gradually. The AHA/ACSM guidelines recommend using similar guidelines for persons over the age of 65 as mentioned above, with one important modification—use of the Rating of Perceived Exertion (RPE; 0–10) for determination of intensity instead of MET level. Specifically, a moderate intensity is considered an RPE of 5 to 6 out of 10 and vigorous intensity is considered a 7 to 8 out of 10 (Nelson et al. 2007). Previously sedentary elderly individuals may be more comfortable initiating an exercise program with some supervision, which allows them to become accustomed to this new level of activity in a safe environment. Group exercise may be especially appealing to older persons. The new guidelines recommend that, with the specific inclusion of resistance training 2 (or more) nonconsecutive days/week, using 8 to 10 major muscle groups and 1 set of 10 to 15 repetitions at a moderate intensity as based on the RPE scale (5–6 out of 10). Moreover, the updated guidelines recommend that older individuals should perform flexibility and balance (e.g., dancing) exercises a minimum of 10 minutes, 3 times per week, to prevent age-related loss of range of motion (and, hence, prevent falls) (Nelson et al., 2007; DHHS-PAAC, 2008).

Affective Disorders

Exercise is an effective although underused intervention for individuals with affective disorders. There is considerable evidence supporting the positive effects of exercise in combating depression and anxiety (By-rne & Byrne, 1993). There are fewer, if any, side effects when compared with pharmacotherapy, and exercise is often more cost-effective than psychotherapy and pharmacotherapy (Yaffe, 1981). Although most studies have evaluated the effects of aerobic activity as the intervention, anaerobic activity has also been shown to be beneficial in alleviating depression. This suggests that improvement in mood is associated with exercise in general, rather than increased aerobic capacity (Doyne et al., 1987).

Heart Disease

Cardiac (exercise) rehabilitation is a common intervention prescribed for those with CHD, providing a safe environment for the initiation of an exercise program. Programs usually have several phases and are tailored to the specific needs, limitations, and characteristics of individual patients, helping them resume active and productive lives (Foster & Tamboli, 1992; Hamm & Leon, 1992; Leon et al., 2005). Exercise has multiple protective mechanisms that contribute to reduction of CHD risk, including antiatherosclerotic, antiarrhythmic, anti-ischemic, and antithrombotic effects (Leon et al.).

Exercise training has been shown to improve symptom-limited exercise capacity in CHD patients, primarily as a result of peripheral hemodynamic adaptations (Ferguson et al., 1982; Juneau, Geneau, Marchand, & Brosseau, 1991; Wenger, 1993). Patients with CHD have a low skeletal muscle oxidative capacity, which is significantly improved with training, despite relatively low workloads and exercise intensities, consistent with other non–heart disease populations (Ferguson et al.). Prior to training, patients with CHD are often unable to perform activities of daily living (ADLs) without symptoms. Exercise-trained CHD patients function further above the ischemic threshold in performing ADLs and thus require a lower percentage of maximal effort to perform activities. This increases stamina and endurance and helps to maintain independence (Wenger). Even patients with heart failure, who typically have very poor cardiac function, have found that cardiac rehabilitation improves their exercise tolerance (Koch, Douard, & Broustet, 1992; Sullivan, 1994).

Peripheral Arterial Disease

Peripheral arterial disease (PAD), a prevalent atherosclerotic occlusive disease, limits functional capacity and is related to decreased quality of life. Individuals with PAD typically experience exercise-induced ischemic pain in the lower extremities, known as claudication. Exercise training is one of the most effective interventions available for the treatment of claudication due to PAD (Hiatt, Regensteiner, Hargarten, Wolfel, & Brass, 1990; Regensteiner, Steiner, & Hiatt, 1996). Exercise training has been shown to improve walking distance up to 180% (Regensteiner, 1997; Regensteiner & Hiatt, 1995). Prior to program initiation, an exercise prescription should be generated based on a graded exercise test and patients should start training at 50% of their functional capacity (Ekers & Hirsch, 1999). During a typical session, patients will exercise at a moderate pace until they experience moderate-to-severe claudication. At that point they will rest until the pain subsides. This exercise/rest pattern is repeated throughout the exercise session (Hiatt et al.). The most effective exercise programs for the treatment of claudication include the following components: the patient should exercise to the point of almost maximal claudication; the exercise session should be at least 30 minutes in length, with at least 3 sessions per week; and the exercise program should continue for at least 6 months, with intermittent walking as the most effective mode of exercise (Gardner & Poehlman, 1995).

Measurement of Effectiveness

The appropriate measure of the effectiveness of an exercise intervention depends on the specific exercise prescribed and the goals of the intervention. Changes in atherosclerotic risk factors (i.e., cholesterol levels, triglycerides, insulin sensitivity, waist circumference, BP, and body mass index) may be measured if cardiovascular health is the primary outcome of the exercise program. If cardiovascular fitness is the targeted outcome, an aerobic exercise program would be prescribed and improvements in the cardiovascular system such as increased cardiac output, VO_2, and improved local circulation would be used to determine the effectiveness of the intervention (Fletcher et al., 2001; Halfman & Hojnacki, 1981). Cardiovascular response to submaximal exercise may provide further information and may be even more beneficial in assessing the impact on quality of life, as most ADLs are performed at submaximal intensity. Exercise prescribed to improve function may use parameters such as improved joint mobility, prevention or reduction of osteoporosis, and improved strength in determining exercise effectiveness (Benison & Hogstel, 1986).

Assessment may also include changes in physical functioning and disability, ability to perform ADLs, changes in symptoms and activity tolerance, and other variables that reflect the individual's ability to function in daily life. Lower intensity programs, which may not demonstrate great changes in maximal exercise capacity, might produce sufficient changes in these outcome variables to make a difference in the individual's quality of life. Such programs would be especially appropriate in elderly and very sedentary individuals, where low intensity exercise can produce a modest increase in fitness and more significant improvements in function (Belman & Gaesser, 1991; Foster, Hume, Byrnes, Dickenson, & Chatfield, 1989). Development and implementation of programs designed to meet the specific needs of patients can help maximize functional and quality-of-life outcomes.

Precautions

Before initiating an exercise program, preparticipation screening procedures are recommended. These include such questionnaires as the Physical Activity Readiness Questionnaire (PAR-Q), designed to identify potential patients in need of medical advice prior to exercising (Canadian Society for Exercise Physiology, 1994). If a patient is identified as having potential or actual medical concerns, it is advisable that a graded exercise test be performed. The American College of Sports Medicine recommends that a graded exercise test be performed for any individual with more than two risk factors for CHD. This is done to rule out any potential contraindications to exercise and to provide a tool for determining initial exercise intensity (ACSM, 2006; Fletcher et al., 2001).

To avoid injury, it is important to begin an exercise program slowly, to follow safety guidelines, and to exercise consistently, several times per week. Potential exercise-related injuries include muscle and joint pain, cramps, blisters, shin splints, low back pain, tendonitis, and other sprains or muscle strains. The most commonly reported adverse event of exercise is musculoskeletal injury; approximately 25% of adults between 20 and 85 years of age reported an injury occurring at least once during 1 year (Hootman et al., 2002). It is possible that some of these are misclassified as injuries instead of muscle soreness due to a rapid increase in volume or intensity of training without proper knowledge of the principles of training.

The AHA (1995) has listed general guidelines to help ensure exercise safety. These include: (a) stretching the muscles and tendons prior to beginning exercise; (b) wearing appropriate footwear; (c) exercising on a surface with some "give" to it, especially during high-impact activities; and (d) learning the exercise properly and continuing good form even with increased speed or intensity. Should exercise-related injuries occur, they can usually be treated with one or a combination of therapies, including rest, ice, compression, and elevation (AHA).

Previously sedentary elderly individuals and those with chronic disease, especially heart disease, should consult a physician prior to initiating an exercise program, to ensure that an appropriate exercise prescription is given. The warning signs of heart disease should be spelled out prior to initiation of an exercise program, especially to those in high-risk categories.

CULTURAL APPLICATIONS

The benefits of exercise and physical activity appear to be equal across gender and race, however this topic remains poorly studied and recommendations are primarily based on assumptions that findings in one population will carry over to another population. It should be mentioned that there exist cultural preferences, including religious and ethnic preferences, in the use of exercise and physical activity. Although there has been little systematic investigation regarding these preferences, their potential influence should be considered when prescribing exercise and physical activity. For example, with certain ethnicities, it may be beneficial to modify an exercise program to allow exercise with a garment that covers the body.

The use of alternate exercise techniques has gained popularity during the past few decades, especially among older adults. These forms of physical activity include meditative forms of movement in the practice of *qigong* and its specific forms such as *tai chi* and yoga (discussed in separate chapters in this book). Within these alternate forms of physical activity, numerous styles and movements have been reported, but the overarching theme of this form of physical activity remains the same. Although the evidence base for this type of exercise is less than for structured Western-style exercise (e.g., walking), it appears that these alternate forms of physical activity may provide health benefits, especially in improving balance and lowering fear of falling. However, it should be noted that most reported studies have been small and have employed a large variation of these techniques.

Other cultures have also been able to incorporate daily physical activity as part of their usual routine either by necessity or by choice. For example, European countries have facilitated walking and cycling as modes of transportation by incorporating walkways and bicycle lanes in city planning. It should be noted here that these forms of transportation are also culturally accepted as the primary modes of transportation, whereas in the USA this is commonly not the case. There is a clear need for future city planning to incorporate safe, accessible, and enjoyable walkways and bicycle lanes for the American population to be able to incorporate daily physical activity in their lives and gain the health benefits associated with increased physical activity levels. This will help change the cultural perspective of physical activity in the USA and support walking and/or bicycling as a preferred mode of transportation.

AREAS IN WHICH FUTURE RESEARCH IS NEEDED

There are many gaps in our knowledge related to exercise, its measurement, the benefits, and methods to improve exercise adherence. Specific areas of needed research include:

- Development of measures of exercise behavior that are valid and reliable in different populations and with various levels of activity
- Investigations of cultural and ethnic differences in physical activity and response to exercise
- Investigations of the benefit of exercise in persons with disabilities, including mental and physical disabilities
- Development and testing of specific interventions to increase exercise adherence in multiple populations
- Assessment of the impact of exercise interventions in multiple populations through controlled longitudinal studies
- Development of strategies to increase lifelong physical activity and exercise

SELECTED EXERCISE INFORMATION WEB SITES

General Guidelines and Information

- U.S. Department of Health and Human Services, Physical Activity Guidelines: http://www.health.gov/paguidelines

- President's Council on Physical Fitness and Sports: http://www.fitness.gov
- Centers for Disease Control and Prevention (CDC): http://www.cdc.gov/physicalactivity
- U.S. Department of Agriculture, Center for Nutrition Policy and Promotion: http://www.mypyramid.gov/pyramid/physical_activity.html

Guidelines and Information Pertaining to Individuals and Families

- CDC, Preventing Falls Among Older Adults: http://www.cdc.gov/ncipc/duip/preventadultfalls.htm—promotes physical activity as part of the approach to reducing falls and fall-related injuries among older adults.
- National Institutes of Health: http://nihseniorhealth.gov/exercise/toc.html
- Exercise and Physical Activity: Your Everyday Guide from the National Institute on Aging: http://www.nia.nih.gov/HealthInformation/Publications/ExerciseGuide.
- Office of the Surgeon General: http://www.surgeongeneral.gov/obesityprevention/index.html
- President's Council on Physical Fitness and Sports: http://www.presidentschallenge.org
- President's Council on Physical Fitness and Sports: http://www.fitness.gov

Schools

- CDC, Division of Adolescent and School Health: http://www.cdc.gov/HealthyYouth/physicalactivity

Communities

- Administration on Aging: http://www.aoa.gov
- CDC, Division of Nutrition, Physical Activity, and Obesity: http://www.cdc.gov/nccdphp/dnpa/physical/index.htm
- Federal Highway Administration: http://www.fhwa.dot.gov/environment/bikeped/index.htm

- Environmental Protection Agency: http://www.epa.gov/aging/bhc/index.htm
- National Institutes of Health: http://www.nhlbi.nih.gov/health/public/heart/obesity/wecan
- National Park Service: http://www.nps.gov/ncrc/programs/rtca/helpfultools/ht_publication s.html

Health Care

- U.S. Preventive Services Task Force—counseling recommendations about promoting physical activity, focused on behavioral counseling services delivered in primary care practices: http://www.ahrq.gov/clinic/uspstf/uspsphys.htm

Worksites

- CDC, Healthier Worksite Initiative: http://www.cdc.gov/nccdphp/dnpa/hwi/index.htm

REFERENCES

American College of Sports Medicine. (2006). *Guidelines for graded exercise testing and exercise prescription* (7th ed.) Baltimore, MD: Lippincott, Williams & Willkins.

American Heart Association. (1995). *Your heart: An owner's manual.* Englewood Cliffs, NJ: Prentice Hall.

Andersen, R. E., Crespo, C. J., Bartlett, S. J., Cheskin, L. J., & Pratt, M. (1998). Relationship of physical activity and television watching with body weight and level of fatness among children: Results from the Third National Health and Nutrition Examination Survey. *Journal of the American Medical Association, 279,* 938–942.

Astrand, P., Rodahl, K., Dahl, K., & Stromme, B. (2004). *Textbook of work physiology* (4th ed.). Champaign, IL: Human Kinetics.

Balady, G., & Weiner, D. (1992). Physiology of exercise in normal individuals and patients with coronary heart disease. In N. Wenger & H. Hellerstein (Eds.), *Rehabilitation of the coronary patient* (pp. 103–122). New York: Churchill Livingstone.

Bassett, C., McClamrock, E., & Schmelzer, M. (1982). A 10-week exercise program for senior citizens. *Geriatric Nursing, 3,* 103–105.

Belman, M., & Gaesser, G. (1991). Exercise training below and above the lactate threshold in the elderly. *Medicine and Science in Sports and Exercise, 23,* 562–568.

Benison, B., & Hogstel, M. O. (1986). Aging and movement therapy: Essential interventions for the immobile elderly. *Journal of Gerontological Nursing, 12*(12), 8–16.

Blumenthal, J., Schocken, D., Needles, T., & Hindle, P. (1982). Psychological and physiological effects of physical conditioning on the elderly. *Journal of Psychosomatic Medicine 26*, 505–510.

Byrne, A., & Byrne, D. G. (1993). The effect of exercise on depression, anxiety and other mood states: A review. *Journal of Psychosomatic Research, 37*, 565–574.

Canadian Society for Exercise Physiology. (1994). *PAR-Q and you: A questionnaire for people aged 15 to 69*. Ottawa, ON: Health Canada.

Coyle, E. F., Martin, W. H., Sincacore, D. R., Joyner, M. J., Hagberg, J. M., & Holloszy, J. O. (1984). Time course of loss of adaptation after stopping prolonged intense endurance training. *Journal of Applied Physiology, 57*, 1857–1864.

Crews, D., & Landers, D. (1987). A meta-analytic review of aerobic fitness and reactivity to psychosocial stressors. *Medicine and Science in Sports and Exercise, 19*(Suppl.), S114–S120.

Dalsky, O., Stocke, K., Ehsani, A., Slatopolsky, E., Lee, W., & Birge, S. (1988). Weight-bearing exercise training and lumbar bone mineral content in post-menopausal women. *Annals of Internal Medicine, 108*, 824–829.

Doyne, E. J., Osip-Klein, D. J., Bowman, E. D., Osborn, K. M., McDougall-Wilson, I. B., & Neimeyer, R. A. (1987). Running versus weight-lifting in the treatment of depression. *Journal of Consulting and Clinical Psychology, 55*(5), 748–754.

Ekers, M. A., & Hirsch, A. T. (1999). Vascular medicine and vascular rehabilitation. In V. Fahey (Ed.), *Vascular nursing* (3rd ed., pp. 188–211). Philadelphia: Saunders.

Ferguson, R., Taylor, A., Cote, P., Charlebois, J., Dinelle, Y., Perionnet, F., et al. (1982). Skeletal muscle and cardiac changes with training in patients with angina pectoris. *American Journal of Physiology, 243*, H830–H836.

Fleg, J., & Lakatta, E. (1986). Prevalence and significance of post exercise hypotension in apparently healthy subjects. *American Journal of Cardiology, 57*(15), 1380–1384.

Fletcher, G. (1982). *Exercise in the practice of medicine*. Mount Kisco, NY: Futura.

Fletcher, G. F., Balady, G. J., Amsterdam, E. A., Chaitman, B., Eckel, R., Fleg, J., et al. (2001). Exercise standards for testing and training: A statement for healthcare professionals from the American Heart Association. *Circulation, 104*, 1694–1740.

Fletcher, G. F., Balady, G., Blair, S., Blumenthal, J., Casperson, C., Chairman, B., et al. (1996). Statement on exercise: Benefits and recommendations for physical activity programs for all Americans. *American Heart Association Scientific Statement*. Retrieved February 3, 2009, from http//www.americanheart.org/Scientific/ statements/1996/ 0815_exp.html

Foster, C., & Tamboli, H. (1992). Exercise prescription in the rehabilitation of patients following coronary artery bypass graft surgery and coronary angioplasty. In R. Shephard & H. Miller (Eds.), *Exercise and the heart in health and disease* (pp. 283–298). New York: Marcel Dekker.

Foster, V., Hume, G., Byrnes, W., Dickenson, A., & Chatfield, S. (1989). Endurance training for elderly women: Moderate vs. low intensity. *Journal of Gerontology, 44*(6), M184–M178.

Gardner, A. W., & Poehlman, E. T. (1995). Exercise rehabilitation programs for the treatment of claudication pain: A meta-analysis. *Journal of the American Medical Association, 274*(12), 975–980.

Gavin, J. (1988). Psychological issues in exercise prescription. *Sports Medicine, 6*, 1–10.

Halfman, M., & Hojnacki, L. (1981). Exercise and the maintenance of health. *Topics in Clinical Nursing, 3*(2), 1–10.

Hamm, L., & Leon, A. (1992). Exercise training for the coronary patient. In N. Wenger & H. Hellerstein (Eds.), *Rehabilitation of the coronary patient* (pp. 367–402). New York: Churchill Livingstone.

Haskell, W. L., Lee, I. M., Pate, R. R., Powell, K. E., Blair, S. N., Franklin, B. A., et al. (2007). Physical activity and public health: Updated recommendation for adults from the American College of Sports Medicine and the American Heart Association. *Circulation, 116*, 1081–1093.

Hargraves, M. (1995). Exercise metabolism. In M. Hargraves (Ed.), *Exercise metabolism* (pp. 41–73). Champaign, IL: Human Kinetics.

Hiatt, W. R., Regensteiner, J. G., Hargarten, M. E., Wolfel, E. E., & Brass, E. P. (1990). Benefit of exercise conditioning for patients with peripheral arterial disease. *Circulation, 81*(2), 602–609.

Hootman, J. M., Macera, C. A., Ainsworth, B. E., Addy, C. L., Martin, M., & Blair, S. N. (2002). Epidemiology of musculoskeletal injuries among sedentary and physically active adults. *Medicine and Science in Sports and Exercise, 34*(5), 838–844.

Institute of Medicine Report. (2005). Retrieved February 3, 2009, from www.iom.edu/report. asp?id=4340

Juneau, M., Geneau, S., Marchand, C., & Brosseau, R. (1991). Cardiac rehabilitation after coronary artery bypass surgery. *Cardiovascular Clinics, 12*(2), 25–42.

Kisner, C., & Colby, L. (1996). *Therapeutic exercise: Foundations and techniques* (3rd ed.). Philadelphia: Davis.

Koch, M., Douard, H., & Broustet, J-P. (1992). The benefit of graded physical exercise in chronic heart failure. *Chest, 101*(5 Suppl.), 231S–235S.

Kujala, U. M., Kapiro, J., Sarna, S., & Koskenvuo, M. (1998). Relationship of leisure-time physical activity and mortality: The Finnish twin cohort. *Journal of the American Medical Association, 279*(6), 440–444.

Leon, A. S., Franklin, B. A., Costa, F., Balady, G. J., Berra, K. A., Stewart, K. J., et al. (2005). Cardiac rehabilitation and secondary prevention of coronary heart disease. *Circulation, 111*, 369–376.

Mazzeo, R. S., Cavanagh, P., Evans, W. J., Evans, W. J., Fiatarone, M., Hagberg, J., et al. (1998). Exercise and physical activity for older adults: American College of Sports Medicine position stand. *Medicine and Science in Sports and Exercise, 30*(6), 992–1008.

McKenzie, T. L., Nader, P. R., Strikmiller, P. K., Yang, M., Stone, E. J., Perry, C. L., et al. (1996). School physical education: Effect of the child and adolescent trial for cardiovascular health. *Preventive Medicine, 25*(4), 423–431.

Nelson, M. E., Rejeski, J. E., Blair, S. N., Duncan, P. W., Judge, J. O., King, A. C., et al. (2007). Physical activity and public health in older adults: Recommendation from the American College of Sports Medicine and the American Heart Association. *Circulation, 116*, 1094–1105.

Paffenbarger, R. S., Hyde, R. T., Wing, A. L., Lee, I. M., Jung, D. L., & Kampert, J. B. (1993). The association of changes in physical activity level and other lifestyle characteristics with mortality among men. *New England Journal of Medicine, 328*(8), 538–545.

Pender, N. (1996). *Health promotion in nursing practice* (3rd ed.). Stamford, CT: Appleton & Lange.

Regensteiner, J. G. (1997). Exercise in the treatment of claudication: Assessment and treatment of functional impairment. *Vascular Medicine, 2*(3), 238–242.

Regensteiner, J. G., & Hiatt, W. R. (1995). Exercise rehabilitation for patients with peripheral arterial disease. *Exercise and Sport Sciences Reviews, 23,* 1–24.

Regensteiner, J. G., Steiner, J. F., & Hiatt, W. R. (1996). Exercise training improves functional status in patients with peripheral arterial disease. *Journal of Vascular Surgery, 23*(1), 104–115.

Robergs, R., Ghiasvand, F., & Parker D. (2004). Biochemistry of exercise-induced metabolic acidosis. *American Journal of Physiology. Regulatory, Integrative, and Comparative Physiology, 287,* R502–R516.

Rowell, L. (1993). *Human cardiovascular control.* New York: Oxford University Press.

Saltin, B., Blomqvist, G., Mitchell, J. H., Johnson, R. L., Wildenthal, K., & Chapman, C. B. (1968). Response to exercise after bed rest and after training. *Circulation, 38*(Suppl. 5), VII1–VII78.

Sherman, S. D., D'Agostino, R. B., Cobb, J. L., & Kannel, W. B. (1994). Physical activity and mortality in women in the Framingham Heart Study. *American Heart Journal, 128*(5), 879–884.

Smith, E., & Reddan, W. (1976). Physical activity—a modality for bone accretion in the aged. *American Journal of Roentgenology, 126,* 1297.

Sullivan, M. (1994). New trends in cardiac rehabilitation in patients with chronic heart failure. *Progress in Cardiovascular Nursing, 9*(1), 13–21.

Thompson, P. D., Buchner, D., Pina, I. L., Balady, G. J., Williams, M. A., Marcus, B. H., et al. (2003). Exercise and physical activity in the prevention and treatment of atherosclerotic cardiovascular disease: American Heart Association scientific statement. *Circulation, 107,* 3109–3116.

U.S. Department of Health and Human Services. (2000, November). *Healthy people 2010: Understanding and improving public health* (2nd ed.). Washington, DC: U.S. Government Printing Office. [Available online at: http://www.healthypeople.gov/Publications/]

U.S. Department of Health and Human Services, Physical Activity Advisory Committee. (2008). *Physical Activity Guidelines Advisory Committee Report, 2008.* Washington, DC: USDHHS/PAAC. [Available online at: http://www.health.gov/paguidelines/guidelines/default.aspx]

U.S. Department of Transportation. (1994). *National bicycling and walking study: Transportation choices for a changing America* (Pub. FH10A PD 94-023). Washington, DC: Federal Highway Administration.

U.S. Surgeon General. (1996). *Report on physical activity and health.* Retrieved February 3, 2009, from http://www.cde.800/nccdphd/sgr/mm.htm

Wenger, N. (1993). Modern coronary rehabilitation: New concepts in care. *Postgraduate Medicine, 94*(2), 131–141.

Westerblad, H., Allen, D., & Lannergren, J. (2002). Muscle fatigue: Lactic acid or inorganic phosphate the major cause? *News in Physiological Science, 17,* 17–21.

Williams, M. A., Haskell, W. L., Ades, P. A., Amsterdam, E. A., Bittner, V., Franklin, B. A., et al. (2007). Resistance exercise in individuals with and without cardiovascular disease: 2007 update: A scientific statement from the American Heart Association Council on Clinical Cardiology and council on Nutrition Physical Acivity, and Metabolism. *Circulation, 116,* 572–584.

Yaffe, M. (1981). Sport and mental health. *Journal of Biosocial Science Supplement, 7,* 83–95.

24

Tai Chi

KUEI-MIN CHEN

Because of the pressures of work, many people do not get proper exercise, which may lead to mental strain, nervous breakdown, or inefficiency in their daily work (Cheng, 1994). Good health is essential and how to acquire and maintain a strong mind and body is a vital concern. It is commonly recognized that proper physical exercise is an excellent method for keeping a person's entire being fit and healthy. However, it is not easy to find an exercise that suits people of all ages (Cheng).

Tai Chi is one intervention that is receiving increasing attention in many professions: nurses, physicians, occupational therapists, physical therapists, and recreational therapists. It is a manipulative and body-based therapy that can heighten individuals' awareness of their bodies and take advantage of their body structure for expressing feelings and ideas. Gradually, individuals become more aware of their total being, and harmony is enhanced.

DEFINITION

Tai Chi, which means "supreme ultimate," is a traditional Chinese martial art (Koh, 1981) and a mind–body exercise. It involves a series of fluid, continuous, graceful, dance-like postures and the performance of movements known as forms (Smalheiser, 1984). The graceful body movements engage continuous body and trunk rotation, flexion/extension of the hips and knees, postural alignment, and the coordination of the arms, which are integrated by mind concentration, the balanced shifting of body weight, muscle relaxation, and breath control. They are performed in a slow, rhythmic, and well-controlled manner (Plummer, 1983).

There are several styles of Tai Chi that are currently practiced: Chen (quick and slow large movements), Yang (slow large movements), Wu (mid-paced, compact movements), and Sun (quick, compact movements) (Jou, 1983). Each style has a characteristic protocol that differs from the other styles in the postures or forms included, the order in which they appear, the pace at which movements are executed, and the level of difficulty; yet, the basic principles are the same (Yang, 1991). For example, one significant difference between Chen and Yang styles is that Yang movements are relaxed, evenly paced, and graceful. It is the most popular Tai Chi practiced by older adults (Jou). In comparison, the Chen style is characterized by alternating slow, gentle movements with quick and vigorous ones, and restrained and controlled actions, which reflect a more martial origin (Yang). Most Tai Chi movements were named after animals, such as "white crane spreads its wings" and "grasp the bird's tail" (Koh, 1981).

There are a few simplified forms of the ancient Tai Chi. For example, the Simplified Tai-Chi Exercise Program (STEP), developed by Chen, Chen, and Huang (2006), encompasses three phases: warm-up, Tai Chi exercises, and cool-down. In the warm-up phase, nine exercises are designed to loosen the body from head to toe; the second phase includes 12 easy-to-learn and easy-to-perform Tai Chi movements; three activities during the cool-down phase help the body to return to a pre-intervention state of rest. STEP differs from traditional Tai Chi styles in that it incorporates fewer leg movements, fewer knee bends, and less complicated hand gestures. It was specifically designed for older adults suffering from chronic illness (Chen, Chen, & Huang).

SCIENTIFIC BASIS

Tai Chi practice is closely linked to Chinese medical theory, in which the vital life energy, *chi* (or *qi*), is thought to circulate throughout the body in discrete channels called meridians. Using correct postures and adequate relaxation, the principle of Tai Chi is to promote the free flow of *chi* throughout the body, which improves the health of an individual. The movements of Tai Chi are regulated by the timing of deep breathing and the movement of the diaphragm. It offers a balanced exercise to the muscles and joints of various parts of the body (Cheng, 1994). In addition, a peaceful state of mind and spiritual dedication to each movement during the exercise ensure that the central nervous system is given sufficient training and is consequently toned up with time as the exercise continues. A strong central nervous system is the basic condition of a healthy body and the various organs depend largely on the soundness of the central nervous system (Cheng).

INTERVENTION

In Eastern countries such as Taiwan, it is common and popular for older adults to practice Tai Chi as a group in the early morning in parks or on the athletic grounds of elementary schools. Tai Chi practice groups are usually led by masters who are pleased to share its essence with others. People who are interested in Tai Chi are welcome to join the groups and learn the movements from these masters. In Western countries, there is a growing interest in the practice of Tai Chi. Various Tai Chi clubs are available to the public through community centers, health clinics, or private organizations. General information is widespread through Web sites, books, and videos. Tai Chi is a convenient exercise that can be practiced in any place, at any time, and without any equipment.

Techniques

As mentioned earlier, although various styles of Tai Chi are currently practiced, the underlying practice principles are the same. In Schaller's study (1996), five essential principles of movement were identified:

- Hand and leg movement should be synchronous.
- The emphasis should be on a soft, relaxed rather than a hard, tense position.
- Moves should be practiced with a quiet and open mind.

- The soles of the feet should be rooted to the ground with the knees bent in a low stance and the primary focus of awareness within the lower abdomen.
- The physical force should be rooted in the feet, passed up through the legs as weight is shifted, and distributed by the pivoting of the waist.

In the physical performance, an individual must relax and think of nothing else before starting. The movements should be slow and rhythmic with natural breathing. Every action becomes easy and smooth, the waist turns freely, and the feelings of comfort and relaxation are gradually developed (Cheng, 1994). In its spiritual aspect, Tai Chi is an exercise that produces harmony of body and mind. Each movement should be guided by thought instead of physical strength. For instance, to lift up the hands, an individual must first have the necessary mental concentration, and then the hands can be raised slowly in a proper manner. Hence, the breathing will become deeper and the body will be strengthened (Cheng).

Guidelines for Use

The steps for performing the movement called "around the platter" are presented in Exhibit 24.1.

Various videotapes on Tai Chi are also available through local video rental stores. The following books and/or DVDs are useful for learning Tai Chi:

- *Sunset Tai Chi* (Rones, 2007) demonstrates practical approach to Tai Chi that can correct stress-related illness.
- *Complete Book of Tai Chi* (Kit, 2002) provides information about Tai Chi and its various forms.
- *Tai Chi for Beginners and the 24 Forms* (Lam & Kaye, 2006) is both a book and a companion DVD that provides information and visual guides to performing Tai Chi forms. The authors also publish books specific to the use of Tai Chi in persons with a variety of disease conditions.
- *Tai Chi: Transcendent Art* (Cheng, 1994) demonstrates each Tai Chi movement through pictures and graphs.

Exhibit 24.1

Procedure for Performing "Around the Platter"

1. Hands are held at chest level, wrists slightly bent and elbows close to sides. Fingers are spread apart. Legs are slightly apart and bent with the left in front of the right. Weight is equally distributed between legs.
2. Begin to rock forward, shifting weight to the left leg with hands moving to the left. (Imagine a round platter at the chest level, and the hands circling around the platter from left to right.)
3. As most of the weight shifts to the left leg and the hands are directly in front of the body, the left heel comes off the ground. As the hands move right of midline, the weight begins to shift to the right leg. When the hands have completed a full circle (held at chest level), most of the weight is on the right leg and the right toe is off the ground.
4. This movement can be repeated 6–9 times and then repeated again going from right to left.

Note: Adapted from Stone (1994).

Additional information can be found through the following useful Web links:

- www.supply.com/lee/tcclinks.html—provides links to more than a hundred other Web sites on Tai Chi and related topics
- http://sunflower.signet.com.sg/~limttk/index.htm—is a valuable site with complete historical and background information on Tai Chi

Measurement of Outcomes

According to Plummer (1983), mind concentration and breathing control are two of the major tenets of Tai Chi practice. When practicing Tai Chi with a peaceful, focused mind and incorporating smooth breathing into each movement, a person will experience physical and psychological relaxation, which leads to enhanced well-being, both physically and psychologically (Plummer). With this conceptual framework in mind, the measurement of the effects of Tai Chi could be for both physical and psychological well-being. Based on the literature, which will be discussed in detail later, more studies were done to measure the physical outcomes of Tai Chi practice (such as cardiovascular func-

Exhibit 24.2

Selecting a Tai Chi Class

1. If possible, find a studio or organization that specializes in Tai Chi.
2. Find an experienced teacher (6–10 years of experience) who demonstrates and verbally explains the movements. Ask to observe a class before joining.
3. Find a class with fewer than 20 students.
4. Avoid purchasing any special clothing or equipment.

Note: Adapted from Downs (1992).

tioning) with little emphasis on psychological well-being outcomes (such as mood states).

Precautions for Use

Tai Chi is unique for its slow graceful movements with low impact, low velocity, and minimal orthopedic complications and is a suitable conditioning exercise for older adults (Chen, Yen, Fetzer, Lo, & Lam, 2008). Although many research studies have shown the benefits of Tai Chi, there are some contraindications to its practice, such as an acute stage of angina, ventricular arrhythmia, or myocardial ischemia. The instructor and the learner have to be aware of those contraindications and an initial assessment is necessary to determine an individual's exercise tolerance and other limitations (Forge, 1997). While learning Tai Chi, a novice should be periodically evaluated in terms of progress, program adherence, cognitive response, muscular strength, balance, and level of flexibility at fairly regular (e.g., 4-week) intervals for the first 60 to 90 days of participation in such a program and, if progress is considered satisfactory, at 6-month intervals thereafter (Forge). It is strongly recommended that one learn Tai Chi from an experienced master who is able to teach the movements based on individual needs and physical tolerance. Recommendations for choosing a class are found in Exhibit 24.2.

USES

Tai Chi is especially appropriate for older adults or for patients with chronic diseases because of its low intensity, steady rhythm, and low physical and mental tension (Xu & Fan, 1988). It has been shown to enhance cardiovascular and respiratory functions, improve health-related fitness, and promote positive health status (Lan, Lai, Chen, & Wong, 1998). In addition, practicing Tai Chi has been effective in lowering blood pressure (Thornton, Sykes, & Tang, 2004; Tsai et al., 2003; Wolf, Barnhart, Kutner, McNeely, Coogler, & Xu, 2003). Studies also indicated that Tai Chi increases postural stability, enhances balance (Chen, Lin, et al., 2008; Thornton et al., 2004; Tsang & Hui-Chan, 2004), and improves muscle strength and endurance (Chen, Lin, et al., 2008), which leads to a reduction in the risk of falls (Hainsworth, 2004). Tai Chi also plays an important role in symptom control of chronic illnesses such as osteoarthritis (Chen, Yen, et al., 2008). Chen and Yen (2002) summarized experimental studies on the effects of Tai Chi on symptom control in patients with various chronic illnesses. Most results indicated that Tai Chi was beneficial for cardiovascular diseases, arthritis, chronic obstructive pulmonary disease, and low back pain. In addition, studies have indicated that Tai Chi practice may also provide psychological benefits, such as enhanced positive mood states (Chen, Snyder, & Krichbaum, 2001) and quality of sleep (Chen, Li, et al., 2007; Li et al., 2004). Researchers have suggested that Tai Chi could be incorporated into community programs or senior center activities to promote the well-being of community-dwelling elders. It could also be included as one of the activities in nursing homes or in rehabilitation programs in hospital settings (Chen, Hsu, Chen, Tseng, 2007; Hung & Chen, 2007).

CULTURAL ASPECTS

Tai Chi is based on the Eastern philosophy of *qi*. Tai Chi is taught and practiced in the West. Two quite distinct applications of its use in the West include "*Chi*-running" and "*Chi*-walking." Dreyer and Dreyer (2004) detail how applying the principles of Tai Chi to running results in fewer injuries and more enjoyment. The four principles underlying its application to running are:

- Find your center in your body.
- Sense your center in your feelings.

- See your center in your mind.
- Be centered in your spirit (Dreyer & Dreyer, p. 34).

Movement and effort are balanced in six directions: left to right, up to down, and front to back. The same principles that apply to forms in Tai Chi are applied. For example, as the front of the body moves forward, the complement moves to the back.

After applying the principles of Tai Chi to running, Dreyer and Dreyer focused on their use in the most commonly used exercise: walking. The key elements are aligning shoulders, hips, and ankles in a vertical line; engaging the body core by leveling the pelvis and leading with the upper body; creating balance throughout the body during the walk; selecting the focus for mindful practice; and, eventually, using the principles during the entire walk (Dreyer & Dreyer, 2006).

For the fast-paced Western lifestyle, applying the principles of Tai Chi to two very active forms of exercise will require practice. For persons desiring more healthy and holistic outcomes from running or walking, *Chi*-walking or *Chi*-running may provide the benefit desired.

FUTURE RESEARCH

Overall, practicing Tai Chi appropriately has various benefits, as evidenced in the literature, and it is highly recommended for the appropriate populations. More studies about the effects of Tai Chi from a nursing perspective are needed in order to provide guidance to nurses in its use with various populations (Chen & Snyder, 1999). Some questions for further research include:

1. Which populations, especially children, can most benefit from practicing Tai Chi and are there conditions that would preclude its use?
2. What is the nature of stability or change in the well-being status of elders who practice Tai Chi?
3. What are the differences on well-being outcomes of beginners (people who are just starting to learn Tai Chi movements), practitioners (people who have practiced Tai Chi regularly for more than a year), and masters (people who have practiced Tai

Chi regularly for more than a decade and are licensed by the National Tai Chi Association to be instructors)?

REFERENCES

Chen, C. H., & Yen, M. F. (2002). The effects of Tai Chi on symptom control in patients with chronic illness. *The Journal of Nursing, 49*(5), 22–27.

Chen, C. H., Yen, M., Fetzer, S., Lo, L. H., & Lam, P. (2008). The effects of Tai Chi exercise on elders with osteoarthritis: A longitudinal study. *Asian Nursing Research, 2*, 235–241.

Chen, K. M., Chen, W. T., & Huang, M. F. (2006). Development of the Simplified Tai-Chi Exercise Program (STEP) for the frail older adults. *Complementary Therapies in Medicine, 14*, 200–206.

Chen, K. M., Hsu, Y. C., Chen, W. T., & Tzeng, H. F. (2007). Well-being of institutionalized elders after Yang-style Tai Chi practice. *Journal of Clinical Nursing, 16*, 845–852.

Chen, K. M., Li, C. H., Lin, J. N., Chen, W. T., Lin, H. S., & Wu, H. C. (2007). A feasible method to enhance and maintain the health of elderly living in long-term care facilities through long-term, simplified Tai-Chi exercises. *Journal of Nursing Research, 15*(2), 156–164.

Chen, K. M., Lin, J. N., Lin, H. S., Wu, H. C., Chen, W. T., Li, C. H., et al. (2008). The effects of a Simplified Tai-Chi Exercise Program (STEP) on the physical health of older adults living in long-term care facilities: A single group design with multiple time points. *International Journal of Nursing Studies, 45*, 501–507.

Chen, K. M., Snyder, M., & Krichbaum, K. (2001). Tai Chi and well-being of Taiwanese community-dwelling elders. *Clinical Gerontologist, 24*(3/4), 137–156.

Chen, K. M., & Snyder, M. (1999). A research-based use of Tai Chi/movement therapy as a nursing intervention. *Journal of Holistic Nursing, 17*, 267–279.

Cheng, T. H. (1994). *Tai Chi: Transcendent art*. Hong Kong: The Hong Kong Tai Chi Association.

Downs, L. B. (1992). Tai chi. *Modern Maturity, 35*(4), 60–64.

Dreyer, D., & Dreyer, K. (2004). *Chi running*. New York: Simon & Schuster.

Dreyer, D., & Dreyer, K. (2006). *Chi walking*. New York: Simon & Schuster.

Forge, R. L. (1997). Mind–body fitness: Encouraging prospects for primary and secondary prevention. *Journal of Cardiovascular Nursing, 11*(3), 53–65.

Hainsworth, T. (2004). The role of exercise in falls prevention for older patients. *Nursing Times, 100*(18), 28–29.

Hung, S. M., & Chen, K. M. (2007). Effects of the Simplified Tai-Chi Exercise Program in promoting the health of the urban elderly. *Journal of Evidence-Based Nursing, 3*(3), 225–235.

Jou, T. H. (1983). *The tao of tai chi chuan: Way to rejuvenation* (3rd ed.). Piscataway, NJ: Tai Chi Foundation.

Kit, W. K. (2002). *The complete book of tai chi chuan*. Boston, MA: Tuttle.

Koh, T. C. (1981). Tai chi chuan. *American Journal of Chinese Medicine, 9*, 15–22.

Lam, P., & Kaye, N. (2006). *Tai Chi for beginners and the 24 forms*. New South Wales, Australia: Limelight.

Lan, C., Lai, J. S., Chen, S. Y., & Wong, M. K. (1998). 12-month tai chi training in the elderly: Its effect on health fitness. *Medicine and Science in Sports and Exercise, 30,* 345–351.

Li, F., Fisher, K. J., Harmer, P., Irbe, D., Tearse, R. G., & Weimer, C. (2004). Tai chi and self-rated quality of sleep and daytime sleepiness in older adults: A randomized controlled trial. *Journal of the American Geriatrics Society, 52,* 892–900.

Plummer, J. P. (1983). Acupuncture and tai chi chuan (Chinese shadow boxing): Body/mind therapies affecting homeostasis. In Y. Lau & J. P. Fowler (Eds.), *The scientific basis of traditional Chinese medicine: Selected papers* (pp. 22–36). Hong Kong: Medical Society.

Rones, R. (2007). *Sunset tai chi.* Wolfeboro, NH: Yang's Martial Arts Association.

Schaller, K. J. (1996). Tai chi chih: An exercise option for older adults. *Journal of Gerontological Nursing, 22*(10), 12–17.

Smalheiser, M. (1984). Tai chi chuan in China today. *Tai Chi Chuan: Perspectives of the Way and Its Movement, 1,* 3–5.

Stone, J. F. (1994). *Tai chi chih: Joy through movement.* Fort Yates, ND: Good Karma.

Thornton, E. W., Sykes, K. S., & Tang, W. K. (2004). Health benefits of Tai Chi exercise: Improved balance and blood pressure in middle-aged women. *Health Promotion International, 19,* 33–38.

Tsai, J. C., Wang, W. H., Chan, P., Lin, L. J., Wang, C. H., Tomlinson, B., et al. (2003). The beneficial effects of Tai Chi Chuan on blood pressure and lipid profile and anxiety status in a randomized controlled trial. *Journal of Alternative & Complementary Medicine, 9,* 747–754.

Tsang, W. W., & Hui-Chan, C. W. (2004). Effects of exercise on joint sense and balance in elderly men: Tai chi versus golf. *Medicine & Science in Sports & Exercise, 36,* 658–667.

Wolf, S. L., Barnhart, H. X., Kutner, N. G., McNeely, E., Coogler, C., & Xu, T. (2003). Selected as the best paper in the 1990s: Reducing frailty and falls in older persons: An investigation of Tai Chi and computerized balance training. *Journal of the American Geriatric Society, 51,* 1794–1803.

Xu, S. W., & Fan, Z. H. (1988). Physiological studies of tai ji quan in China. *Medicine Sport Science, 28,* 70–80.

Yang, Z. (1991). *Yang style Taijiquan* (2nd ed.). Beijing: Morning Glory.

25

Relaxation Therapies

ELIZABETH L. PESTKA
SUSAN M. BEE
MICHELE M. EVANS

Relaxation therapies are used to reduce muscle tension in the body. Relaxation has been shown to manage stress, offer pain relief, and promote health. Different types of therapies range from the simple and easily implemented diaphragmatic breathing to more complex methods, such as *Gua Sha*, that require a skilled provider. Using a combination of relaxation therapies with patients is a common practice in the health care field.

DEFINITIONS

Relaxation is reducing the tension that resides in muscles. Learning to relax can reduce the destructive effects and symptoms of stress-induced illnesses and improve a person's quality of life. Teaching relaxation therapies to patients allows them to become more active partners in their own health care.

Diaphragmatic breathing (DB), or relaxed deep breathing, is the utilization of the diaphragm when taking a breath. The purpose of relaxed breathing is to slow down the breathing and to reduce the use of shoulder, neck, and upper chest muscles, so as to breathe more

Exhibit 25.1

Insstruction for Self-Guided Autogenic Training

Autogenic training consists of a warm-up period of breathing and progressively learning six phases of relaxation, which all together may take several months to fully master. Upon completion, a person will progress through:

Warm-up: Focus on slowly exhaling each breath

Phase I: Attention to heaviness of arms and legs

Phase II: Attention to the warmth of the arms and legs

Phase III: Attention to calming the heart

Phase IV: Attention to breathing so that it is rhythmic

Phase V: Attention to stomach to achieve warmth and softness

Phase VI: Attention to the forehead being cool

Completion: Feel supremely calm. To maintain proficiency, once-a-day practice is recommended.

efficiently. This type of breathing improves oxygenation to the entire body.

Progressive muscle relaxation (PMR) is the tensing and releasing of successive muscle groups. This was first introduced by Jacobson (1938) and is still used widely today. A person's attention is drawn to discriminating between the feelings experienced when a muscle group is relaxed and when it is tensed.

Autogenic training (AT) is a relaxation method that uses both imagery and body awareness to reduce stress and muscle tension. This technique was developed and published by the German neurologist Schultz (Shultz & Luthe, 1959) and addresses autonomic sensations which lead to muscle relaxation (see Exhibit 25.1).

SCIENTIFIC BASIS

Real and perceived events and thoughts can create stress, which activates the sympathetic nervous system. This begins a cascade of physical and chemical reactions. The heart rate increases, blood pressure rises, respirations become shallow, pupils dilate, and the muscles tense as the body prepares to cope when the person perceives a real or imaginary stressor. This is often called the "fight or flight" response. The parasympathetic nervous system is known as the "rest and digest" or "rest and restore" response. When one response is activated, the other is quiet. Prolonged activation of the sympathetic nervous system over time can have deleterious effects on the body. The desired outcome of relaxation strategies is the mitigation of persisting high levels of stress and activation of the parasympathetic nervous system or the maintenance of a relaxed state.

When a person breathes, the body takes in oxygen and releases carbon dioxide. If the body detects an imbalance in these two gases, it signals for changes in breathing that may lead to fast, shallow breathing, called hyperventilation, oftentimes in response to stressful events or pain. Diaphragmatic breathing is a relaxation technique in which the person expands the diaphragm to the maximum extent possible to improve oxygenation to the entire body. It is a learned skill, and practice is required for optimal benefit.

Jacobson (1938) reported that PMR decreased the body's oxygen consumption, metabolic rate, respiratory rate, muscle tension, premature ventricular contractions, and systolic and diastolic blood pressure, and increased alpha brain waves. Subsequent studies have validated Jacobson's findings.

Autogenic training (AT) reduces excessive autonomic arousal. In addition, it is effective in raising low levels of autonomic functions such as a low heart rate. It is known as a self-regulatory model. AT may not only affect the sympathetic tone, but may also activate the parasympathetic system as well. The increase in parasympathetic dominance results in peripheral vasodilation and increased feelings of warmth and heaviness in the body.

INTERVENTION

Relaxation means more than simply having peace of mind or resting. It means eliminating tension from the body and mind. Learning relaxation skills or therapies requires focus on mind–body connections, such as when muscles are tensed, and practicing ways to relax the muscles to improve overall health and wellness.

Exhibit 25.2

Instructions for Diaphragmatic (Deep) Breathing

Sit comfortably with feet flat on the floor.

Loosen tight clothing around abdomen and waist.

May place hands in lap or at sides.

Breathe in slowly (through nose, if possible), allowing abdomen to expand with inhalation.

Exhale at normal rate.

May use pursed-lip breathing, which is creating a very small opening between lips through which to breathe out.

Succinct information on diaphragmatic deep breathing can be found at http:naturalhealth perspective.com/resilience/deep-breathing.html

Techniques

Diaphragnatic Breathing Technique

Diaphragmatic breathing can be used before and during stressful situations, such as a painful medical procedure, or for overall health enhancement. It is a relatively simple relaxation technique that can be used in any health care setting and does not require extensive training on the part of the instructor. After demonstrating deep breathing, the nurse observes the patient and provides suggestions for achieving improved results. The person learning DB is encouraged to practice relaxed breathing throughout the day until it becomes a natural way of breathing. For best effect, he/she should practice this technique frequently when he/she is neither anxious nor short of breath. Guidelines for DB are found in Exhibit 25.2.

Progressive Muscle Relaxation

Numerous techniques for muscle relaxation have been developed since Jacobson publicized his technique in 1938. Often the techniques include attention to breathing (Schaffer & Yucha, 2004). The instructor assists the individual to identify a place that is quiet and restful in which to practice relaxation. A comfortable chair, bed, or couch that provides support for the body is ideal. Clothing should be loose and not restrictive; shoes, glasses, and contact lenses should be removed. The person may wish to use the bathroom before practicing muscle relaxation.

The PMR technique developed by Bernstein and Borkovec (1973) is widely used. They combined the 108 muscles and muscle groups of Jacobson's original technique into the initial tensing and relaxing of 16 muscle groups. Subsequently the number of groups is reduced to 7 and then to 4 (Exhibit 25.3). Although Bernstein and Borkovec included instructions for tensing muscles of the feet, those are not included in Exhibit 25.3 because spasms in the foot may result when tensing these muscles. The ultimate goal is to achieve muscle relaxation throughout the body without initially having to tense the muscles. Through practice, the person acquires a mental image of how the muscles feel when they are relaxed and is able to relax them by using this image.

Education on the scientific basis for the use of PMR is provided during the first session. Stressors, the impact of stress on the body, and the signs and symptoms of high levels of stress are discussed. Descriptions and demonstrations for achieving tension of each muscle group are given, and the person then practices tensing each of the muscle groups.

After progressing through all the muscle groups, the instructor asks the patient to identify whether tension remains in any of them. The instructor observes the patient, to assess for general relaxation, focusing on slowed, deeper breathing; arms relaxed and shoulders forward; and feet apart with toes pointing out. Two or three minutes are provided at the conclusion of the session for the patient to enjoy the feelings associated with relaxation. Terminating relaxation is done gradually. The instructor counts backward from four to one. An opportunity is provided for the patient to ask questions or discuss the feelings experienced.

Bernstein and Borkovec proposed using 10 sessions to teach PMR. However, in many studies instruction has been limited to fewer sessions with positive results (Peck, 1997; Sloman, Brown, Aldana, & Chu, 1995). A critical factor in determining the number of teaching sessions needed is ensuring that a person has mastered relaxing the muscle groups and has integrated PMR into his/her lifestyle.

An essential factor in the effectiveness of PMR and other relaxation techniques is daily practice. At least one 15-minute practice session per day is recommended. Schaffer and Yucha (2004) suggest two 10-minute

Exhibit 25.3

Guidelines for 14 Muscle Group Progressive Muscle Relaxation

General Information:

Instruct persons to tense a specific muscle group when they hear "tense" and to release the tension when they hear "relax." Tension is held for 7 seconds.

Draw attention to the feeling of tension and relaxation.

When muscles are relaxed, attention is drawn to the differences between the two states.

Tensing Specific Muscle Groups:

Dominant hand and forearm: Make a tight fist and hold it.

Dominant upper arm: Push elbow down against the arm of the chair.

   Repeat instructions for the nondominant arm.

Forehead: Lift eyebrows as high as possible.

Central face (cheeks, nose, eyes): Squint eyes and wrinkle nose.

Lower face and jaw: Clench teeth and widen mouth.

Neck: Pull chin down toward chest but do not touch chest.

Chest, shoulders, and upper back: Take deep breath and hold it, pull shoulder blades back.

Abdomen: Pull stomach in and try to protect it.

Dominant thigh: Lift leg and hold it straight out.

Dominant calf: Point toes toward ceiling.

   Repeat instructions for nondominant side.

Note: Adapted from Bernstein and Borkovec (1973).

sessions. Helping patients find a time of day to practice relaxation is an important component of instruction. Often an audiotape of the instructions is provided for home practice. Persons are also instructed to use the relaxation technique any time they feel tense or before an event that may cause them to become anxious and tense. For comprehensive instructions on PMR, refer to http://www.guidetopsychology.com/pmr.htm

Autogenic Training

Autogenic training is a relaxation method that is self-generated or self-guided, using relaxation phrases. A health care provider familiar with the therapy can recommend the therapy and provide assistance with learning the method. It is increasing in use worldwide. The intent is to create a feeling of warmth and heaviness throughout the body while the person experiences a profound state of physical relaxation, and of good physical and mental health. The person needs to practice AT alone in a quiet place. It is best practiced before eating. Removing shoes and weaing loose clothing facilitates achieving relaxation. The focus is intently on the inner experiences to the exclusion of external events. When a person finishes a session, they should relax with their eyes closed for a few seconds, and then get up slowly.

More information about AT and its use in achieving relaxation can be found at http://www.guidetopsychology.com/autogen.htm.

Measurement of Outcomes

Although findings from many studies have shown positive outcomes from the use of relaxation techniques, positive results have not been reported in all of the studies reviewed. Reasons for the differences in outcomes may relate to the wide variation in the types of relaxation techniques, the length and type of instruction, the degree of mastery of the technique, and irregular or sporadic use of the technique.

A variety of outcomes has been used to measure the efficacy of relaxation techniques. Physiological measurements that are often used include respiratory rate, heart rate, and blood pressure. Electromyogram readings are occasionally taken to determine the degree of tension in the specific muscle groups. Practitioners need to be alert to underlying pathologies or concurrent medication use, which may interfere with reduction in physiological parameters. Some studies have focused on measuring immune system responses, such as T and B cell markers, leukocytes, and cortisol level.

Anxiety is the most frequently used subjective measure of PMR. The State-Trait Anxiety Inventory (STAI) of Spielberger, Gorsuch, Luschene, Vagg, and Jacobs (1983) has been widely used. Persons' self-reports about feelings of relaxation have been included in many studies, because satisfaction is a good indicator of whether a person will continue to use an intervention. Reports of reduction of pain, increased comfort, and improved sleep are other results that have been used to measure the effects of relaxation techniques.

Precautions

Although relaxation techniques have been used with multiple populations and have been proven to be an effective therapy for nurses to use, some cautions should be observed. It is important for practitioners to know whether patients practice the relaxation techniques on a regular basis, as this may affect the pharmacokinetics of medications. Adjustment in doses may be indicated.

Relaxation of muscles may produce a hypotensive state. People are instructed to remain seated for a few minutes after practice. Movement in place and gradual resumption of activities helps in raising the blood pressure. Taking a person's blood pressure at the conclusion of teaching sessions helps in identifying those who are prone to hypotensive states after muscle relaxation and AT.

Some persons with chronic pain have reported a heightened awareness of pain following the tensing and relaxing of muscles. Concentrating on tensing and relaxing of muscles may draw attention to the pain rather than to the muscle sensation. A good assessment of individuals is needed to determine whether negative outcomes are occurring.

Children below school age lack the discipline needed to learn and practice AT. Also, those with mental retardation, acute central nervous system disorders, or uncontrolled psychosis may be unable to process the in-depth instructions (Linden 2007). In some patients, AT may produce the side effects of anxiety, sadness, resurfaced memories, and suppressed thoughts, or reawakened pain sensation from old illnesses or injuries. These effects may stem from disinhibition of various cortical processes resulting from the autogenic formulas and the focus on body sensations (Lehrer, 2009).

USES

A certain degree of motivation is required to benefit from any relaxation therapy. Relaxation takes time, and patients often lose motivation to continue. The nurse has the opportunity to encourage scheduled times

Exhibit 25.4

Studies Supporting Use of Relaxation Therapies

Therapy	Health Condition	Study Authors
DB	Chronic pain	Schmidt et al., 2008
DB	Stem cell transplantation	Kim & Kim, 2005
PMR	Hypertension	Sheu et al., 2003; Kaushik, Kaushik, Mahajan, & Rajesh, 2006; Yung et al., 2001
PMR	Cancer (decrease nausea and vomiting, pain, and depression)	Campos de Carvalho, Titareli Merizio Martins, & Benedita dos Santos, 2007; Molassiotis, Yung, Yam, Chan, & Mok, 2002; Sloman, 2002; Kwekkeboom et al., 2008; Sloman et al., 1995
PMR	Chronic obstructive pulmonary disease	Chang et al., 2004
PMR	Asthma	Nickel et al., 2006
PMR	Osteoarthritis	Baird & Sand, 2004
PMR	Insomnia	Richardson, 2003
PMR	Headache	Fichtel & Larrson, 2001
PMR	Stress	Pawlow & Jones, 2002
PMR	Postoperative pain	dePaula, deCarvalho, & dos Santos, 2002; Good et al., 2002
AT	Cancer (stress)	Hidderly & Holt, 2004
AT	Chest pain	Asbury, Kanji, Ernst, Barbir, & Collins, 2009
AT	Multiple sclerosis	Sutherland, Andersen, & Morris, 2005
AT	Posttraumatic stress disorder	Mitani et al., 2006
Gua Sha	Pain	Nielsen et al., 2007

AT = autogenic training; DB = diaphragmatic breathing; PMR = progressive muscle relaxation.

for the patient to practice. Promoting an understanding of the anticipated positive benefits of the therapy is critical.

Relaxation therapies have been used to achieve a variety of outcomes in diverse populations. Exhibit 25.4 lists conditions and populations in which these techniques have been used. Their use in reduction of stress, relief of pain, and health promotion in specific conditions will be discussed.

Reduction of Anxiety and Stress

As noted in Exhibit 25.4, relaxation therapies have been effective in reducing the stress associated with a number of conditions. DB exercises reduced anxiety and depression in stem cell transplantation patients as measured by the State-Trait Anxiety Inventory and Beck Depression Inventory (Kim & Kim, 2005). Sloman's study (1995) found that 92% of the patients with cancer who were taught PMR reported that relaxation occurred, and 90% noted that they would continue to use the therapy. In a subsequent study, Sloman (2002) reported a reduction in depression and anxiety in patients with advanced stages of cancer. One research team (Mitani, Fujjita, Sakamoto, & Shirakawa, 2006) reported that following AT a group of patients with posttraumatic stress disorder showed a significant decline in cardiac sympathetic nervous activity and a significant increase in cardiac parasympathetic nervous activity. Relaxation techniques can be used both to decrease and prevent stress.

Pain

Relaxation therapies have been used extensively in the management of many types of pain. Muscle tension increases the perception of pain, so lessening anxiety and tension may help in reducing it. Schmidt, Hooten, Kerkvliet, Reid, & Joyner (2008) reported that three 10-minute sessions of DB each day in chronic pain patients were associated with significant changes in a number of areas of physiological and psychological functioning. Results indicated significant improvements in fatigue, pain management, self-efficacy, and changes in pain severity. Mean pain severity scores changed from 4.56 to 3.78 ($p < .05$) on a 0–10 rating scale. Using a treatment of listening twice a day to an audiotaped PMR script resulted in a significant reduction in pain and improvement in mobility in a group of patients with osteoarthritis (Baird & Sand, 2004). In a study by Kwekkeboom, Hau, Wanta, and Bumpus (2008), cancer patients reported their perception of the effectiveness of PMR on reducing the intensity of their pain even more than their pain scores indicated. They identified that patients benefited from active involvement in their own pain management.

Health Promotion

Nursing has been at the forefront in teaching patients about health promotion practices. Reducing and managing stress is an important health promotion strategy. Relaxation therapies are a prime way of preventing or reducing stress. Although relaxation therapies may not reduce heart rate and blood pressure in those who have readings within the normal range, use of these techniques on a regular basis by healthy persons may help to prevent the development of hypertension. Progressive muscle relaxation was found to decrease both systolic and diastolic blood pressure and heart rate in those with essential hypertension; and these indices decreased more as they continued to practice (Sheu, Irvin, Lin, & Mar, 2003; Yung., French, & Leung, 2001). Thus, muscle relaxation techniques can be used in conjunction with hypertensive medications in persons with high blood pressure.

CULTURAL ASPECTS

Numerous relaxation techniques are used in cultures across the globe. One of these is *Gua Sha*, or spooning, an East Asian relaxation technique. *Gua Sha* involves the application of friction to increase circulation to promote healing and pain relief by scraping an affected area with the blunt edge of a coin, spoon, or water buffalo horn.

In many Asian systems of medicine, pain is defined as a form of stasis. *Gua Sha* increases microcirculation locally to a treated area. Extravasated blood and metabolic waste that are collected in the muscle tissue are released, reducing muscle strain and tension. *Gua Sha* is used in the treatment and prevention of fever and respiratory and digestive complaints, as well as stiffness and tightness of muscles, or any illness that disrupts the flow of blood or *Qi* (Nielson et al., 2007).

In performing *Gua Sha*, oil is applied to the affected area of skin, and cutaneous stimulation is applied in strokes by a round-edged instrument. This action results in the appearance of small red petechiae, called "*sha*," which will fade in 2 to 3 days. *Gua Sha* is applied primarily on the neck, back, shoulders, buttocks, limbs, and occasionally on the chest and abdomen. A trained traditional medicine practitioner should be consulted to administer *Gua Sha* (Nielson et al., 2007). The Web site www.guasha.com provides helpful information about this therapy.

A body of research documenting the effectiveness of *Gua Sha* is beginning to appear in the literature. Nielsen et al. (2007) reported on *Gua Sha* in a Western journal. In the study, each subject experienced immediate decrease in myalgia both in the site treated and, in some cases, other distal sites after receiving *Gua Sha* treatment. Some pain relief persisted until the follow-up visit 2 to 3 days after the treatment.

FUTURE RESEARCH

Relaxation therapies have been used singly and in combination with other therapies. A scientific body of knowledge is emerging to guide the use of these therapies in practice, but considerably more research is necessary. Following are several areas in which studies are needed:

1. As the focus of health care becomes more individualized, it is important to identify relaxation therapies that will be effective for each person based on their genetic information, cultural background, and lifestyle preferences. Studies connecting phenotype with genotype will be informative.
2. A combination of therapies has been used in a number of studies. Some studies used excellent designs to compare the efficacy of each technique. However, numerous other studies fail to differentiate the effects from each therapy. Attention to study design in relaxation therapy studies is needed.
3. Sheu and colleagues (2003) found continuing improvement over a month's period of practice. In the majority of studies, however, the effects of relaxation therapies have been evaluated immediately following administration of the intervention. Longitudinal studies are needed to determine long-term effects.

REFERENCES

Asbury, E., Kanji, N., Ernst, E., Barbir, M., & Collins, P. (2009). Autogenic training to manage symptomatology in women with chest pain and normal coronary arteries. *Menopause, 16*(1), 1–6.

Baird, C., & Sand, L. (2004). A pilot study of the effectiveness of guided imagery with progressive muscle relaxation to reduce chronic pain and mobility difficulties of osteoarthritis. *Pain Management Nursing, 5*(3), 97–104.

Bernstein, D., & Borkovec, T. (1973). *Progressive relaxation training.* Champaign, IL: Research Press.

Campos de Carvalho, E., Titareli Merizio Martins, F., & Benedita dos Santos, C. (2007). A pilot study of a relaxation technique for management of nausea and vomiting in patients receiving cancer chemotherapy. *Cancer Nursing, 30*(2), 163–167.

Chang, B., Jones, D., Hendricks, A., Boehmer, U., Locastro, J., & Slawsky, M. (2004). Relaxation response for Veterans Affairs patients with congestive heart failure: Results from a qualitative study within a clinical trial. *Preventive Cardiology, 7*(2), 64–70.

dePaula, A., deCarvalho, E., & dos Santos, C. (2002). The use of the "progressive relaxation" technique for pain relief in gynecology and obstetrics. *Revista Latino-Americana de Enfermagen, 10*, 654–659.

Fichtel, A., & Larrson, B. (2001). Does relaxation treatment have differential effects on migraine and tension-type headache in adolescents? *Headache, 41*, 290–296.

Good, M., Anderson, G., Stanton-Hicks, M., Grass, J., & Makii, M. (2002). Relaxation and music reduce pain after gynecologic surgery. *Pain Management Nursing, 3*, 61–70.

Hidderly, M., & Holt, M. (2004). A pilot randomized trial assessing the effects of autogenic training in early stage cancer patients in relation to psychological status and immune system responses. *European Journal of Oncology Nursing, 8*, 61–65.

Jacobson, E. (1938). *Progressive relaxation.* Chicago: University of Chicago Press.

Kaushik, R., Kaushik, R., Mahajan, S., & Rajesh, V. (2006). Effects of mental relaxation and slow breathing in essential hypertension. *Complementary Therapies in Medicine, 14*, 120–126.

Kim, S., & Kim, H. (2005). Effects of a relaxation breathing exercise on anxiety, depression, and leukocyte in hemopoietic stem cell transplantation patients. *Cancer Nursing, 28*(1), 79–83.

Kwekkeboom, K., Hau, H., Wanta, B., & Bumpus, M. (2008). Patients' perceptions of the effectiveness of guided imagery and progressive muscle relaxation interventions used of cancer pain. *Complementary Therapies in Clinical Practice, 14*, 185–194.

Lehrer, P. (2009). An expert speaks. In L. Freeman (Ed.), *Mosby's complementary and alternative medicine: A research-based approach* (3rd ed., pp. 148–150). St. Louis, MO: Mosby Elsevier.

Linden, W. (2007). *Autogenic training.* New York: Guilford.

Mitani, S., Fujita, M., Sakamoto, S., & Shirakawa, T. (2006). Effect of autogenic training on cardiac autonomic nervous activity in high-risk fire service workers for posttraumatic stress disorder. *Journal of Psychosomatic Research, 60*, 439–444.

Molassiotis, A., Yung, H., Yam, B., Chan, F., & Mok, T. (2002). The effectiveness of progressive muscle relaxation training in managing chemotherapy-induced nausea and vomiting in Chinese breast cancer patients: A randomized controlled trial. *Supportive Care in Cancer, 10*, 237–246.

Nickel, C., Lahmann, C., Muehlbacher, M., Gil, F., Kaplan, P., Buschmann, W., et al. (2006). Pregnant women with bronchial asthma benefit from progressive muscle relaxation: A randomized, prospective, controlled trial. *Psychotherapy and Psychometrics, 75*, 237–243.

Nielsen, A., Knoblauch, N., Gustav, J., Dobos, G., Michalsen, A., & Kaptchuk, T. (2007). The effect of Gua Sha treatment on the microcirculation of surface tissue: A pilot study in healthy subjects. *Explore, 3*(5), 456–466.

Pawlow, L., & Jones, G. (2002). The impact of abbreviated progressive muscle relaxation on salivary cortisol. *Biological Psychology, 60*, 1–16.

Peck, S. (1997). The effectiveness of therapeutic touch for decreasing pain in elders with degenerative arthritis. *Journal of Holistic Nursing, 15*(2), 13–26.

Richardson, S. (2003). Effects of relaxation and imagery on the sleep of critically ill adults. *Dimensions of Critical Care Nursing, 22*, 182–190.

Schaffer, S.D., & Yucha, C. B. (2004). Relaxation & pain management: The relaxation response can play a role in managing chronic and acute pain. *American Journal of Nursing, 104*(8), 75–82.

Schmidt, J., Hooten, W., Kerkvliet, J., Reid, K., & Joyner, M. (2008). Psychological and physiological correlates of a brief intervention to enhance self-regulation in chronic pain [Abstract]. *Journal of Pain, 9*(4), 55.

Schultz, J. H., & Luthe, W. (1959). *Autogenic training: A psycho-physiological approach in psychotherapy.* New York: Grune and Statton.

Sheu, S., Irvin, B. L., Lin, H. S., & Mar, C. L. (2003). Effects of progressive muscle relaxation on blood pressure and psychosocial status of clients with essential hypertension. *Holistic Nursing Practice, 17*(1), 41–47.

Sloman, R. (2002). Relaxation and imagery for anxiety and depression control in community patients with advanced cancer. *Cancer Nursing, 25*, 432–435.

Sloman, R., Brown, R., Aldana, E., & Chu, E. (1995). The use of relaxation for promotion of comfort and pain relief in persons with advanced cancer. *Contemporary Nurse, 3*(1), 6–12.

Spielberger, C., Gorsuch, R., Luschene, R., Vagg, P., & Jacobs, G. (1983). *Manual for STAI.* Palo Alto, CA: Consulting Psychological Press.

Sutherland, G., Andersen, M., & Morris, T. (2005). Relaxation and health-related quality of life in multiple schlerosis: The example of autogenic training. *Journal of Behavioral Medicine, 28*(3), 249–256.

Yung, P., French, P., & Leung, B. (2001). Relaxation training as complementary therapy for mild hypertension control and the implications of evidence-based medicine. *Complementary Therapies in Nursing & Midwifery, 7*, 59–65.

Biologically Based Therapies

OVERVIEW

Biologically based therapies are the most popular of the complementary therapies according to the NCCAM (2009). More than 90 million Americans use at least one herbal preparation. Additionally, "nutraceuticals" (additives, vitamins, and special diets) are used by many Americans. A person encounters reference to these therapies when just paging through a magazine or watching television, as there are frequent articles and ads highlighting specific biological therapies. The authors have placed aromatherapy in the "biologically based" category because it uses essential oils, which are naturally occurring plant substances. NCCAM also places therapies such as laetrile and shark cartilage in the category of biologically based therapy.

Although research on herbs is relatively sparse in the United States, a significant amount has been conducted in other countries, particularly Germany. The chapter on herbal preparations details concerns about the use of herbal preparations in the United States. Suggestions are given to increase safety in the use of herbs. Because of the growing percentage of Americans using herbal preparations, it is incumbent on nurses to be familiar with herbal preparations such as St. John's wort, echinacea, chamomile, kava kava, ginkgo biloba, and saw palmetto. Assessing a patient's use of herbal preparations is important, since many herbal-medication interactions have been identified.

Although nurses ordinarily will not be in a position to prescribe or recommend specific nutraceuticals to patients, the wide use of this group of biologically based therapies requires that nurses have knowledge about them. Much information is available to the public about food additives, vitamins, and special diets, and knowing about a patient's use of these products will assist the health care team in devising a safe plan of care.

As with many of the other biologically based therapies, the essential oils used in aromatherapy have a much wider use in other countries than in the United States. Much of the research on essential oils has been conducted in France and England, and it is only in recent years that aromatherapy has been introduced into health facilities in the United States. Essential oils can be taken internally, but this mode of administration is not within the purview of nurses.

Many of the lists of herbal preparations and other biologically based therapies refer to products common in the Western world. Little attention has been given to herbal preparations and biologically based therapies used in other health systems such as TCM and health care systems of indigenous cultures. The increasing number of first-generation Americans from countries who have traditionally used herbal preparations indigenous to their ancestral cultures requires that health professionals expand their knowledge about herbs and other biologically based therapies, so as to avoid herb–drug interactions and other complications.

Practices such as drinking holy water (from Catholic shrines such as those in Lourdes, France or Knock, Ireland) or mihaya (a traditional healing drink found in Sudan in which sacred verses from the Koran are washed with water) could be placed in this category or in the energy category. Persons in these traditions fervently believe that these waters possess healing properties.

As with other complementary therapies, research on biologically based therapies is increasing. It is more difficult to conduct research on herbal preparations used in other cultures, because each preparation is a mixture of herbs based on the individual characteristics of the patient and the nature of condition or illness. Research on the use of essential oils is beginning to show the efficacy of some of these compounds. As scientists explore the rain forests and deserts for new natural products, the products in this category will continue to increase.

REFERENCES

National Center of Complementary and Alternative Medicine. (2009). *The use of complementary and alternative medicine in the United States.* Retrieved February 27, 2009, from http://nccam.nih/news/camstats2007/camsurvey_fs1.htm

26 Aromatherapy

LINDA L. HALCÓN

Aromatherapy is a relatively recent addition to nursing care in the United States, although it has been accepted as part of nursing in Switzerland, Germany, Australia, Canada, and the United Kingdom—and even as a medical specialty in France for many years. This modality is particularly well suited to nursing, because it incorporates the therapeutic value of sensory experience (i.e., smell) and often includes the use of touch in the delivery of care. It also builds upon a rich heritage of botanical therapies within nursing practice (Libster, 2002).

Aromatherapy originates in herbal or botanical medicine. There is evidence of plant distillation dating back 5,000 years. In ancient times, essential oils and other aromatic plant products were used throughout much of the world. In ancient Egypt and the Middle East, they were used in embalming, incense, perfumery, and healing. The therapeutic applications of essential oils were recorded as part of Greek and Roman medicine, and essential oils have been used in Ayurvedic medicine in the Indian subcontinent and in traditional Chinese medicine for over a thousand years. With the expansion of trade and improvements in distillation methods, essential oils became common elements of herbal medicine and perfumery in Europe during the Middle Ages (Keville & Green, 2009). In the late 1800's, scientists noted the association between environmental exposure to plant essential oils and the prevention of disease, and microbiologists conducted studies showing the in vitro activity of certain plant oils against microorganisms (Battaglia, 2003).

The development of clinical aromatherapy within the context of modern Western health science began in France just prior to World War I, when chemist Maurice Gattefossé was healed of a near-gangrenous wound with lavender essential oil. He subsequently championed its use for battle wounds during World Wars I and II. Physician Jean Valnet and nurse Marguerite Maury followed in promoting the therapeutic value of essential oils in Europe, and in the 1930's interest in the anti-infective value of essential oils from native plants began to appear in the European and Australian medical literature (Price, & Price, 1999). The use of essential oils continued sporadically as a nonconventional treatment modality in the West until the recent explosion of interest in botanical medicines, when its use became more visible and widespread. Eisenberg and colleagues (1998) reported that 5.6% of 2,055 adults surveyed indicated that they used aromatherapy. More recent large surveys to estimate the overall prevalence of complementary therapies have not included aromatherapy as a separate modality (Tindle, Davis, Phillips, & Eisenberg, 2005; Barnes, Bloom, & Nahin, 2008). Surveys of special populations, however, suggest its continuing and increasing use by the public (Crawford, Cincotta, Lim, & Powell, 2006; Sinha & Efron, 2005).

DEFINITION

There are many operant definitions of aromatherapy, and some of them contribute to common misconceptions. The word *aromatherapy* can lead people to believe that it simply involves smelling scents (Schnaubelt, 1999), but this is incorrect. Styles (1997) defined aromatherapy as the use of essential oils for therapeutic purposes that encompass mind, body, and spirit, a broad definition that is consistent with holistic nursing practice. Clinical aromatherapy in nursing is defined as the use of essential oils for expected and measurable health outcomes (Buckle, 2000). Because aromatherapy clinical research is still in its infancy in the United States, the evidence base for using aromatherapy in nursing practice sometimes may be difficult to establish. It is important to remember that the widespread use of synthetic scents in household and personal products is not considered aromatherapy.

Essential oils are obtained from a variety of plants throughout the world, but not all plants produce essential oils. Depending on the plant, the essential oil may be found in flowers, leaves, bark, wood, roots, seeds, or peels. Most essential oils are obtained by steam distillation of a specific plant material. Steam-distilled essential oils are concentrated substances made up of the oil-soluble, lower-molecular-weight chemical constituents found in the source plant material. Essential oils from citrus fruit peels are usually obtained by expression (similar to grating or grinding). Carbon dioxide extraction is increasingly accepted by scientists and practitioners as a legitimate method for obtaining essential oils; however, other types of solvent extraction generally are not accepted for clinical use. Expressed and CO_2 extracted essential oils contain a broader range of the chemicals present in the plant material. Essential oils do not necessarily have the same medicinal properties as the plants from which they are derived.

SCIENTIFIC BASIS

Essential oils processed by any of the above methods are highly volatile, complex mixtures of organic chemicals consisting of terpenes and terpenic compounds. The chemistry of an essential oil largely determines its therapeutic properties. There are 60 to 300 separate chemicals in each essential oil, with the proportions of the constituents within plant species varying naturally, depending on a host of genetic and environmental factors. Knowing the plant species, the chemotype, the part of the plant used, the country of origin, and the method of essential oil extraction can provide an indication of the essential oil's chemical constituents using readily accessible aromatherapy reference books.

The pharmacologic activity of essential oils begins upon entry to the body through the olfactory, respiratory, gastrointestinal, or integumentary systems. All body systems can be affected once the chemical molecules making up essential oils reach the circulatory and nervous systems. The compounds within an essential oil find their way into the bloodstream however they are applied (Tisserand & Balacs, 1995). Inhaled aromas have the fastest effect, although compounds absorbed through massage can be detected in the blood within 20 minutes (Jager, Bauchbauer, Jirovetz, & Fritzer, 1979).

When inhaled, the many different molecules in each essential oil act as olfactory stimulants that travel via the nose to the olfactory bulb, and from there impulses travel to the limbic system of the brain. Of the limbic system regions, the amygdala and the hippocampus are of particular importance in the processing of aromas. The amygdala governs emotional responses. The hippocampus is involved in the formation and retrieval of explicit memories. The limbic system interacts with the cerebral cortex, contributing to the relationship between thoughts and feelings; it is directly connected to those parts of the brain that control heart rate, blood pressure, breathing, stress levels, and hormone levels (Kiecolt-Glaser et al., 2007). Although inhalation of essential oils is largely thought to be associated with olfaction, some molecules from any vapor inhaled will travel to the lungs, where they can have an immediate effect on breathing and can be absorbed into the circulatory system. Tisserand and Balacs (1995) gave the example of the effect of *Lavandula angustifolia* (true lavender), thought to reduce the effect of external emotional stimuli by increasing gamma-aminobutyric acid (GABA), which in turn inhibits neurons in the amygdala, producing a sedative effect similar to that of diazepam (Tisserand, 1988).

Essential oils are absorbed through the skin by diffusion, with the epidermis and fat layer acting as a reservoir before the components of the essential oils reach the dermis and the bloodstream. Topically applied essential oil preparations are absorbed rapidly through the skin; some have been used to enhance the dermal penetration of pharmaceuticals (Williams & Barry, 1989). The rate and extent of penetration and absorption can vary depending on multiple factors, such as the part of the body treated, the condition of the skin, the age of the patient, and the carrier or vehicle for the essential oil. Massage can enhance dermal penetration through heat and friction. Essential oils are excreted from the body through respiration, kidneys, and insensate loss.

INTERVENTION

The choice of application method—inhalation, topical application, ingestion—depends on the condition being treated or the desired effect, the nurse's knowledge and practice parameters, the available or desired time for the action to occur, the targeted outcome, the chemical components of the essential oil, and the preferences and psychological needs of the patient.

Although essential oils are not always pleasant smelling, inhalation is one of the simplest and most direct application methods. With this method, one to five drops of an essential oil can be placed on a tissue or floated on hot water in a bowl and then inhaled for 5 to 10 minutes. Other inhalation techniques include the use of burners, nebulizers, and vaporizers that can be operated by heat, battery, or electricity and may or may not include the use of water. Larger, portable aroma-inhalation systems are available commercially to provide controlled release of essential oils into rooms of any size.

Inhalation effects as well as skin effects are also experienced when essential oils are used in a bath. Four to six drops of the essential oil are dissolved first in a teaspoon of whole milk, rubbing alcohol, or carrier oil (cold-pressed) and then placed in the bath water. Because essential oils are not soluble in water, they would float on the top of the water if used without such a dispersant and this could result in an uneven and possibly too concentrated treatment. The essential oil bath should last about 10 to 15 minutes. Essential oils can also be dissolved in salts (e.g., Epsom salts); this can be soothing to muscles and joints. One such recipe for bath salts consists of 1 tablespoon of baking soda, 2 tablespoons of Epsom salts, and 3 tablespoons of sea salt with 4 to 6 drops of essential oils mixed throughout. Salts should be added to the bath water just before immersion and after agitating the water to disperse them.

Compresses can be a useful method for applying essential oils to treat skin conditions or minor injuries. To prepare a compress, add 4 to 6 drops of essential oil to warm water. Soak a soft cotton cloth in the mixture, wring it out, and apply the cloth to the affected area, contusion, or abrasion. Cover the compress with plastic wrap to retain moisture, place a towel over the plastic wrap, and keep it in place for as long as desired (up to 4 hours). The use of very warm water can enhance the absorption of some of the components of essential oils (Buckle, 2003).

Massage also can facilitate absorption of essential oils through the skin and can reduce the patient's perceived stress, thus enhancing the healing process and possibly communication as well. To create a mixture for massage, dilute one to two drops of an essential oil in a teaspoon

(5 mL) of cold-pressed vegetable oil, organic and scent-free cream, or gel. Mixtures for massage are generally 1 to 5% essential oil concentration (Tisserand & Balacs, 1995).

Essential oils should not be used undiluted on mucous membranes; even on intact skin they are generally used in concentrations seldom exceeding 10%. When used to treat conditions such as vaginal infections, essential oils preparations can be created or purchased as pessaries or suppositories. Only essential oils high in alcohols, such as tea tree, are appropriate in pessaries; alcohols are less likely to cause skin irritation. If essential oils are applied via tampons, they should be changed regularly (Buckle, 2003). Oral thrush (candidiasis) in adults also can be treated with diluted essential oils by the swish-and-spit method, taking care not to swallow (Jandourek, Vaishampayan, & Vazquez, 1998).

General Guidelines for Use of Essential Oils

There are general safety guidelines for essential oils that nurses should be aware of for patient education and in practice. These include:

- Store essential oils away from open flames; they are volatile and highly flammable.
- Store essential oils in a cool place away from sunlight; use amber or blue-colored glass containers. Close the container immediately after use. Essential oils can oxidize in the presence of heat, light, and oxygen, changing their chemistry, and thus their actions, in unpredictable ways.
- Be aware that essential oils can stain clothing and textiles and that undiluted essential oils can degrade some plastics. Take appropriate precautions.
- Keep essential oils away from children and pets unless you are well-versed in clinical aromatherapy. The literature is full of case studies of adverse reactions or deaths related to improper applications or accidental ingestion in small children and pets.
- Use essential oils from reputable suppliers. Seek the advice of a trained aromatherapist or the recommendation of a knowledgeable clinical provider. If using essential oils in clinical or research settings, test results verifying the chemical constituency should be obtained.

- Special care is needed when using essential oils with or around persons who have a history of severe asthma or multiple allergies. Be sure to ask.
- Despite the relative safety of essential oils when used properly, sensitization and skin irritation can occur with topical application. In these cases, any residual essential oil solution should be removed and its use should be discontinued. Most such reactions resolve without treatment; however a health care provider should be consulted if discomfort/itching is severe or persists.
- If an essential oil gets into the eyes, rinse it out with milk or carrier oil first and then with water.

Measurement of Outcomes

Selection of suitable methods to assess aromatherapy treatment effects will depend on the problem for which essential oils are used and the targeted outcomes. For example, if lavender is used to promote sleep, measures might include changes in sleep patterns or comparison of signs and symptoms of insomnia between a treated group and another group that is similar in all ways other than the treatment. For psychological conditions such as depression or anxiety, many reliable survey instruments are available and they can be further validated by adding physiological measures such as cortisol levels or skin temperature. For infectious disease outcomes, standard laboratory tests can be used to measure the effect of treatment on microbial load. Other useful measures could include digital photography, pain scales, quality-of-life scales, or tests of cognitive performance. Using established measurement tools where possible is helpful in facilitating interpretation and comparing the effects of essential oils with those of other approaches.

Precautions

Aromatherapy is a very safe complementary therapy if it is used with knowledge and within accepted guidelines. Many essential oils have been tested by the food and beverage industry for use as flavorings and preservatives, and much research has been carried out by the perfume and tobacco industries. Most of the essential oils commonly used in clinical aromatherapy have been given GRAS (generally regarded as safe) status. However, nurses should not administer essential oils orally, as this is outside a nurse's scope of practice, and poisonings have been documented (Jacobs & Hornfeldt, 1994). A list of contraindicated essential oils can be found in training manuals; both novices and more experienced practitioners should consult these lists. Many essential oils should not be used during early pregnancy and should only be used cautiously in later pregnancy. Nurses need to be aware of essential oils that can cause photosensitivity, such as bergamot (*Citrus bergamia*) and other citrus oils (Clark & Wilkinson, 1998), and they should provide appropriate patient education and protection when these are used.

Essential oils are very concentrated and potent compounds, and in most cases they must be diluted in carrier oils for topical use. Tea tree (*Melaleuca alternifolia*) and lavender (*Lavandula angustifolia*) are among the few exceptions to this rule. These essential oils can be used full strength on minor cuts, abrasions, and small burns.

Some essential oils are known to be carcinogenic and others are contraindicated in persons with specific conditions. Essential oils can potentiate or decrease the effects of medications (Tisserand & Balacs, 1995). Extra care is needed when using essential oils with patients receiving chemotherapy because they may affect the absorption rate of cancer-treating drugs (Williams & Barry, 1989). In short, it cannot be assumed that all essential oils are safe in all situations simply because they are *natural*.

Product identity confusion is another potential threat to safety. Essential oils should not be confused with herbal extracts, which are completely different chemical mixtures, and they cannot be used interchangeably. Besides their chemical dissimilarities, herbal extracts and teas are usually taken internally, whereas essential oils are not. Nurses share responsibility for ensuring product integrity when essential oils are used in clinical practice. Chemical testing of those essential oils used in patient care should be incorporated into ongoing quality assurance/quality control programs.

Nurses using essential oils regularly should protect themselves from unintended effects. Because essential oils are volatile, their molecules will be inhaled by those applying them as well as by patients. It has been demonstrated that hand dermatitis is associated with long-term unprotected use of lotions and other products containing essential oils (Crawford, Katz, Ellis, & James, 2004).

Table 26.1

COMMON AND BOTANICAL NAMES OF ESSENTIAL OILS COMMONLY USED IN AROMATHERAPY

COMMON NAME	BOTANICAL NAME
Basil	*Ocimum basilicum*
Chamomile, German	*Matricaria recutita*
Chamomile, Roman	*Chamaemelum nobile*
Clary sage	*Salvia sclarea*
Eucalyptus	*Eucalyptus globulus*
Ginger	*Zingiber officinale*
Lavender, true	*Lavandula officinalis* or *L. angustifolia*
Lemon	*Citrus limon*
Peppermint	*Mentha piperita*
Rose	*Rosa damascena*
Sandalwood	*Santalum album*
Tea tree	*Melaleuca alternifolia*

Perhaps one of the greatest risks in aromatherapy is using an incorrect essential oil for a particular health outcome. This could stem from a nurse's lack of knowledge of plant taxonomy. Many essential oils have familiar common names such as lavender, rose, and rosemary, but it is important to know the full botanical name. For example, "lavender" is a common name that covers *three different kinds* of lavender *and* a number of hybrid plants. The genus of lavender is *Lavandula*, and all lavenders begin with this word. *Lavandula angustifolia* is one of the most widely used and researched essential oils and is recognized as a relaxant. The other two species used in aromatherapy have very different properties. *Lavandula latifolia* (spike lavender) is a stimulant and expectorant; *Lavandula stoechas* is antimicrobial and not safe to use for long periods of time. Nurses who use aromatherapy clinically must know the full botanical name of an essential oil they intend to use. The botanical names of commonly used essential oils are found in Table 26.1.

Credentialing

Currently there is no recognized national certification exam for aromatherapists and no governing body. The Aromatherapy Registration

Council, a nonprofit entity that was established in 2000, administers a national exam and can provide the public with a list of registered aromatherapy practitioners. Nurses and health professionals wishing to use aromatherapy in their practice should check with their licensing bodies; nurses, specifically, should check with their state board of nursing. Many states allow nurses to use aromatherapy in their practice if they have received specialized education. There are many different courses available and health professionals should choose one that is relevant to their own clinical practice. The largest aromatherapy professional organization in the United States is the National Association of Holistic Aromatherapy. There are no requirements in the United States at this time for a person administering aromatherapy to be certified or accredited; however, Canadian nurses have established criteria for practice. The length of training programs in aromatherapy may range from one weekend to several years. Generally, it is not necessary to be a health professional to enroll in these educational programs. Despite the lack of uniform credentialing, it is no longer unusual for hospitals and other clinical settings to include aromatherapy services, and nurses must insist that policies and procedures include good quality assurance and quality control.

USES

Many health outcomes that fall within the domain of nursing practice can be addressed with essential oils, either alone or combined with other approaches. Essential oils can affect people psychologically and physically. They can increase or decrease sympathetic activity in humans, affecting blood pressure, plasma adrenaline, and plasma catecholamine levels (Haze, Sakai, & Gozu, 2002). The effect of essential oil odors can be relaxing or stimulating, depending on the individual's previous experiences, likes and dislikes, and the chemistry of the essential oil used; therefore, it is important to explore patient preference and the purpose for which the oil is being used when selecting essential oils for therapeutic purposes.

Essential oils are used therapeutically to address almost any symptom or body system, and there are many texts describing their use and recommending particular essential oils for specific conditions. It would be difficult to identify evidence other than case studies or historical anecdotes for some of these uses, and this has hindered the adoption of aromatherapy in clinical settings. The main current applications of essential oils in conventional health care settings are to help address pain, anxiety, nausea, sleeplessness, or agitation, and to prevent or treat infections. Nurse midwives have long incorporated essential oils into their practices, notably to reduce pain and aid relaxation during and after childbirth (Allaire, Moos, & Wells, 2000; Burns, Blamey, Ersser, Barnetson, & Lloyd, 2000). In long-term-care and hospital settings, essential oils are increasingly used to help reduce anxiety and agitation in patients with or without dementia (Bowles, Griffiths, Quirk, & Croot, 2002; Gray & Clair, 2002; Morris, 2008), promote sleep and reduce nighttime sedation (Hardy, Kirk-Smith, & Stretch, 1995), and promote wound healing (Kerr, 2002). Aromatherapy has been used to address acute or chronic pain (Ghelardini, Galeotti, Salvatore, & Mazzanti, 1999), fatigue and nausea (Tate, 1997), infection control (Gravett, 2001), and mood and cognition (Morris, 2002; Imura, Misao, & Ushijima, 2006). The literature includes other studies reporting the use of essential oils in the treatment of head lice (Veal, 1996) and as an aid to smoking cessation (Rose & Behm, 1994).

There is considerable and growing international literature on the use of plant essential oils against pathogenic microorganisms. The efficacy of essential oils in the treatment and prevention of infectious diseases has important implications for patient health as well as institutional disinfection and hygiene (Harkenthal, Reichling, Geiss, & Saller, 1999; Edwards-Jones, Buck, Shawcross, Dawson, & Dunn, 2004), especially with the increase in resistance bacteria (Hammer, Carson, & Riley, 2008). Methicillin-resistant *Staphylococcus aureus* and other microorganisms have been found to be sensitive to tea tree oil (*Melaleuca alternifolia*) (Halcón & Milkus, 2004; Bagg, Jackson, Sweeney, Ramage, & Davies, A., 2006; Carson, Hammer, Messager, & Riley, 2005). Preliminary work suggests that essential oils may also be effective in other difficult-to-treat infections (Sherry, Sivananthan, Warnke, & Eslick, 2003).

Aromatherapy is one of the complementary therapies most used for children and adolescents (Simpson & Roman, 2001). Despite the many aromatherapy products on the market for babies, it is recommended that essential oils be used cautiously, if at all, in infants, except for specific purposes. Many accidental poisonings of young children have been reported, illustrating the importance of keeping essential oils out of reach in bottles with integral drop dispensers and of knowing their safety profiles (Tisserand & Balacs, 1995). Essential oils are being used in pediatric oncology settings for nausea and fatigue. They have also been used to treat head lice and acne (Enshaieh, Jooya, Siadat, & Iraji, 2007) and to help with infantile colic (fennel seed) (Alexandrovich,, Rakovitskaya, Kolmo, Sidorova, & Shushunov, 2003). Nurses who are knowledgeable about essential oils can introduce them in pediatric practice and remain within safety guidelines.

CULTURAL APSECTS

There are regional, cultural, and religious traditions and preferences for the types of essential oils used therapeutically. For example, Ayurvedic practices include many essential oils that are produced in the Indian subcontinent, including those from sandalwood, jasmine, and other floral or spicy aromatic plants. The Middle East and Africa are the sources of such oils as frankincense, myrrh, ylang ylang, ravensara, and others. In Europe and much of the United States, essential oil production focuses on herbs or flowers that grow and thrive in temperate climates, such as peppermint, lavender, and basil. Citrus oils are produced in countries with warmer climates. However, the lines are not as distinct as in earlier times when the procurement of essential oils was limited to native and local plants. Plants are routinely transported and grown in non-native regions, and the essential oils most commonly used for therapeutic purposes are now readily available throughout the world, obtainable through global trade and Internet sales.

Cultural plant-healing traditions often have been altered and adopted by newcomers. The case of Australian tea tree oil provides an example of adaptation of cultural and regional health practices over time. *Melaleuca alternifolia* grows in one area of Australia as a native plant, and it was used as an herbal anti-infective medicine by Aboriginal peoples for centuries. Over 200 species of the genus *Melaleuca* are native to Australia, and only a few have been explored for modern medicinal uses as essential oils (Weiss, 1997). *Melaleuca alternifolia* is one of many plants referred to as "tea tree" in Australia and New Zealand; hence the importance of relying on Latin names for identification. The healing properties of this plant were noted by European explorers and settlers and at some point the foliage was distilled to produce a very concentrated antiseptic substance referred to as "tea tree oil." Since the early 1900's there has been intermittent interest in tea tree oil on the part of the medical community. This interest has expanded in recent years, partly through partnerships between the Australian government and the private agricultural sector to expand tea tree oil's economic impact. Both public and private funding was provided for excellent scientific research on the antimicrobial properties of tea tree oil, subsequently added to by health care researchers and scientists around the world. Extensive information can be found at the Web site of the Tea Tree Oil Research Group, University of Western Australia (http:// www.tto.bcs.uwa.edu.au/TTO_home). Tea tree is now an important plantation crop, and the antimicrobial properties of tea tree oil (*M. alternifolia*) are somewhat known in Western biomedical health care settings, but more widely so by the public. Affordable pure essential oil or health products with tea tree oil as a major ingredient are available worldwide, benefiting the Australian agricultural sector and health care.

The growing interest in discovery of new plant medicines that have health applications or profit possibilities has fueled expanded research on essential oils. It is important to note, however, that much of this research is aimed at improved food preservation and resultant prevention of food-borne illness or insects and parasites (Singh et al., 2008; Samarasekera, Weerasinghe, & Hemalal, 2008). As new essential oils are produced and tested for their health and environmental applications (Dongmo et al., 2008; Baik et al., 2008), their production can provide international trade opportunities and improved agricultural sustainability in addition to usually very affordable natural medicines. Geographical sources of some essential oils with current and historic cultural significance are shown in Table 26.2.

FUTURE RESEARCH

Aromatherapy researchers face several unique challenges. First, it is exceedingly difficult to conduct aromatherapy randomized controlled trials, the gold standard for quantitative research, because of the difficulty of blinding research subjects and staff to odor. Some researchers have attempted to use specialized masks to eliminate smell for participants, while others have used alternate and supposedly nontherapeutic

Table 26.2

MAJOR SOURCES OF COMMON ESSENTIAL OILS

COMMON NAME	BOTANICAL NAME	MAJOR SOURCE
Basil	*Ocimum basilicum*	France, Italy, Egypt, Bulgaria, Hungary, USA
Bergamot	*Citrus bergamia*	Italy, Ivory Coast, Guinea, Morocco, Corsica
Chamomile, German	Matricaria recutita	Hungary, former Yugoslavia, Bulgaria, Russia, Belgium, Spain
Chamomile, Roman	*Chamaemelum nobile*	England, Belgium, France, Hungary, USA
Cypress	*Cupressus sempervirens*	France, Italy and region, N. Africa, Spain, Portugal, Balkans, Morocco
Eucalyptus (there are many other species [spp.] of eucalyptus used medicinally)	*Eucalyptus globulus*	Australia, Spain, Portugal, Brazil, USA, Russia, China
Frankincense	*Boswellia carteri*	Somalia, Ethiopia, China, Arabia
Ginger	*Zingiber officinale*	India, China, S.E. Asia, Australia, tropical Africa, Indonesia, Japan
Jasmine (other spp. of Jasminum also are called jasmine)	*Jasminum grandiflorum*	India, Mediterranean countries, Iran, Afghanistan, China
Juniper Berry	*Juniperus communis*	Italy, Austria, Czech Rep., Hungary, Croatia, Serbia, France, Germany, Canada
Lavender, true	*Lavandula angustifolia*	France, Bulgaria, Australia, Argentina, England, Hungary, Japan, Morocco, Italy, Algeria, India, Russia, USA
Lemon	*Citrus limon*	Cultivated worldwide
Lemongrass, W. Indian	*Cymbopogon citratus*	Guatemala, Madagascar, Comoros, Brazil, Malaysia, Vietnam
Lemongrass, E. Indian	*Cymbopogon flexuosus*	India

Table 26.2 *(continued)*

COMMON NAME	BOTANICAL NAME	MAJOR SOURCE
Marjoram, Sweet	*Origanum majorana*	France, Tunisia, Morocco, Italy, Hungary, Bulgaria, Poland, Germany, Turkey
Melissa	*Melissa officinalis*	France, Germany, Italy, Spain, Hungary, Egypt, Ireland
Myrrh	*Commiphora myrrha*	N.E. Africa, S.E. Asia
Orange, Sweet	*Citrus sinensis*	Israel, Brazil, North America, Australia
Patchouli	*Pogostemon cablin*	Indonesia, Philippines, Malaysia, China, India, Caribbean, West Africa
Peppermint	*Mentha piperita*	USA, Argentina, Brazil, France, Italy, Morocco, bulgaria, Holland, Spain, Germany, England, India, Australia
Rose (Damask Rose)	*Rosa damascena*	Bulgaria, France, Morocco, Turkey, Italy, China
Rosemary	*Rosmarinus officinalis*	Spain, France, Tunisia
Sage	*Salvia officinalis*	Bosnia, USA., Bulgaria, Turkey, Malta, France, Germany, China
Sandalwood	*Santalum album* (other *Santalum* spp. also are named sandalwood)	Tropical Asia (India, Sri Lanka, Malysia, Indonesia, Taiwan)
Tea tree	*Melaleuca alternifolia*	Australia (other *Melaleuca* and *Leptospermum* spp. grown in Australia and New Zealand are also called tea tree)

From Battaglia (2003) and Lawless (1995).

smells for control groups. These approaches can improve study methods, but still have limitations.

Another research challenge is presented by the essential oils themselves due to their natural chemical variation. Pure and genuine essential oils cannot be truly standardized because each batch varies depending on growing conditions, plant stresses, harvesting and processing differences, and even storage factors. When using essential oils in research or clinical practice, it is essential to obtain chemical testing and verify that the specific batch used meets the standard ranges of the major constituents. Yet another research challenge is the use of blends versus single essential oils. There is evidence of synergistic and antagonistic effects when different oils are combined, making it more difficult to identify therapeutic elements. Finally, many studies test essential oil mixtures applied topically via massage, making it difficult to separate the effect of massage from that of the essential oil. Nurses should be aware of these research challenges when evaluating the evidence base for aromatherapy in practice.

There is a large body of unpublished research on the therapeutic effects of essential oils, much of it proprietary and conducted by the food, cosmetics, and flavoring industries. There is also a large volume of scientific research published in languages other than English, notably from Japan, China, India, and Europe. Despite a growing body of research in English-speaking countries, there remains a dearth of studies in English and a great need for additional research. Studies are needed to test the efficacy of essential oils already in common use and extend the practice of aromatherapy in clinical settings where, for some conditions and individuals, it may be a cost-effective alternative or adjunct therapy with fewer side effects than pharmaceuticals and other biomedical treatments.

The following are Web sites that nurses may find helpful in identifying more about essential oils:

National Association of Holistic Aromatherapists: www.naha.org

Aromatherapy Registration Council:
www.aromatherapycouncil.org

REFERENCES

Alexandrovich, I., Rakovitskaya, O., Kolmo, E., Sidorova, T., & Shushunov, S. (2003). The effect of fennel (*Foeniculum vulgare*) seed oil emulsion in infantile colic: A randomized, placebo-controlled study. *Alternative Therapies, 9*(4), 58–61.

Allaire, A., Moos, M., & Wells, S. (2000). Complementary and alternative medicine in pregnancy: A survey of North Carolina certified nurse-midwives. *Obstetrics & Gynecology, 95*(1), 19–23.

Bagg, J., Jackson, M., Sweeney, M., Ramage, G., & Davies, A. (2006). Susceptibility to *Melaleuca alternifolia* (tea tree) oil of yeasts isolated from the mouths of patients with advanced cancer. *Oral Oncology, 42,* 487–492.

Baik, J., Kim, S., Lee, J., Oh, T., Kim J., Lee, N., et al. (2008). Chemical composition and biological activities of essential oils extracted from Korean endemic citrus species. *Journal of Microbiology and Biotechnology, 18*(1), 74–79.

Barnes, P.M., Bloom, B., & Nahin, R. (2008). *CDC National Health Statistics Report #12. Complementary and alternative medicine use among adults and children:* United States 2007. Retrieved December 10, 2008, from http://www.CDC.gov

Battaglia, S. (2003). *The complete guide to aromatherapy* (2nd ed.). Brisbane: International Centre of Holistic Aromatherapy.

Bowles, E. J., Griffiths, M., Quirk, L., & Croot, K. (2002). Effects of essential oils and touch on resistance to nursing care procedures and other dementia-related behaviours in a residential care facility. *International Journal of Aromatherapy, 12*(1), 22–29.

Buckle, J. (2000). The "M" technique. *Massage and Bodywork, 15,* 52–64.

Buckle, J. (2003). *Clinical aromatherapy: Essential oils in practice* (2nd ed.). New York: Churchill Livingstone.

Burns, E. E., Blamey, C., Ersser, S. J., Barnetson, L., & Lloyd, A. J. (2000). An investigation into the use of aromatherapy in intrapartum midwifery practice. *Journal of Alternative and Complementary Therapies, 6*(2), 141–147.

Carson, C., Hammer, K., Messager, S., & Riley, T. (2005). Tea tree oil: A potential alternative for the management of methicillin-resistant *Staphylococcus aureus* (MRSA). *Australian Infection Control, 10*(1), 32–34.

Clark, S., & Wilkinson, S. (1998). Phototoxic contact dermatitis from 5-methoxypsoralen in aromatherapy oil. *Contact Dermatitis, 38,* 289.

Crawford, G., Cincotta, D., Lim, A., & Powell, C. (2006). A cross-sectional survey of complementary and alternative medicine use by children and adolescents attending the University Hospital of Wales. *BMC Complementary and Alternative Medicine, 6,* 16.

Crawford, G., Katz, K., Ellis, E., & James, W. (2004). Use of aromatherapy products and increased risk of hand dermatitis in massage therapists. *Archives of Dermatology, 140*(8), 991–996.

Dongmo, P., Tchoumbougnang, F., Sonwa, E., Kenfack, S., Zollo, P., & Menut, C. (2008). Antioxidant and anti-inflammatory potential of essential oils of some *Zanthoxylum* (Rutaceae) of Cameroon. *International Journal of Essential Oil Therapeutics, 2,* 82–88.

Edwards-Jones, V., Buck, R., Shawcross, S., Dawson, M., & Dunn, K. (2004). The effect of essential oils on methicillin-resistant *Staphylococcus aureus* using a dressing model. *Burns, 30*(8), 772–777.

Eisenberg, D. M., Davis, R. B., Ettner, S. L., Appel, S., Wilkey, S., Van Rompay, M. I., et al. (1998). Trends in alternative medicine in the USA, 1990–1997: Results of a follow-up national survey. *Journal of the American Medical Association, 280,* 784–787.

Enshaieh, S., Jooya, A., Siadat, A., & Iraji, F. (2007). The efficacy of 5% topical tea tree oil gel in mild to moderate acne vulgaris: A randomized, double-blind placebo-controlled study. *Indian Journal of Dermatology, Venereology and Leprology, 73*(1), 22–25.

Ghelardini, C., Galeotti, N., Salvatore, G., & Mazzanti, G. (1999). Local anaesthetic activity of the essential oil of Lavandula angustifolia. *Planta Medica, 65*, 700–703.

Gravett, P. (2001). Aromatherapy treatment for patients with Hickman Line infection following high-dose chemotherapy. *International Journal of Aromatherapy, 11*(1), 18–19.

Gray, S., & Clair, A. (2002). Influence of aromatherapy on medication administration to residential-care residents with dementia and behavioral challenges. *American Journal of Alzheimer's Disease and Other Dementias, 17*(3), 169–173.

Halcon, L., & Milkus, K. (2004). *Staphylococcus aureus* and wounds: A review of tea tree oil (*Melaleuca alternifolia*) as a promising antibiotic. *American Journal of Infection Control, 3*, 402–408.

Hammer, K. A., Carson, C. F., & Riley, T. V. (2008). Frequencies of resistance to *Melaleuca alternifolia* (tea tree) oil and rifampicin in *Staphylococcus aureus, Staphylococcus epidermidis* and *Enterococcus faecalis. International Journal of Antimicrobial Agents, 32*(2), 170–173.

Hardy, M., Kirk-Smith, M., & Stretch, D. (1995). Replacement of drug treatment for insomnia by ambient odor. *Lancet, 346*, 701.

Harkenthal, M., Reichling, J., Geiss, H., & Saller, R. (1999). Comparative study on the *in vitro* antibacterial activity of Australian tea tree oil, cajuput oil, niaouli oil, manuka oil, kanuka oil, and eucalyptus oil. *Pharmazie, 54*(6), 460–463.

Haze, S., Sakai, K., & Gozu, Y. (2002). Effects of fragrance inhalation on sympathetic activity in normal adults. *Japanese Journal of Pharmacology, 90*, 247–253.

Imura, M., Misao, H. & Ushijima, H. (2006). The psychological effects of aromatherapy-massage in healthy postpartum mothers. *Journal of Midwifery & Women's Health, 51*(2), e21–e27.

Jacobs, M., & Hornfeldt, C. (1994). Melaleuca oil poisoning. *Clinical Toxicology, 32*(4), 461–464.

Jager, W., Bauchbauer, G., Jirovetz, L., & Fritzer, M. (1979). Percutaneous absorption of lavender oil from a massage oil. *Journal of Social Cosmetology Chemistry, 43*(1), 49–54.

Jandourek, A., Vaishampayan, J., & Vazquez, J. (1998). Efficacy of melaleuca oral solution for the treatment of fluconazole refractory oral candidiasis in AIDS patients. *AIDS, 12*(9), 1033–1037.

Kerr, J. (2002). Research project—using essential oils in wound care for the elderly. *Aromatherapy Today, 23*, 14–19.

Keville, K., & Green, M. (2009). *Aromatherapy: A complete guide to the healing art* (2nd ed). Berkeley, CA: Crossing Press.

Kiecolt-Glaser, J., Graham, J., Malarkey, W., Porter, K., Lemeshow, S., & Glaser, R. (2007). Olfactory influences on mood and autonomic, endocrine, and immune function. *Psychoneuroendocrinology, 11*(15), 765–772.

Lawless, J. (1995). *The illustrated encyclopedia of essential oils*. London: Element Books.

Libster, M. (2002). *Delmar's integrative herb guide for nurses*. Victoria, Australia: Delmar Thompson Learning.

Morris, N. (2002). The effects of lavender (*Lavandula angustifolium*) baths on psychological well-being: Two exploratory randomized control trials. *Complementary Therapies in Medicine, 10*, 223–228.

Morris, N. (2008). The effects of lavender (*Lavandula angustifolia*) essential oil baths on stress and anxiety. *International Journal of Clinical Aromatherapy, 5*(1), 3–7.

Price, S., & Price L. (1999). *Aromatherapy for health professionals* (2nd ed.). Edinburgh: Churchill Livingstone.

Rose, J., & Behm, F. (1994). Inhalation of vapor from black pepper extract reduces smoking withdrawal symptoms. *Drug and Alcohol Dependence, 34,* 225–229.

Samarasekera, R., Weerasinghe, I., & Hemalal, K. (2008). Insecticidal activity of menthol derivatives against mosquitoes. *Pest Management Science, 64*(3), 290–295.

Schnaubelt, K. (1999). *Medical aromatherapy.* Berkeley, CA: Frog Ltd.

Sherry, E., Sivananthan, S., Warnke, P., & Eslick, G. (2003). Topical phytochemicals used to salvage the gangrenous lower limbs of type 1 diabetic patients. *Diabetes Research and Clinical Practice, 62*(1), 65–66.

Simpson, N., & Roman, K. (2001). Complementary medicine use in children: Extent and reasons. A population based study. *British Journal of General Practice, 51*(472), 914–916.

Singh, G., Kiran, S., Marimuthu, P., de Lampasona, M., de Heluani, C., & Catalan, C. (2008). Chemistry, biocidal and antioxidant activities of essential oil and oleoresins from *Piper cubeba* (seed). *International Journal of Essential Oil Therapeutics, 2,* 50–59.

Sinha, D., & Efron, D. (2005). Complementary and alternative medicine use in children: Extent and reasons. A population based study. *British Journal of General Practice, 51*(472), 914–916.

Styles, J. (1997). The use of aromatherapy in hospitalized children with HIV. *Complementary Therapies in Nursing, 3,* 16–20.

Tate, S. (1997). Peppermint oil, a treatment for postoperative nausea. *Journal of Advanced Nursing, 26,* 543–549.

Tindle, H., Davis, R., Phillips, R., & Eisenberg, D. (2005). Trends in the use of complementary and alternative medicine by U.S. adults: 1997–2002. *Alternative Therapies in Health and Medicine, 11,* 42–49.

Tisserand, R. (1988). Lavender beats benzodiazepines. *International Journal of Aromatherapy, 1*(2), 1–2.

Tisserand, R., & Balacs, T. (1995). *Essential oil safety.* London: Churchill Livingstone.

Veal, L. (1996). The potential effectiveness of essential oils as a treatment for head lice, *Pediculus humanis capitus. Complementary Therapies in Nursing and Midwifery, 2*(4), 97–101.

Weiss, E. (1997). *Essential oil crops.* Cambridge, UK: CAB International.

Williams, A., & Barry, B. (1989). Essential oils as novel skin penetration enhancers. *International Journal of Pharmaceutics, 57,* R7–R9.

27 Herbal Medicines

GREGORY A. PLOTNIKOFF

Herbs and related natural products such as spices are the oldest and most widely used form of medicine in the world. The use of herbs for the treatment of disease and the promotion of well-being can be traced back in many cultures at least 2,500 years. However, herbal medicines are not restricted to historical use. Today, in addition to aspirin, digoxin, and antibiotics, numerous plant-derived medications are available, including anticholinergic agents, anticoagulants, antihypertensives, and antineoplastic agents. In fact, of the top 150 pharmaceuticals in 1995, no less than 86 contained at least one major active compound from natural sources. These represented only 35 of the estimated 2 million extant plant species (Grifo, 1997).

The most comprehensive and reliable data on the use of herbal medicine comes from the 2007 National Health Interview Survey (NHIS), a survey of 23,300 adults and 9,400 adults on behalf of a child in their household. Use of natural products, including herbs, for medicinal purposes was documented in 17.7% of the American population (Barnes, Bloom, & Nahin, 2008).

The high prevalence of use in all regions of the United States and across all ages, genders, ethnicities, and medical diagnoses means that health professionals must address herbal medicine use in all patient encounters (Arcury et al., 2006; Cherniack et al., 2008). In the 2002 NHIS study, 55% of adults believed that use of complementary and alternative medicines (CAM) would support health when used in combination with conventional medical treatments (Barnes, Powell-Griner, McFann, & Nahin, 2004). This is significant. Use of herbal medicines may not be disclosed unless specifically requested by the nurse, pharmacist, or physician. Even in 2008, as many as 62.5% of regular herbal medicine users also used prescription medicines, but only 33% routinely reported their use to their care provider (Archer & Boyle, 2008). The 2004 Council for Responsible Nutrition survey of 1,000 randomly selected U.S. adults documented that 90% looked to health care professionals, including nurses, for guidance in herbal medicine use (Ward & Blumenthal, 2005). Thus, herbal medicine warrants significant attention by all nurses.

DEFINITION

Herbal medicines, or plant-based therapies, continue to occupy a place of central importance in the world's many healing traditions. These include the use of single herbs in many Western traditions and multiple-herb combinations in traditional Asian medical systems. Frequently, herbs are part of an overarching belief system that may involve spiritual or metaphysical components. Herbal medicines are often included in the work of shamans and other traditional healers who serve as intermediaries with the spirit world. Herbal medicines are also a tool in traditional Asian medicine and are used, like acupuncture, to open blocked channels (meridians) for the free flow of *qi* (life spirit or force).

Herbal medicines, also known as botanicals or phytotherapies, are one component of the range of natural products sold in the United States as dietary supplements. These include fungi-based products (mycotherapies); essential oils (aromatherapies); and vitamin, mineral, and nutritional therapies (nutraceuticals). Since the passage of the Dietary Supplement Health and Education Act of 1994 (DSHEA), these biological modifiers have been available over-the-counter as dietary supplements. Though neither food nor drug, these substances are still regulated by the Food and Drug Administration (FDA), but with less stringent requirements. Unlike foods and drugs, dietary supplements can be sold based on evidence of safety in the possession of the manufacturer and can only be removed from the market if the FDA can prove them unsafe under ordinary conditions of use.

Under DSHEA, herbal medicines can be sold for "stimulating, maintaining, supporting, regulating and promoting health" rather than for treating disease. As dietary supplements rather than drugs, herbal medicines cannot claim to restore normal (or correct abnormal) function. Additionally, herbs cannot claim to "diagnose, treat, prevent, cure, or mitigate" (DSHEA, 1994). Herbal medicine companies can assert that their product supports cardiovascular health but not that it lowers cholesterol. To do so would suggest that the product is intended for treating a disease (hypercholesterolemia) and is therefore subject to FDA pharmaceutical regulations.

This has raised questions about what constitutes a disease. The FDA originally defined a disease as any deviation, impairment, or interruption of the normal structure or function of any part, organ, or system of the body that is manifested by a characteristic set of one or more signs and symptoms. This definition generated many concerns. "Normal structure" appeared to be normed to a 30-year-old male and therefore did not account for gender or aging. For example, are menopause and menstrual cramps diseases? With no signs or symptoms, is hypercholesterolemia a disease or a risk factor? After significant public outcry, the FDA adopted the definition of disease found in the Nutrition Labeling and Health Act of 1989. Disease is currently considered damage to an organ, part, structure, or system of the body such that it does not function properly (e.g., cardiovascular disease) or a state of health leading to such (e.g., hypertension).

SCIENTIFIC BASIS

Significant research has been done using Western biomedical/scientific models on numerous single herbal agents. Beginning in 1978, the German government's *Bundesgesunheitsamt* (Federal Health Agency) began evaluating the safety and efficacy of phytomedicines. The health professionals charged with doing so, known as the Commission E, met until 1994 and evaluated 300 herbal medicines, of which they recognized 190 as suitable for medicinal use. The complete reports have been translated and are available from the American Botanical Council (2000).

Beginning in 1996, significant meta-analyses and review articles of single herb products began appearing on a regular basis in leading

Western medical journals. These are readily accessible via the National Library of Medicine's PubMed Web site (http://www.ncbi.nlm.nih.gov/PubMed/). Compiling data from similar studies for analysis (meta-analysis) is complicated by the fact that many studies published to date have left out important information, including naming the specific plant species studied (e.g., echinacea versus *Echinacea purpurea, E. pallida,* or *E. augustofolia*), the parts used (stems, leaves, or roots), the form (pressed juice, powdered whole extract, aqueous extract, ethanol extract, or aqueous-ethanol extract), and the formulation (stated proportions of water to alcohol or specifically extracted fractions and concentrations).

Standardization of herbal medicines is crucial both for scientific study and consumer protection. Standardization is equated with reproducibility, guaranteed potency, quality of active ingredients, and documentable effectiveness. However, with herbal medicines, standardization presents several problems. First, the active ingredient may not be known. Second, there may be more than one active ingredient. Third, both content and activity of an herbal medicine may be related to the means of extraction and processing. This significantly complicates both research and counseling for health professionals and consumers.

An increasing number of health care professionals are studying the effects of these substances. With an increase in the FDA's involvement, we can look forward to a more reliable herb market. Increased knowledge of herbal indications may increase the safety and efficacy of herbal therapies for patients.

INTERVENTION

Technique

Herbal medicines and dietary supplements need to be addressed in clinical settings in the same manner one addresses pharmaceutical agents. Every health professional needs to be aware of the wide use of herbal medicines and other dietary supplements. Efficient and effective patient advocacy means including questions on alternative therapies as a standard part of each patient interview. Reasonable questions include: *Are you using any herbs? Vitamins? Dietary supplements?* Follow-up questions include: *What dose? What source? What directions are you following? Why are you taking it?* Asking about the source of information can be quite helpful, as in, *"Are you working with any other health professionals?"* As with all good interviewing, listening for understanding rather than agreement or disagreement enhances the therapeutic alliance. In addition to knowing the type of herb used, the dose of each herb, and the intended purpose of each herb, gathering information regarding the duration of herb use will also be helpful in assessing patients and providing safe and effective care.

Unfortunately, professionals often do not ask such questions and up to 69% of CAM-using patients do not volunteer such information (Graham et al., 2005). This "don't ask, don't tell" policy makes no sense in patient care. All health professionals need to create a safe environment that is conducive to patients' open sharing of important information such as herbal use or use of other complementary/alternative therapies without fear of ridicule or other negative responses. "Ask, then ask again" is a practice policy foundational to safe and effective patient care.

Precautions

A common misconception regarding herbal medicines is that herbs have no side effects because they are "natural." However, herbs do indeed have side effects and may be toxic or poisonous if not used appropriately. Consider the toxicity of such widely used natural products as coffee, cocaine, and tobacco. Another dilemma is patient use of herbs in lieu of their prescribed medications. Although herbs may be a good option in particular cases and conditions, the decision to decline medications should be based upon fully informed judgments in partnership with a health professional.

Interviewing for herbal medicine use is crucial for identifying those patients at risk for interactions with prescription medications or for excessive bleeding in surgery. Patients with special risks of drug interactions include those taking the following pharmaceutical agents: anticoagulants, hypoglycemics, antidepressants, sedative-hypnotics, antihypertensives, and medications with narrow therapeutic windows such as digoxin and theophylline.

Pregnancy, lactation, breastfeeding, and child care are special topics in herbal medicine use. For these situations, the most authoritative

Exhibit 27.1

References for Pregnancy, Breastfeeding, Lactation, and Children

Hale, T. W. (2004). *Medications and Mother's Milk: A Manual of Lactational Pharmacology,* 11th edition. Amarillo, TX: Pharmasoft Medical Publishers.

Humphrey, S. (2004). *The Nursing Mother's Herbal.* Minneapolis, MN: Fairview Press.

Kemper, K. J. (2002). *The Holistic Pediatrician,* 2nd Edition. New York: Perennial Currents.

Romm, A. J. (2003). *The Natural Pregnancy Book.* Berkeley, CA: Ten Speed Press.

references are cited in Exhibit 27.1. In the absence of clinical trial data, use is guided by historical experience or breast milk analysis. Herbs that increase breast milk production, such as fenugreek, are frequently recommended by International Board of Certified Lactation Consultants (IBCLC).

Nursing skills include the ability to counsel. Exhibit 27.2 lists key teaching points regarding herbal medicines. Herbal therapies are only safe if herbs are prepared in the right way and used for the right indication, in the right amounts, for the right duration, and with appropriate monitoring. Potential herb–herb and herb–drug interactions should be considered when patients are using herbal products. The lack of national standards in the collection and preparation of herbal products complicates this field in the United States. Because many herbs have potential or actual risks that need to be recognized, it is important for health providers to have reliable and accessible sources of information to prevent adverse herb-related reactions and also to identify and manage complications of herbal therapies; Exhibit 27.2 cites selected reputable herbal references.

All serious adverse reactions should be reported to the FDA through the MedWatch program at 1-800-332-1088 or at http://www.fda.gov/medwatch. An example of a complication associated with herbal therapy is illustrated in the case of the use of *Ma huang* (Ephedra), marketed in the United States until recently as a major ingredient in formulations for weight reduction. Because use of this herb had been linked to numerous adverse cardiovascular events, including stroke, myocardial infarction, and sudden death (Haller & Benowitz, 2000), the FDA banned sales of this herb in April of 2004.

Exhibit 27.2

Herbal References and Resources

American Botanical Council: www.herbalgram.org

American Nutraceutical Association: www.americanutra.com

The U.S. FDA Center for Food Safety and Applied Nutrition—a link to report adverse events: www.cfsan.fda.gov/~dms/aems.html

National Center for Complementary and Alternative Medicine: www.nccam.nih.gov

Herb Research Foundation: www.herbs.org

Herbal Medicine—The Expanded Commission E Monographs (2000). Blumenthal, Goldberg, and Brinckmann (Eds.). Austin, TX: American Botanical Council.

Nurses Herbal Medicine Handbook (2001). Lippincott Williams & Wilkins, 2001.

HerbalGram magazine—published quarterly by the American Botanical Council and the Herb Research Foundation: www.herbalgram.org

Tarascon Pocket Pharmacopoeia—contains a section on herbal and alternative therapies and has a PDA version that may be downloaded for a free trial: www.tarascon.com

Micromedex Alternative Medicine Database—an authoritative, full-text drug information resource; includes alternative medicine and is one of the most comprehensive resources for herbal medicine: www.library.ucsf.edu/db/micromedex.html

USES

Given the volume and variety of products, herbal medicine knowledge relevant for nursing practice cannot be summarized quickly. This chapter will now address three of the most important herbs from an evidence-based perspective. The reader will note that there is a significant range in scientific data available on each and the theoretical risks should be acknowledged and carefully considered both by patients and health professionals. Further, the clinical knowledge related to combining herbal products with prescription and nonprescription drugs is only in the developmental stages; much remains to be known about interactions and side effects.

Chronic illness (such as cancer or autoimmune disease or chronic pain), surgery, and use of prescription medications are three situations in which herbal medicine reviews by nurses are important. Echinacea does stimulate the immune system, but this is not necessarily a positive effect. Ginkgo biloba's pharmacologic activity places people at risk in

Exhibit 27.3

> **Five Key Patient Learning Points**
>
> Just because it is natural does not mean it is safe.
>
> Just because it is safe does not mean it is effective.
>
> Labels may not equal contents.
>
> Self-diagnosis and self-treatment can result in self-malpractice.
>
> Herbs are never a replacement for an emergency room.

surgery. Saint John's wort is effective for depression but can render many prescription medications ineffective or even toxic. Readers should be aware that many herbs have a sufficient evidence base and potential as alternatives to Western medicine. However, herbal medicine in the United States is a very broad and multicultural phenomenon; it is difficult to know all products used by or all products of potential benefit to patients. Readers should be aware that there are reputable clinical resources readily accessible for assistance in informed decision making (see Exhibit 27.3).

Echinacea (*Echinacea augustofolia, E. pallida, E. purpurea*)

Echinacea is the most commonly used herbal medicine in the United States, used by persons of all ages, genders, and ethnicities. This includes 19.8% of herbal medicine-using adults and 37.2% of herbal medicine-using children (Barnes et al., 2008). North American gardens commonly contain Echinacea, also known as the purple coneflower. It was traditionally used by Native Americans and early settlers as a remedy for infections and for healing wounds. Several components, particularly the alkamides and caffeic acid derivatives, have clear pharmacologic activity (Barnes, Anderson, Gibbons, & Phillipson, 2005). In vitro research suggests an immunostimulatory effect principally by macrophage, polymorphonuclear leukocyte, and natural killer cell activation (Barrett, 2003). Monocyte secretion of tumor necrosis factor-alpha (TNF-á) is particularly stimulated (Senchina et al., 2005). However, the therapeutic effectiveness of echinacea has not been established.

Echinacea is promoted in the United States for the prevention and treatment of the common cold. In Europe, it is used topically for wound healing and intravenously for immunostimulation. Several methodologically valid clinical studies have been published in recent years with unimpressive results, suggesting that Echinacea is not effective for the treatment or prevention of upper respiratory illness for adults. A 2006 meta-analysis by the prestigious Cochrane Collaborative stated that the Echinacea products used in clinical trials differed greatly but that preparations based on the aerial parts of *Echinacea purpurea* may be effective for the early treatment of colds (Linde, Barrett, Bauer, Wölkart, & Melchart, 2006). A follow up meta-analysis of 14 randomized, controlled trials documented that Echinacea decreased the odds of developing a common cold by 58% and reduced the duration of symptoms by 1.4 days (Shah, Sander, White, Rinaldi, & Coleman, 2007).

Echinacea has a good safety profile but has been associated (very infrequently) with gastric upset, rashes, and severe allergic reactions. Echinacea is not recommended for persons with allergies to members of the *Asteraceae* family (formerly termed *Compositae*), which includes ragweed, daisies, thistles, and chamomile. More importantly, nonspecific immunostimulation may exacerbate preexisting autoimmune disease or precipitate autoimmune disease in genetically predisposed persons (Lee & Werth, 2004). Tumor necrosis factor-alpha and interleukin-1 are pro-inflammatory cytokines, and recent evidence demonstrates that anti-TNF and anti–interleukin-1 therapies are effective for autoimmune diseases, including Crohn's disease and rheumatoid arthritis. Echinacea cannot be recommended for people with other chronic immunologic diseases, including multiple sclerosis, lupus, and HIV.

There are no verifiable reports of drug–herb interactions with any Echinacea product. *E. purpurea* products have a low potential for generating any cytopchrome P450 drug–herb intereactions (Freeman & Spelman, 2008).

The LD_{50} of intravenously administered echinacea juice is 50 mL/ kg in mice and rats. Regular oral administration to mice at levels greater than proposed human therapeutic doses has failed to demonstrate toxic effects (Mengs, Clare, & Poiley, 1991). However, one study has suggested that repeated daily doses suppress the immune response (Coeugniet & Elek, 1987). The German government's Commission E recommends that use be limited to 8 weeks. Use of Echinacea for more than 8 weeks is associated with higher risk of neutropenia (Blumenthal et al., 1998).

Ginkgo (*Ginkgo biloba*)

Ginkgo is the number-one-selling herb in Europe for improvement of blood flow and enhancement of cognition. Clinically, ginkgo is used for circulatory problems such as peripheral artery disease (Pittler & Ernst, 2005), impotence (Sikora, 1989), and "cerebral insufficiency" (Kleijnen & Knipschild, 1992a). The German government's Commission E also approved its use for dementia syndromes with memory deficits, disturbances in concentration, depressive emotional conditions, dizziness, tinnitus, and headaches.

The *Cochrane Review* in 2007 stated that ginkgo appears safe with no excess side effects, compared with placebo. Benefits were seen at doses of 200 mg/day beginning at 12 weeks. However, they noted that, because of variability in trial design and quality, the evidence for predictable and clinically significant benefit is unconvincing (Birks & Grimley Evans, 2007). A follow-up systematic review noted that in all studies with active controls, ginkgo was at least as effective as the pharmaceutical intervention (May, Lit, Xue, Yang, Zhang Owens, et al., 2009). An additional review found that of seven studies with relatively high external validity and good overall quality, five showed a positive result in more than 50% of parameters measured (Bornhöft, Maxion-Bergemann, & Matthiessen, 2008).

European studies published in 1994 and 1996 demonstrated ginkgo's effectiveness in slowing or reversing dementia (Hofferberth, 1994; Kanowski, Herrmann, Stephan, Wierich, & Horr, 1996). A study published in 1997 confirmed these findings for patients with Alzheimer's disease and multi-infarct dementia in an American trial with 309 subjects (LeBars et al., 1997).

Recently, intriguing data have been published that suggest possible use of ginkgo in Parkinson's disease (Ahmad et al., 2005; Kim, Lee, Lee, & Kim, 2004) and diabetic retinopathy (Huang, Jeng, Kao, Yu, & Liu, 2004). Additionally, there is interest in its use for cell phone users (Ilhan et al., 2004) and stressed adults (Walesiuk, Trofimiuk, & Braszko, 2005). However, larger trials are still needed to confirm such therapeutic benefit. Additionally, there is no convincing evidence that ginkgo enhances cognitive function in healthy young people (Canter & Ernst, 2007).

Ginkgo's leaf extracts are used in Europe both orally and intravenously for treatment of Alzheimer's dementia, multi-infarct dementia, peripheral vascular disease, and vertigo (Kaufmann, 2002; Li, Ma, Scherban, & Tam, 2002). Ginkgo's active ingredients are terpene trilactones (6%; specifically, ginkgolides and bilobalide) and flavanoid glycosides (24%), which are the bases for standardized leaf extracts. Ginkgo's mechanism of action is believed to be its in vitro antioxidative, antiplatelet, antihypoxic, antiedemic, hemorrheologic, and microcirculatory actions (Mahadevan & Park, 2008). It is more effective than beta-carotene and vitamin E as an oxidative scavenger and inhibitor of lipid peroxidation of cellular membranes (Pietschmann, Kuklinski, & Otterstein, 1992) and stimulates the release of nitric oxide (Chen, Salwinski, & Lee, 1997). Ginkgo is also a potent antagonist of platelet-activating factor (Engelsen, Nielson, & Winther, 2002) and thus inhibits platelet aggregation and promotes clot breakdown. Ginkgo in the central nervous system (CNS) inhibits production of pro-inflammatory cytokines and upregulates anti-inflammatory cytokines (Jiao, Rui, Li, Yang, & Qiu, 2005). These properties may result in neuroprotective and ischemia reperfusion–protective effects (Oyama, Chikahisa, Ueha, Kanemaru, & Noda, 1996; Sener et al., 2005; Shen & Zhou, 1995).

Side effects with ginkgo are uncommon. They include gastrointestinal discomfort, headache, and dizziness. Because of its antiplatelet effect, however, there has been reported widely a risk of significant bleeding when ginkgo is used with anticoagulants and other antiplatelet agents (Bebbington, Kulkarni, & Roberts, 2005; Matthews, 1998; Rosenblatt & Mindel, 1997; Rowin & Lewis, 1996). The most recent studies on ginkgo and platelet activity in vivo do not support concerns for perioperative bleeding or potentiation of anticoagulant or antiplatelet drugs (Beckert, Concannon, Henry, Smith & Puckett, 2007; Bone, 2008). At this time, most surgeons request that ginkgo be discontinued 10 days prior to surgery and not restarted until the surgical wound has healed sufficiently to allow for aspirin use.

Saint John's Wort (*Hypericum perforatum*)

Saint John's wort, one of the world's top-selling herbs, has been used for centuries in Europe as a sedative and as a balm for skin injuries.

Since 1996, it has been widely promoted in the United States as a wonder drug for depression or as "nature's Prozac." Today, it is often used to treat mild-to-moderate depression, anxiety, and sleep disorders.

In vitro studies have shown that *Hypericum* extract inhibits the neuronal uptake of the neurotransmitters serotonin, noradrenaline, dopamine, gamma-aminobutyric acid (GABA), and L-glutamate (Muller, Rolli, Schafer, & Hafner, 1997). No in vivo MAO-inhibiting activity has been demonstrated with *Hypericum*.

Three significant reviews appeared in 2008 that demonstrated positive effects for *Hypericum* (Carpenter, Crigger, Kugler, & Loya, 2008; Kasper et al., 2008; Linde, Berner, & Kriston, 2008). In the *Cochrane Review* meta-analysis of 29 trials with 5,489 patients, 18 comparisons with placebo and 17 comparisons with prescription antidepressants were included. For 9 large trials, the response rate compared with placebo was 1.28 (95% CI: 1.10 to 1.49) and for 9 smaller trials, the response rate ratio was 1.87 (95% CI: 1.22–2.87). The review team concluded that St. John's Wort extracts are superior to placebo and similarly effective as standard prescription antidepressants with fewer side effects (Linde et al., 2008).

There is no one active ingredient in St. John's Wort. Bioactive components include the napthodianthones hypericin and pseudohypericin and the phloroglucionols hyperforin and adhyperforin. Ginkgo also contains many flavanoids (Butterweck & Schmidt, 2007).

The most serious toxicity associated with St. John's wort is the negative interactions with prescription drugs. Saint John's wort is a potent inducer of both P-glycoprotein and cytochrome P450 (CYP) 3A4, the hepatic enzyme involved in the metabolism of more than 50% of all prescription drugs (Zhou & Lai, 2008). Significant interactions include anticancer agents (imatinib and irinotecan), anti-HIV drugs (indinavir, lamivudine, and nevirapine), anit-inflammatory drugs (ibuprofen and fexofenadine), antibiotics/antifungals (erythromycin and voriconazole), cardiac medications (digoxin, ivabradine, warfarin, verapamil, nifedipine, atorvastatin, pravastatin, and talinolol), CNS agents (amitryptiline, buspirone, phenytoin, methadone, midazolam, alprazolam, and sertraline), diabetes medications (tolbutamide and gliclazide), and immunosuppressants (cyclosporine and tacrolimus), as well as oral contraceptives, proton pump inhibitors, and theophylline (Di, Li, Xue, & Zhou, 2008). Hence, the use of Saint John's wort can be life-threatening for people requiring prescription medications. Because of its long half-life, the herb should be discontinued at least 5 days prior to initiation of any of the above medications, and close monitoring of drug levels may be indicated. Additional theoretical concerns include the risk of photosensitivity or the precipitation of a serotonergic crisis in interaction with other prescription antidepressants.

CULTURAL APPLICATIONS

The practice of Western herbalism parallels that of Western pharmaceutical interventions. One herb with a defined pharmacologic activity can be applied to a given patient with a given medical diagnosis. Successful treatment is understood as relief or eradication of the offending symptoms. Herbal medicines differ from pharmaceuticals in that, unlike plant-derived medications such as digoxin, single active agents are not identified, isolated, purified, and concentrated for human use. There is a presumed synergy of multiple bioactive components. Rigorous scientific studies are thus much more difficult to conduct than for pharmaceuticals.

In sharp contrast to the North American experience, traditional Asian herbal traditions use formulas containing multiple herbs that are customized for the patient and often for unmeasurable constitutional states and nonquantifiable outcomes. Up to 12 ingredients can exist in these formulas. Ingredients can include plants, mushrooms, and minerals. In Chinese formulas, animal parts are often included.

Of particular interest may be Japan's Kampo tradition. Today, in Japan, medical students are routinely taught to prescribe 148 ancient, multiherb formulas that are approved by Japan's equivalent of the FDA and covered by their national health plan. Approximately 70% of all physicians do prescribe these multiherb formulas, including nearly 100% of Japanese gynecologists. Diagnosis is made by physical exam of tongue, pulse, and abdomen. Diagnoses can be very subjective, such as *katakori* (literally, frozen shoulder, but patients have full range of motion) and *hiesho* (cold condition with normal body temperatures). There is no 1:1 correlation between a condition such as *hiesho* and a formula. Several formulas exist and are used for multiple conditions. The correct formula is based on the patient's history, physical exam, and response to initial treatment (Plotnikoff, Watanabe, & Yashiro, 2008).

FUTURE RESEARCH

Before even Western single-herb medicines can be more widely accepted by the conventional allopathic medical system, more randomized, double-blind, placebo-controlled trials are needed in the United States. The NIH's National Center for Complementary and Alternative Medicine (NCCAM) has funded and will continue to fund such clinical trials of herbal therapies. Promising understudied areas of study for herbal therapies include:

1. Numerous herbs for perimenopausal hot flash management
2. Milk thistle for hepatoprotection in the presence of hepatotoxic agents
3. Feverfew to augment breast milk production
4. Numerous medicinal mushrooms for adjunctive cancer therapy

Additionally, significant efforts are needed to identify the most promising herbal supports for chemotherapy and radiation therapy as well as for asthma and heart disease.

Western medicine has yet to explore the potential benefits from the world's many healing traditions that use customized combinations of herbs. To research these will require a new paradigm, one that accounts for potential synergy and counterbalancing activities of multiple ingredients. Although intriguing preliminary data exist for many dietary supplements, the historic paucity of funding mechanisms in these areas has meant that scientific support for the use of many commercial products lags significantly behind consumer marketing efforts.

REFERENCES

Ahmad, M., Saleem, S., Ahmad, A., Yousuf, S., Ansari, M. A., Khan, M. B., et al. (2005). Ginkgo biloba affords dose-dependent protection against 6-hydroxydopamine-induced parkinsonism in rats: Neurobehavioral, neuro-chemical and immunohistochemical evidence. *Journal of Neurochemistry, 93,* 94–104.

American Botanical Council. (2000). *Herbal medicine: Expanded commission E monographs.* Austin, TX: American Botanical Council.

Archer, E. L., & Boyle, D. K. (2008). Herb and supplement use among the retail population of an independent, urban herb store. *Journal of Holistic Nursing, 26,* 27–35.

Arcury, T. A., Suerken, C. K., Brzywacz, J. G., Bell, R. A., Lang, W., & Quandt, S. A. (2006). Complementary and alternative medicine use among older adults: Ethnic variation. *Ethnic Diseases, 16,* 723–31.

Barnes, J., Anderson, L. A., Gibbons, S., & Phillipson, J. D. (2005). Echinacea species (*Echinacea angustifolica* (DC.) Hell., *Echinacea pallida* (Nutt.) Nutt., *Echinacea purpurea* (L.) Moench): A review of their chemistry, pharmacology and clinical properties. *Journal of Pharmacy and Pharmacology, 57,* 929–54.

Barnes, P. M., Bloom, B., & Nahin, R. (2008, December 10). Complementary and Alternative Medicine Use Among Adults and Children: United States, 2007. *CDC National Health Statistics Report #12.*

Barnes, P. M., Powell-Griner, E., McFann, K., & Nahin, R. I. (2004). Complementary and alternative medicine use among adults: United States, 2002. *Advance Data, 343,* 1–19.

Barrett, B. (2003). Medicinal properties of Echinacea: A critical review. *Phytomedicine, 10,* 66–86.

Bebbington, A., Kulkarni, R., & Roberts, P. (2005). Ginkgo biloba: Persistent bleeding after total hip arthroplasty caused by herbal self-medication. *Journal of Arthroplasty, 20,* 125–126.

Beckert, B. W., Concannon, M. J., Henry, S. L., Smith, D. S., & Puckett, C. L. (2007). The effect of herbal medicines on platelet function: An in vivo experiment and review of the literature. *Plastic and Reconstructive Surgery, 120,* 2044–2050.

Birks, J., & Grimley Evans, J. (2007, April 18). Ginkgo biloba for cognitive impairment and dementia. *Cochrane Database of Systematic Reviews,* CD003120.

Blumenthal, M., Busse, W. R, Goldberg, A., et al. (1998). *The complete German Commission E monographs.* American Botanical Council, Austin, TX.

Bone, K. M. (2008). Potential interaction of Ginkgo biloba leaf with antiplatelet or anticoagulant drugs: What is the evidence? *Molecular Nutrition and Food Research, 52,* 764–771.

Bornhöft, G., Maxion-Bergemann, S., & Matthiessen, P. F. (2008). Die Rolle der externen Validität bei der Beurteilung klinischer Studien zur Demenzbehandlung mit Ginkgo-biloba-Extrakten. [External validity of clinical trials for treatment of dementia with ginkgo biloba extracts]. *Zeitschrift für Gerontologie und Geriatrie, 41,* 298–312.

Butterweck, V., & Schmidt, M. (2008). St. John's Wort: Role of active compounds for its mechanism of action and efficacy. *Wiener medizinische Wochenschrift, 157,* 356–361.

Canter, P. H., & Ernst, E. (2007). Ginkgo biloba is not a smart drug: An updated systemic review of randomized clinical trials testing the nootropic effects of G. biloba extracts in healthy people. *Human Psychopharmacology, 22,* 265–278.

Carpenter, C., Crigger, N., Kugler, R., & Loya, A. (2008). Hypericum and nurses: A comprehensive literature review on the efficacy of St. John's Wort in the treatment of depression. *Journal of Holistic Nursing, 26,* 200–207.

Chen, X., Salwinski, S., & Lee, T. J. (1997). Extracts of Ginkgo biloba and ginsenosides exert cerebral vasorelaxation via a nitric oxide pathway. *Clinical Experimental Pharmacology and Physiology, 24,* 958–959.

Cherniack, E. P., Ceron-Fuentes, J., Florez, H., Sandals, L., Rodriguez, O., & Palacios, J. C. (2008). Influence of race and ethnicity on alternative medicine as a self-treatment for common medical conditions in a population of multi-ethnic urban elderly. *Complementary Therapies in Clinical Practice, 14,* 116–123.

Coeugniet, E. G., & Elek, E. (1987). Immunomodulation with Viscum album and Echinacea purpurea extracts. *Onkologie, 10*(Suppl. 3), 27.

Di, Y. M., Li, C. G., Xue, C. C. & Zhou, S. F. (2008). Clinical drugs that interact with St. John's wort and implication in drug development. *Current Pharmacology Design, 14,* 1723–1742.

Dietary Supplement Health & Education Act of 1994, Public Law 103-417, 103rd Congress of the United States of America.

Engelsen, J., Nielson, J. D., & Winther, K. (2002). Effect of coenzyme Q10 and Ginkgo Biloba on warfarin dosage in stable, long-term warfarin treated outpatients: A randomized double blind placebo-crossover trial. *Thrombosis & Haemostatis, 87*(6), 1075–1076.

Freeman, C., & Spelman, K. (2008). A critical evaluation of drug interactions with Echinacea spp. *Molecular Nutrition and Food Research, 52,* 789–798.

Graham, R. E., Ahn, A. C., Davis, R. B., O'Connor, B. B., Eisenberg, D. M., & Phillips, R. S. (2005). Use of complementary and alternative medical therapies among racial and ethinic minority adults: results from the 2002 National Health Interview Survey. *Journal of the National Medical Association, 97,* 535–545.

Grifo, F. (1997). *Biodiversity and human health.* Washington, DC: Island Press.

Haller, C. A., & Benowitz, N. L. (2000). Adverse cardiovascular and central nervous system events associated with dietary supplements containing ephedra alkaloids. *New England Journal of Medicine, 343*(25), 1833–1838.

Hofferberth, B. (1994). The efficacy of Egb 761 in patients with senile dementia of the Alzheimer's type: A double-blind, placebo-controlled study on different levels of investigation. *Human Psychopharmacology, 9,* 215–222.

Huang, S. Y., Jeng, C., Kao, S. C., Yu, J. J., & Liu, D. Z. (2004). Improved haemorrheological properties by Ginkgo biloba extract EGb 761 in type 2 diabetes mellitus complicated with retinopathy. *Clinical Nutrition, 23,* 615–621.

Ilhan, A., Gurel, A., Armutcu, F., Kamisli, S., Iraz, M., Akyol, O., et al. (2004). Ginkgo biloba prevents mobile phone-induced oxidative stress in rat brain. *Clinica Chimica Acta, 340,* 153–162.

Jiao, Y. B., Rui, Y. C., Li, T. J., Yang, P. Y., & Qiu, Y. (2005). Expression of proinflammatory and anti-inflammatory cytokines in brain of atherosclerotic rats and effects of Ginkgo biloba extract. *Acta Pharmacologica Sinica, 26,* 835–839.

Kanowski, S., Herrmann, W. M., Stephan, K., Wierich, W., & Horr, R. (1996). Proof of efficacy of the Ginkgo biloba extract Egb 761 in outpatients suffering from mild to moderate primary degenerative dementia of the Alzheimer's type of multi-infarct dementia. *Pharmacopsychiatry, 29,* 47–56.

Kasper, S., Gastpar, M., Müller, W. E., Volz, H. P., Dienel, A., Kieser, M., et al. (2008). Efficacy of St. John's Wort extract WS 5570 in acute treatment of mild depression: A reanalysis of data from controlled clinical trials. *European Archives of Psychiatry and Clinical Neuroscience, 258,* 59–63.

Kaufmann, H. (2002). Treatment of patients with orthostatic hypotension and syncope. *Clinical Neuropharmacology, 25*(3), 133–141.

Kim, M. S., Lee, J. I., Lee, W. Y., & Kim, S. E. (2004). Neuroprotective effect of Ginkgo biloba L. extract in a rat model of Parkinson's disease. *Phytotherapy Research, 18,* 663–666.

Kleijnen, J., & Knipschild, P. (1992a). Ginkgo biloba for cerebral insufficiency. *British Journal of Pharmacology, 34,* 352.

LeBars, P. L., Katz, M. M., Berman, N., Itil, T. M., Freedman, A. M., & Schatz-berg, A. F. (1997). A placebo-controlled, double-blind, randomized trial of an extract of Ginkgo biloba for dementia. *Journal of the American Medical Association, 278,* 1327–1332.

Lee, A. N., & Werth, V. P. (2004). Activation of autoimmunity following use of immunostimulatory herbal supplements. *Archives of Dermatology, 140,* 723–772.

Li, X. F., Ma, M., Scherban, K., & Tam, Y. K. (2002). Liquid chromatography-electrospray mass spectrometric studies of ginkgolides and bilobalide using simultaneous monitoring of proton, ammonium, and sodium adducts. *Analyst, 127,* 641–646.

Linde, K., Barrett, B., Bauer, R., Melchart, D., & Wölkart, K. (2006). Echinacea for preventing and treating the common cold. *Cochrane Database of Systematic Reviews, 1,* CD000530.

Linde, K., Berner, M. M., & Kriston, L. (2008). St. John's Wort for major depression. *Cochrane Database of Systematic Reviews, 4,* CD000448.

Mahadevan, S., & Park, Y. (2008). Multifaceted therapeutic benefits of Ginkgo biloba L.: Chemistry, efficacy, safety and uses. *Journal of Food Science, 73*(1), R14-9.

Matthews, M. K., Jr. (1998). Association of Ginkgo biloba with intracerebral hemorrhage. *Neurology, 50,* 1933–1934.

May, B. H., Lit, M., Xue, C. C., Yang, A. W., Zhang, A. L., Owens, M. D., et al. (2009). Herbal medicine for dementia: A systematic review. *Phytotherapy Research, 23,* 447–459.

Mengs, U., Clare, C. B., & Poiley, J. A. (1991). Toxicity of Echinacea purpurea. Acute, subacute and genotoxicity studies. *Arzneimittel-Frosch, 41,* 1076–1081.

Muller, W. E., Rolli, M., Schafer, C., & Hafner, U. (1997). Effects of Hypericum extract (L160) in biochemical models of antidepressant activity. *Pharmopsychiatry, 30*(Suppl. 2), 102–107.

National Library of Medicine. Retrieved 2005 from *http://www.ncbi.nlm.nih.* gov/Pubmed

Oyama, Y., Chikahisa, L., Ueha, T., Kanemaru, K., & Noda, K. (1996). Ginkgo biloba extract protects brain neurons against oxidative stress induced by hydrogen peroxide. *Brain Research, 712,* 349–352.

Pietschmann, A., Kuklinski, B., & Otterstein, A. (1992). Protection from UV-light-induced oxidative stress by nutritional radical scavengers. *Zeitschrift fur die Gesamte Innere Medizin und Ihre Grenzgebiete, 47*(11), 518–522.

Pittler, M. H., & Ernst, E. (2005). Complementary therapies for peripheral artery disease: Systematic review. *Atherosclerosis, 18,* 1–7.

Plotnikoff, G. A, Watanabe, K., & Yashiro, F. (2008). Kampo: From old wisdom comes new knowledge. *HerbalGram,78,* 46–56.

Rosenblatt, M., & Mindel, J. (1997). Spontaneous hyphema associated with ingestion of Ginkgo biloba extract. *New England Journal of Medicine, 336,* 1108.

Rowin, J., & Lewis, S. L. (1996). Spontaneous bilateral subdural hematomas associated with chronic Ginkgo biloba ingestion have also occurred. *Neurology, 46,* 1775–1776.

Senchina, D. S., McDann, D. A., Asp, J. M., Johnson, J. A., Cunnick, J. E., Kaiser, M. S. et al. (2005). Changes in immunomodulatory properties of Echinacea spp. root infusions and tinctures stored at 4 degrees C for four days. *Clinica Chimica Acta, 355,* 67–82.

Sener, G., Sener, E., Sehirli, O., Ogune, A. V., Cetinel, S., Gedik, N., et al. (2005). Ginkgo biloba extract ameliorates ischemia reperfusion-induced renal injury in rats. *Pharmacology Research,* Epub May 13.

Shah, S. A., Sander, S., White, C. M., Rinaldi, M., & Coleman, C. I. (2007). Evaluation of Echinacea for the prevention and treatment of the common cold: A meta-analysis. *Lancet Infectious Disease 7,* 473–480.

Shen, J. G., & Zhou, D. Y. (1995). Efficiency of Ginkgo biloba extract (Egb 761) in antioxidant protection against myocardial ischemia and re-perfusion injury. *Biochemical Molecular Biological Institute, 35,* 125–134.

Sikora, K. (1989). Complementary medicine and cancer treatment. *Practitioner, 233*(1476), 1285–1286.

U.S. Congress, Senate Committee on Labor and Human Resources. (1989, November 13). *Nutrition Labeling and Education Act of 1989.* [S.1425.] Washington, DC: U.S. Government Printing Office.

U.S. House of Representatives, Committee on Government Reform. (1999, March 25). *Dietary Supplement Health and Education Act: Is the FDA trying to change the intent of Congress?* Washington, DC: U.S. Government Printing Office.

Walesiuk, A., Trofimiuk, E., & Braszko, J. J. (2005). Ginkgo biloba extract diminishes stress-induced memory deficits in rats. *Pharmacology Reporter, 57,* 176–187.

Ward, E., & Blumenthal, M. (2005). Americans confident in dietary supplements according to CRN survey. *HerbalGram, 66,* 64–65.

28 Functional Foods and Nutraceuticals

MELISSA FRISVOLD

In the twenty-first century, the focus of the relationship between eating habits and health is changing from an emphasis on health maintenance through recommended dietary allowances of nutrients, vitamins, and minerals to an emphasis on the use of foods to provide better health, increase vitality, and aid in preventing disease and many chronic illnesses. The connection between food and health is not new. Indeed, the adage "Let food be your medicine and medicine your food" was adopted by Hippocrates (trans. 1932). Today, the philosophy that supports the paradigm of nutraceuticals as functional foods is once again at the forefront.

Despite this ancient wisdom, the use of nutraceuticals and functional foods remains in its infancy in the Western world. It was not until the late 1970s that the trend toward improved physical fitness and overall well-being began. At that time, scientific evidence began to stress the importance of a balanced diet low in saturated fat, sodium, and cholesterol, and higher in fiber. Currently, the use of nutraceuticals, including additives to certain conventional foods, phytochemicals, functional foods, dietary foods and supplements, and medical foods is growing at an astronomical rate. In the past several years, the U.S. Food and Drug Administration (FDA) has worked to examine the possible connections between nutritional products and disease states, including calcium and osteoporosis, sodium and hypertension, lipids and cardiovascular disease, lipids and cancer, and dietary fiber and cardiovascular disease (Gardner, 1994).

With the developing market of functional foods, it is estimated that in 2008 consumers in the United States spent over $129 billion on dietary supplements (*Nutrition Business Journal*, 2008). One can now find calcium added to juices, pasta, rice, dry cereals, and even chocolate and caramel candy products. Many companies are using soy protein isolates in foods ranging from candy bars and salad dressings to infant formulas. Plant stanols and sterols are being added to margarine-like spreads in an effort to reduce total cholesterol and low-density lipoprotein (LDL) levels. Common nutraceuticals receiving broad attention include calcium-fortified fruit drinks and candy; soy protein bars fortified with whey protein; soy protein products and high-fiber cereals; and "snack" bars providing L-arginine, which may improve vascular functioning.

Coverage of all nutraceuticals is beyond the scope of this chapter. There has been a plethora of functional foods developed in recent times and in fact in the past year there were 142 new functional foods or beverages aimed at digestive health and 134 new functional food products for cardiovascular health (Mintel's New Global Products Database, 2009). In the interest of brevity, in this chapter several selected products will be covered in depth. Because the use of nutraceuticals is so prevalent and because their use may impact health and wellness, it is important that nurses know about nutraceuticals and their potential benefits and risks.

DEFINITIONS

To understand the terms *functional food* and *nutraceuticals,* one must understand the definition of foods. The FDA defines foods as "articles used primarily for taste, aroma, or nutritive value" (Federal Food, Drug and Cosmetic Act, 1938, § 210). Historically, the FDA has made several attempts to regulate these products and remove some of them from the market (Kottke, 1998). Functional foods are defined as manufactured foods for which scientifically valid claims can be made. They may be produced by food-processing technologies, traditional breeding, or genetic engineering. Functional foods should safely deliver a long-term health benefit. Accordingly, a functional food may be one of the following:

- A known food to which a functional ingredient from another food is added
- A known food to which a functional ingredient new to the food supply is added
- An entirely new food that contains one or more functional ingredients (Pariza, 1999)

Nutraceutical

Nutraceutical has been defined as "a blend word of nutrition and pharmaceutical, for a substance that may be considered a food or part of a food and that provides medical or health benefits, including the prevention or treatment of disease" (Marshall, 1994, p. 243). These substances pose problems for official medicine regulators. The Japanese, who were among the first to use functional foods, have highlighted three conditions that define a functional food:

- It is a food (not a capsule, tablet, or powder) derived from naturally occurring ingredients.
- It can and should be consumed as part of a daily diet.
- It has a particular function when ingested, serving to regulate a particular body process, such as enhancement of the biological defense mechanism, prevention of a specific disease, recovery from a specific disease, control of physical and mental conditions, and slowing of the aging process (PA Consulting Group, 1990).

According to these definitions, unmodified whole foods such as fruits and vegetables represent the simplest form of a functional food. For example, broccoli, carrots, or tomatoes would be considered functional foods because they contain high levels of physiologically active components such as beta-carotene, lycopene, and sulforaphane. Modified foods, including those that have been fortified with nutrients or enhanced with phytochemicals, are also within the realm of functional foods.

SCIENTIFIC BASIS

During the past century there have been many changes in the types of foods people eat. This reflects the application of scientific findings and technological innovations in the food industry. Although much research has been conducted on nutrition and health and disease, scientific research on the use of nutraceuticals is more limited.

Interest in foodstuffs has generated research to link nutrient and food intake with improvements in health or prevention of disease. More than 200 studies in the epidemiological literature have been reviewed and consistently show an association between a low consumption of fruits and vegetables and the incidence of cancer. The quarter of the population with the lowest dietary intake of fruits and vegetables has roughly twice the rate of cancer as those with the highest intake (Shibamoto, Terao, & Osawa, 1997).

Hasler (2002) suggests that claims about the health benefits of functional foods should be based on sound scientific evidence. For example, resveratrol, which is found in red wine and grape juice, appears to benefit health by causing platelet aggregation reduction, with strong evidence to support this assertion. Conversely, the evidence that catechins (found in green tea) reduce the risk of certain types of cancer is moderate. It would indeed be helpful if reliable, evidence-based sources of information were available to the consumer on all nutraceuticals.

Much scientific research has been conducted on the role of the various products added to normal foods to enhance their ability to inhibit or prevent diseases. Many regard dietary intake as the best means of acquiring necessary nutrients (Kottke, 1998). However, supplementation of nutrients is common. The findings of selected scientific research focused on selected nutraceuticals are summarized below.

Dietary Plant Stanols and Sterols

The cholesterol-lowering potential of dietary plant stanols and sterols has been known for many years. Modifying plant stanols and sterols structurally makes them easily incorporated into fat-containing foods without losing their effectiveness in lowering cholesterol (Cater & Grundy, 1998). Dietary plant stanols and sterols inhibit the absorption of cholesterol in the small intestine, which in turn can lower LDL blood cholesterol. Patients using statin drug therapy may see further decreases in their blood cholesterol levels when using plant sterol and stanol esters (Blair et al., 2000). Recent studies of plant sterol and stanol esters in humans have demonstrated, however, that maximum cholesterol-lowering benefits are achieved at doses of 2 to 3 grams per day (Hendriks, Weststrate, van Vliet, & Meijer, 1999; Jones, Ntanios, Raeini-Sarjaz, & Vanstone, 1999; Jones et al., 2000; Maki et al., 2001).

Plant sterols and their esters are "Generally Recognized As Safe" (GRAS) food-grade substances, a designation indicating that there has been a history of safe intake of these products with no demonstrated harmful health effects found in the research (International Food Information Council, 2003). Overall, the Nutrition Committee of the American Heart Association advises that stanols and sterol esters not be used as a preventive measure in the general population with normal cholesterol levels, in light of limited data regarding any potential risks. They may be used, however, for adults with hypercholesterolemia or adults requiring secondary prevention after an atherosclerotic event (Lichtenstein & Deckelbaum, 2001).

Glucosamine, Chondroitin Sulfate, and Collagen Hydrolysate

According to Kolata (2006), glucosamine and chondrotin are the most popular supplements in the United States. This is despite no scientific basis to support their effective use in osteoarthritis, which is the condition for which they are most widely used and studied. The results of studies, however, have been mixed. The National Institutes of Health conducted a trial on glucosamine and chondrotin and their potential use in arthritis (GAIT). The study's results were inconclusive (Clegg, Red, & Harris, 2006). Meta-analyses by McAlindon, LaValley, Gulin, and Felson (2000) and by Towheed and Hochberg (1997) reviewed clinical trials of glucosamine and chondroitin in the treatment of osteoarthritis. McAlindon and colleagues included 13 double-blind, placebo-controlled trials of more than 4 weeks' duration, testing oral or parenteral glucosamine or chondroitin for treatment of hip or knee arthritis. All 13 studies were classified as positive, demonstrating substantial benefits in treating arthritis when compared with placebo. Towheed and Hochberg reviewed nine randomized, controlled studies of glucosamine sulfate in osteoarthritis. Glucosamine was superior when compared with placebo in seven randomized trials. Two of the randomized trials compared glucosamine sulfate with ibuprofen. In these two trials, glucosamine was superior in one and equivalent in the other.

The literature reflects concern about these specific products. Deal and Moskowitz (1999) underscore that investigators utilizing glucosamine and chondroitin carefully monitor the product manufacturing process because some of the preparations claiming to contain certain doses of these nutraceuticals have significantly less (or none) of the dosages described.

Cost is a factor in the use of these nutraceuticals. The average consumer cost ranges from $35 to $60 per month (Deal & Moskowitz, 1999). In their reviews, the authors emphasize that these agents are neither FDA-evaluated nor recommended for the treatment of osteoarthritis.

Coenzyme Q10

Coenzyme Q10 (CoQ10) is a compound made naturally in the body. It is used by cells to produce energy needed for cell growth and maintenance. It is also used by the body as an antioxidant. Tissue levels of CoQ10 decrease with age. Some studies have suggested that CoQ10 stimulates the immune system and increases resistance to disease (National Cancer Institute, 2002). Several controlled trials of CoQ10 have been performed for the indication of congestive heart failure, and the results have been varied (Khatta et al., 2000). Other therapeutic claims attributed to CoQ10 involve hypertension, impaired immune status, adjuvant therapy for breast cancer, and various neurologic disorders including Huntington's disease and Parkinson's disease. No outcome data describing clinical benefits from CoQ10 could be found in the literature for these conditions.

Probiotics

Probiotics are microorganism supplements intended to improve health or treat a certain disease. Yogurt is an example of a probiotic food source. The organism must have scientifically proven beneficial physiological effects, be safe for human consumption, remain stable in bile and acid, and be able to adhere to the intestinal mucosa. Probiotics protect the intestinal mucosa by competing with pathogens for attachment sites

(Salminen et al., 1998). Lactobacillus is the most widely used and researched probiotic (Kliger & Cohrssen, 2008).

One identified benefit of a probiotic is to improve gastrointestinal health, including prevention/amelioration of diarrhea that is associated with antibiotic use, irritable bowel syndrome, and acute infectious diarrhea (Kligler & Cohrssen, 2008). Two controlled studies were completed by Malin, Suomalainen, Saxelin, and Isolauri (1996) in 9 children with juvenile diabetes and 14 children with Crohn's disease. Use of Lactobacillus GG therapy for 10 days demonstrated an increased immune response in immunoglobulin A of the gut. In a double-blind, randomized, placebo-controlled study of 40 individuals with ulcerative colitis, a mixed-organism probiotic prevented flare-ups of chronic pouchitis (Gionchetti et al., 2000). A meta-review of 143 clinical trials involving 7,500+ subjects revealed no adverse events associated with probiotic use (Naidu, Bidlack, & Clemens, 1999).

INTERVENTION

Many people are using nutraceuticals. Hence, it is important that nurses include assessment of nutraceutical use when they obtain the health history of the patient. Exhibit 28.1 presents guidelines for nurses to use in assessing patients. In addition, Exhibit 28.2 lists reputable sites for information about nutraceuticals.

Measurement of Outcomes

Outcomes of therapy can be assessed in a number of ways, depending on the nutraceutical and the intent of the therapy. For example, blood levels of the nutrient or effect on the target organ (e.g., bone with the use of calcium) could be monitored over time. Also, it is important that potential side effects of the therapy be evaluated in periodic physical assessments and comprehensive histories. Positive or negative changes in subjective health, energy, and symptoms, or those subsequent to changes in nutraceutical use, can also be assessed in individuals as data for tolerance as part of cost–benefit evaluation. Good teaching of nutraceutical principles, intended purpose, and doses and effects of functional foods will result in informed use by clients and greater awareness of intended and adverse effects.

Exhibit 28.1

Guideline: Nutraceutical Assessment Guide for Nurses

■ Screen for nutraceutical use as a routine part of the health assessment interview process. Because surgical complications can arise from nutritional supplement use, their use is often discontinued a few weeks before surgery.

■ Acquire a working knowledge of functional foods and nutraceuticals, which includes benefits/risks, costs, and possible drug interactions.

■ Develop effective communication strategies to ensure that all members of a patient's health care team are aware of any nutraceutical use.

■ Explore the reasons for the use of nutritional supplements and functional foods. Can the same benefits be achieved by using another product that is safer or less expensive?

■ Consider the unique health care needs of various populations. It is important that pregnant women, children, the elderly, and populations with certain medical conditions discuss any nutritional supplementation use with their health care provider.

■ Provide educational resources for patients that are easy to access, timely, evidence-based, and easy to understand.

■ Remember to consult with and refer patients to nutritionists, a very knowledgeable and accessible resource in this promising and rapidly changing area of health and wellness.

Precautions

As stated previously, it is of paramount importance that nutraceutical use be assessed as part of the health history and nutritional assessment. Safe use must be carefully considered (Zeisel, 1999); safe dosage, drug interaction, toxic side effects from overdose, or ineffective clearance should be determined.

A consistent concern expressed in the literature is the lack of regulation of nutraceuticals. Dietary supplements are not formally reviewed for consistency in the manufacturing process and there may be variation in composition from one supplement batch to another (National Cancer Institute, 2002). Hasler (2002) raises concerns about the plethora of "functional" bars, beverages, cereals, and soups enhanced with botanicals that may pose a health risk to certain consumers. Consistent with these concerns, the General Accounting Office in 2000 released a report that raised concerns about the safety of certain foods and the lack of FDA guidance to companies on safety information labeling for consumers (Hasler, 2002). Finally, the American consumer often receives information on these products through less than reliable sources, such as friends, Internet marketing sites, or vitamin store clerks (Morris & Avorn,

Exhibit 28.2

Nutraceutical Internet Sites

American Dietetic Association: www.eatright.org

American Nutraceutical Association: www.ana-jana.org

International Food Safety Council: http://www.ific.org/nutrition/functional/index.cfm

Mayo Clinic: www.mayoclinic.org

National Institutes of Health—National Center for Complementary and Alternative Medicine: http://nccam.nih.gov/

National Institutes of Health—National Library of Medicine: www.ncbi.nlm.nih.gov

National Institutes of Health—Office of Dietary Supplements: http://dietary-supplements.info.nih.gov/

Natural Medicines Comprehensive Database: www.naturaldatabase.com

U.S. Department of Agriculture—Food and Nutrition Information Center: www.nal.usda.gov

U.S. Department of Health and Human Services—Office of Disease Prevention and Health Promotion: www.healthfinder.gov

U.S. Food and Drug Administration—Center for Food Safety and Applied Nutrition: www.cfsan.fda.gov/~dms/supplmnt.html

2003). When all of these factors are taken into consideration, a situation with inherent potential risks is created.

USES

Nutraceuticals have been used to promote health and to prevent and treat illness. Nutraceuticals can be used to target deficiencies, establish optimal nutritional balance, or treat diseases. Because heart disease, cancer, and stroke are leading causes of death in the United States, greater access to nutraceuticals that have been shown to improve risk-factor profiles is desirable. Furthermore, people in the United States and worldwide could benefit from nutraceuticals when there are deficiencies of specific nutrients.

Children/Adolescents

There is a paucity of literature about nutraceutical use in the child/adolescent population. This is a population with unique nutritional needs because this is a time when growth and development occur at a rapid pace. Not only can nutrition during this time impact current health status, it may have implications for lifelong health as well. Consistent with the need for research in this area, the National Institutes of Health (NIH) currently is conducting a pilot study on probiotics in the prevention and treatment of pediatric illness. Further information on this exciting research initiative can be accessed at the NIH Web site listed in Exhibit 28.2.

Heart disease, once thought to be a disease of aging, is now recognized as starting in childhood. One recommended approach to this problem is through dietary interventions that treat dyslipidemia with a low-fat diet supplemented with water-soluble fiber, plant stanols, and plant sterols (Kwiterovich, 2008).

The American Academy of Pediatrics (2001) conducted a survey of its members to determine attitudes, knowledge, and behaviors relative to complementary and alternative therapies (CAM) in their clinical practice, with analysis based on responses from 745 pediatricians. Few of these practitioners had asked their patients or parents about CAM use. Approximately 1 in 5 pediatricians asked specifically about the use of dietary supplements. The findings from this survey will be used to guide the development of educational programs in this area for AAP members.

Women's Health and Nutritional Needs

Throughout their life span, women have unique nutritional needs that place them at risk for nutrition-related diseases and conditions. Nutrition has been shown to have a significant influence on the risk of chronic disease and on the maintenance of optimal health status. Although food should be the first choice in meeting such needs, nutritional supplementation may be necessary (American Dietetic Association, 2001). Following are some examples of increased nutritional needs across the life span:

- An increase in calcium during pregnancy and menopause is necessary.
- Folic acid requirements increase during pregnancy to prevent neural tube defects.
- Iron needs increase during menstruation and pregnancy.

Although acquiring these nutrients through food sources would be ideal, supplementation is often necessary. It is also important to remember that intake of certain nutrients above a certain level can be teratogenic (e.g., too much Vitamin A in the first trimester of pregnancy) and, because many foods are often enriched with vitamins and minerals, it is possible to consume too much.

CULTURAL APPLICATIONS

The influence of culture on both the use and acceptance of functional foods is an important consideration. The attitudes of one's culture mold one's views about everything, including food (McCracken, 1986). A functional food may be more accepted if it is seen as consistent with traditional consumption (Wansink, 2002). For example, soy is widely used in Asian cultures and is considered to be a traditional food source, with customary soy intake being estimated at 30 to 50 grams per day (Cornwell, Cohick, & Raskin, 2004). Hence, the use of soy as a nutraceutical may be more widely and easily accepted by someone in an Asian culture, as this food is already so widely used. In addition, how food itself is viewed within the context of culture may have a strong influence on the use of nutraceuticals and functional foods. In some cultures, food is viewed as providing energy and health (utilitarian), whereas in a hedonistic food culture there is an appreciation of the preparation and a savoring of the taste (Chandon,Wansink, & Laurent, 2000).

FUTURE RESEARCH

Although nutraceuticals have longstanding historical usage, increased interest in these substances to promote health, prevent disease, and treat specific medical conditions is reflected in heightened attention to nutritional science and increased consumption. A consistent theme throughout this chapter has been the need for more research in this area. The book *Complementary and Alternative Medicine in the United States* (Institute of Medicine, 2005) summarizes succinctly what the goal for research in this arena should be: "In terms of medical therapies, a commitment to public welfare is the obligation to generate and provide to health care practitioners, policy makers, and the public access to the best information available on the efficacy of CAM therapies" (p. 169). Consistent with this sentiment, and because there is so much interest and hope in this area, interdisciplinary research teams may explore the following questions:

1. Which of the current nutraceuticals should be incorporated on a regular basis to promote health?
2. Are nutraceuticals cost-effective?
3. What are the side effects associated with short- and long-term use of specific nutraceuticals?
4. Can we increase research in the use of nutraceuticals in the pediatric population?
5. What are innovative ways to educate health care providers about nutraceuticals?
6. Can we discover more effective methods to educate the American health care consumer about the benefits/risks of nutraceuticals?
7. How does culture affect the use of functional foods?

ACKNOWLEDGMENTS

The author wishes to acknowledge and thank Bridget Doyle for her contributions to this chapter in the previous edition.

REFERENCES

American Academy of Pediatrics. (2001). *Periodic Survey #49: Complementary and alternative medicine (CAM) therapies in pediatric practices.* Retrieved May 25, 2005, from http://www.aap.org/research/periodicsurvey/ps49bex.htm

American Dietetic Association. (2001). *Position paper: Nutrition and women's health.* Retrieved May 31, 2005, from http://www.eatright.org/Member/Policy Initiatives/index_21017.cfm

Blair, S. N., Capuzzi, D. M., Gottlieb, S. O., Nguyen, T., Morgan, J. M., & Cater, N. B. (2000). Incremental reduction of serum total cholesterol and low-density lipoprotein cholesterol with the addition of plant stanol ester-containing spread to statin therapy. *American Journal of Cardiology, 86*(1), 46–52.

Castro Cabezas, M., de Vries, J. H., Van Oostrom, A. J., Iestra, J., & van Staveren W. A. (2006). Effects of a stanol-enriched diet on plasma cholesterol and triglycerides in patients treated with statins. *Journal of the American Dietetic Association, 106*(10), 1564–1569.

Chandon, P., Wansink, B., & Laurent, G. (2000). A congruency framework of sales promotion effectiveness. *Journal of Marketing, 64,* 65–81.

Clegg, D., Red, D. J., & Harris, C. L. (2006). Glucosamine, chondroitin sulfate, and the two in combination for painful knee osteoarthritis. *New England Journal of Medicine, 354*(8), 795–808.

Cornwell, T., Cohick, W., & Raskin, I. (2004). Dietary phytoestrogens and health. *Phytochemistry, 65*, 995–1016.

Deal, C. L., & Moskowitz, R. W. (1999). Nutraceuticals as therapeutic agents in osteoarthritis: The role of glucosamine, chondroidin sulfate, and collagen hydroly-sate. *Rheumatic Disease Clinics of North America, 25*(2), 379–953.

Federal Food, Drug and Cosmetic Act. (1938). 52 Stat. 111.21U.S.C. § 210 et seq.

Gardner, J. (1994). The development of the functional food business. In I. Goldberg (Ed.), *Functional foods: Designer foods, pharmafoods, and nutraceuticals* (pp. 472–473). New York: Chapman & Hall.

Gionchetti, P., Rizzello, F., Venturi, A., Brigidi, P., Matteuzzi, D., Bazzocchi, G., et al. (2000). Oral bacteriotherapy as maintenance treatment in patients with chronic pouchitis: A double-blind, placebo-controlled trial. *Gastroenterology, 119*(2), 305–309.

Hasler, C. M. (2002). Functional foods: Benefits, concerns and challenges—a position paper from the American council on science and health. *Journal of Nutrition, 132*, 3772–3781.

Hendriks, J. F., Weststrate, J. A., van Vliet, T., & Meijer, G. W. (1999). Spreads enriched with three different levels of vegetable oil sterols and the degree of cholesterol lowering in normocholesterolaemic and mildly hypercholesterolaemic subjects. *European Journal of Clinical Nutrition, 53*(4), 319–327.

Hippocrates. (1932). *Hippocrates* (W. H. S. Jones, Trans.). Cambridge, MA: Harvard University Press.

Institute of Medicine (2005). *Complementary and alternative medicine in the United States*. Washington, DC: National Academies Press.

International Food Information Council. (2003). *Functional foods fact sheet: Plant stanols and sterols*. Retrieved May 31, 2005, from http://ific.org

Jones, P. J., Ntanios, F. Y., Raeini-Sarjaz, M., & Vanstone, C. A. (1999). Cholesterol-lowering efficacy of a sitostanol-containing phytosterol mixture with a prudent diet in hyperlipidemic men. *American Journal of Clinical Nutrition, 69*(6), 1144–1150.

Jones, P. J., Raeini-Sarjaz, M., Ntanios, F. Y., Vanstone, C. A., Feng, J. Y., & Parsons, W. E. (2000). Modulation of plasma lipid levels and cholesterol kinetics by phytos-terol versus phytostanol esters. *Journal of Lipid Research, 41*(5), 697–705.

Khatta, M., Alexander, B. S., Krichten, C. M., Fisher, M. L., Freudenberger, R., Robinson, S. W., et al. (2000). The effect of coenzyme Q10 in patients with congestive heart failure. *Annals of Internal Medicine, 132*(8), 636–640.

Kligler, B., & Cohrssen, A. (2008). Probiotics. *Complementary & Alternative Medicine, 78*(9), 1073–1078.

Kolata, G. (2006). Supplements fail to stop arthritis pain, study says. *New York Times*. Retrieved December 31, 2008, from http://www.nytimes.com/2006/02/23/health/23arthritis.html

Kottke, M. K. (1998). Scientific and regulatory aspects of nutraceutical products in the United States. *Drug Development and Industrial Pharmacy, 24*(12), 1177–1195.

Kwiterovich, P. (2008). Recognition and management of dyslipidemia in children and adolescents. *Journal of Clinical Endocrinology & Metabolism, 93*(11), 4200–4209.

Lichtenstein, A. H., & Deckelbaum, R. J. (2001). AHA Science Advisory: stanol/ sterol ester-containing foods and blood control levels: A statement for healthcare professionals from the Nutrition Committee of the Council on Nutrition, Physical Activity, and Metabolism of the American Heart Association. *Circulation, 103,* 1177.

Maki, K. C., Davidson, M. H., Umporowicz, D. M., Schaefer, E. J., Dicklin, M. R., & Ingram, K. A. (2001). Lipid responses to plant-sterol-enriched reduced-fat spreads incorporated into a national cholesterol education program step 1 diet. *American Journal of Clinical Nutrition, 74*(1), 33–43.

Malin, M., Suomalainen, H., Saxelin, N., & Isolauri, E. (1996). Promotion of IgA immune response in patients with Crohn's disease by oral bacteriotherapy with lactobacillus GG. *Annals of Nutritional Metabolism, 40,* 137–145.

Marshall, W. E. (1994). Amino acids, peptides and proteins. In I. Goldberg (Ed.), *Functional foods: Designer foods, pharmafoods, and nutraceuticals* (pp. 242–260). New York: Chapman & Hall.

McAlindon, T. E., LaValley, M. P., Gulin, J. P., & Felson, D. T. (2000). Glucosamine and chondroitin for treatment of osteoarthritis: A systematic quality assessment and meta-analysis. *Journal of the American Medical Association, 283*(11), 1483–1484.

McCracken, G. (1986). Culture and consumption: A theoretical account of the structure and movement of the cultural meaning of consumer goods. *Journal of Consumer Research, 13,* 71–84.

Mintel's New Global Database. (2009). Retrieved January 20, 2009, from http://www.mintel.com/gnpd.htm

Morris, C. A., & Avorn, J. (2003). Internet marketing of herbal products. *Journal of the American Medical Association, 290*(11), 1519–1520.

Naidu, A. S., Bidlack, W. R., & Clemens, R. A. (1999). Probiotic spectra of lactic and bacteria. *Critical Reviews in Food Sciences & Nutrition, 39*(1), 13–126.

National Cancer Institute. (2002). *Coenzyme Q10: Questions and answers, cancer facts.* Retrieved May 31, 2005, from http://cis.nci.nih.gov/fact/9-16.htm

National Institutes of Health. (n.d.). *Probiotics for pediatric illnesses.* Retrieved May 31, 2005, from http://grants2.nih.gov/grants/guide/pa-files/PA-05-035 .html

Nutrition Business Journal. (2008). Retrieved January 27, 2009, from http:NBJ's annual industry overview VIII. *Nutrition Business Journal, VIII*(5/6), 2–9.

PA Consulting Group. (1990). *Functional foods: A new global added value market?* London: PA Consulting Group.

Pariza, M. (1999). Functional foods: Technology, functionality and health benefits. *Nutrition Today, 34,* 150–151.

Salminen, S., Bouley, C., Boutron-Ruault, M. C., Cummings, J. H., Franck, A., & Gibson, G. R., et al. (1998). Functional food science and gastrointestinal physiology and function. *British Journal of Nutrition, 80*(Suppl. 1), S147–S171.

Shibamoto, T., Terao, J., & Osawa, T. (Eds.). (1997). *Functional foods for disease prevention. I: Fruits, vegetables, and teas* (ACS Symposium Series 701). Washington, DC: American Chemical Society.

Towheed, T. E., & Hochberg, M. C. (1997). A systematic review of randomized controlled trials of pharmacological therapy in osteoarthritis of the hip. *Journal of Rheumatology, 24,* 349–357.

Wansink, B. (2002). Changing habits on the home front: Lost lessons from World War II research. *Journal of Public Policy Marketing, 21,* 90–99.

Zeisel, S. H. (1999). Regulation of "nutraceuticals." *Science, 285*(5435), 1853–1855.

Practice, Education, and Research

Expansion in the use of complementary therapies has created a need for chapters devoted to their role in nursing practice, education, and research. As noted in the chapters, nurses have assumed leadership roles in making complementary therapies more available to patients in diverse settings and to providing evidence-based guidelines for the use of these therapies.

Although some complementary therapies have been a part of nursing for centuries, the broadening scope of these therapies has necessitated that nurses develop guidelines for their use in practice settings. Key to safe administration of complementary therapies is having nursing students become familiar with complementary therapies and for continuing education offerings to acquaint practicing nurses with new therapies or guidelines for their use. To promote patient safety, state boards of nursing and professional nursing organizations have developed standards and guidelines for nurses' use of complementary therapies.

Nurses are actively involved in research on complementary therapies, either as principal investigators or members of interdisciplinary teams. The budget for the National Center for Complementary/Alternative Therapies (NCCAM) continues to increase. The challenge for health care professionals is making decisions about when sufficient evidence exists to support the use of a therapy in practice settings, particularly identifying possible side effects or conditions for which a therapy should not be used.

Use of complementary therapies will continue to increase. An exciting aspect of complementary therapy use is learning about healing practices that have been used for centuries in other cultures and the role these might have for a broader arena in health care. Nurses will continue to be caring, competent professionals and will search for research on complementary therapies. Nurses must also to be aware of the many therapies that are being used by patients, particularly those who are recent immigrants. Nurses in dedicated service to persons around the globe will also be exposed to the use of complementary therapies by patients.

29 Integrating Complementary Therapies into Nursing Practice

ELIZABETH L. PESTKA
SUSANNE M. CUTSHALL

Although complementary therapies are being more widely used in hospital settings, some resistance to their use by nurses, doctors, and other health professionals still exists. Nurses are oftentimes the leaders in integrating complementary and integrative therapies into practice settings. The concept of holism is fundamental to nursing education and theory and has been described by Libster (2001) as the art of integrative nursing. Because many of the complementary therapies are based on a holistic philosophy, it is logical that nurses would be leaders in incorporating these into patient care.

This chapter provides examples of strategies nurses have used to incorporate complementary therapies into practice settings. Three health care settings in the Midwest will be used to demonstrate the integration of complementary therapies into nursing practice, including one small health campus (Woodwinds Health Campus), one large medical center (Abbott Northwestern), and one multisite medical provider (Mayo Clinic). Additional examples will provide support for nurses who wish to include a variety of complementary therapies in their care.

Woodwinds Health Campus, located in Woodbury, Minnesota, is an 86-bed, not-for-profit facility that opened in 2000. The philosophy of care is based on the creation of an unprecedented healing environment that revolves around the needs of patients and their families, including extensive use of complementary therapies. Woodwinds' vision was to transform the patient care experience. It promises patients compassionate service, holistic care, and a patient-centered care model (Lincoln, 2003). From the spacious main entry to the inviting layout, patients are easily guided to the area of service they need as quickly and comfortably as possible.

Abbott Northwestern Hospital, a part of the Allina Health System, is a 627-bed, tertiary care, not-for-profit hospital, in Minneapolis, Minnesota. The Nursing Department's philosophy at Abbott Northwestern is supported by a patient-centered, holistic framework for practice. In 1999 a complementary and alternative medicine program for cardiovascular inpatients was initiated and has grown into a nationally recognized model for providing integrative care (Sendelbach, Carole, Lapensky, & Kshettry, 2003).

Mayo Clinic, located in Rochester, Minnesota, is a very large tertiary medical center with almost 2,000 hospital beds. The Mayo Clinic Model of Care is based on the core value that the needs of the patient are primary (Mayo Clinic, 2008). Comprehensive individualized care addresses the mind, body, and spirit to promote healing and wellness with complementary therapies integrated into practice. Mayo Clinic was founded in 1889 and has grown into an expansive health care campus that is respected around the world (Clapesattle, 1990).

COMPLEMENTARY THERAPIES AT WOODWINDS HEALTH CARE CENTER

Woodwinds Health Campus offers a variety of healing arts therapies designed to complement medical care. These healing arts therapies are also known as integrative therapies or complementary therapies. Integrative therapies are designed to enhance, not replace, traditional therapeutic measures ordered by a primary provider, such as medications, exercise, and therapy. A variety of complementary therapies are offered to meet the diverse and individualized needs of each patient. Therapies include essential oils, healing touch/energy-based therapies, guided imagery, healing music, acupuncture, acupressure, and massage. For patients to maximize benefit from these options, a *Supporting Your Healing Process* patient education class is offered free of charge to patients, their families, and the community. The class focuses on using the complementary therapies both before surgery and during hospitalization (Woodwinds Health Campus, 2008a).

In addition to complementary therapies offered by the Woodwinds Health Campus, a partnership with Northwestern Health Sciences University provides additional natural care choices, such as chiropractic, acupuncture, massage, and naturopathy at the Natural Care Center. This broadens the range of complementary therapies available so that each patient can select options that will help them most in their healing process (Woodwinds Health Campus, 2008b).

Nurses play an integral role in providing complementary therapies at Woodwinds. Holistic nursing principles are integrated into the vision for the hospital. Woodwinds Health Campus includes components of holistic nursing in job descriptions and ongoing performance evaluations. They continue to attract highly skilled nurses and maintain a low attrition rate and a high level of staff satisfaction. Administration believes that these outcomes are associated with holistic nursing serving as the foundation for practice. The care environment is collaborative and individual contributions are honored, with nurses providing input on how the holistic care model continues to be implemented (Lincoln, 2003).

Education for all nurses at Woodwinds includes holistic nursing–related courses; one focuses on healing touch and the second includes training in other complementary/alternative modalities, such as music therapy, guided imagery, and use of essential oils. In addition, nurses are required to complete at least three educational contact hours annually in holistic nursing. Nurses are expected to use what they have learned in these courses in the care provided to each patient (Lincoln, 2003).

Nurses are encouraged to utilize complementary therapies themselves. They are able to utilize the many healing spaces in the Integrative Services area at Woodwinds to enhance their own well-being. They can take "spirit breaks" to rejuvenate themselves during their work shifts. Using integrative therapies becomes an aspect of the lives of nurses employed at Woodwinds (Lincoln, 2003).

COMPLEMENTARY THERAPIES AT ABBOTT NORTHWESTERN HOSPITAL

Abbott Northwestern Hospital, in collaboration with the Minneapolis Heart Institute, identified a mission to provide an exceptional health care experience and established a holistic nursing framework for practice. The prevalence of the public's use of complementary/alternative therapies identified in the literature, along with an increasing number of patient and family requests for these interventions, motivated Abbott Northwestern Hospital to initiate an inpatient cardiovascular integrative therapy program in 1999. This initial innovative program, called *Healing the Hearts*, included such therapeutic interventions as music and massage (Sendelbach et al., 2003).

With initial success and institutional support, along with continuing education for providers, the inpatient cardiovascular integrative therapy program developed into a national model for not only inpatient care but also for outpatient care, research, and education. The current Penny George Institute for Health and Healing has expanded to offer services that include holistic nursing consultations, acupressure, acupuncture, guided imagery, healing touch, massage therapy, music therapy, reflexology, and other relaxation and stress-reduction techniques (Allina Hospital & Clinics, 2008). The outpatient Institute for Health and Healing offers the same inpatient services with additional services that include: aromatherapy, biofeedback, energy healing, therapeutic yoga, herbal consultation, integrative medicine consultations, nutritional counseling, spiritual guidance, and exercise therapy.

The holistic nurse clinicians and other members of the integrative therapy team provide ongoing education to the staff at Abbott Northwestern. Education programs are focused on conventional and complementary care, promoting self-managed health and wellness, community education classes, nurse training programs, and local health care conferences. Research to measure patient outcomes and identify best practices is also a key to expanding this innovative model. Nurses are involved with ongoing clinical trials, using integrative therapies and data analysis to provide evidence for integrating complementary/alternative therapies into clinical practice.

Nursing involvement is critical to the ongoing success of these programs. In 2001 an Integrative Practice Advisory Board was established and one of the three key areas identified for growth was to further develop holistic nursing to complement the interventions received by patients. The interventions were assessed to be congruent with the nursing department's philosophy and the cornerstones of the patient care model. Work was also focused on enhancing a total healing environment which includes developing positive and collaborative relationships between nurses and physicians, as this has been shown to influence patient outcomes (Sendelbach et al., 2003).

COMPLEMENTARY THERAPIES AT MAYO CLINIC

The Mayo Nursing Care Model is based on the nursing theory of human caring proposed by Dr. Jean Watson. In this model every patient is honored as a unique person with potential to heal holistically, and is nurtured by the intentional presence of a nurse who connects with the patient "in the moment," expressing care through words, actions, and empathy (Mayo Clinic, 2007). Nurses across the continuum of care include complementary therapies as part of the holistic healing process.

All nurses are encouraged to include complementary therapies as part of ongoing pain management. One of the policy statements in the procedure guideline on pain management states that complementary interventions such as relaxation techniques, imagery, and music therapy are incorporated in the pain management plan when appropriate.(Mayo Clinic, 2008). Identification of resources to support use of complementary therapies for pain management has been included in departmental orientation for nurses new to the organization and ongoing staff-development sessions.

Many patients have ineffective coping skills that hinder healing. Nurses have patient education resources available to assist in teaching about complementary therapies to enhance coping abilities. A patient education booklet, *Coping Strategies: Exploring Complementary Therapies* (Mayo Foundation for Medical Education and Research, 1998), is given to patients. It provides an overview of coping strategies that may complement health care needs and treatments. The complementary therapies described include art therapy, exercise, humor, imagery, journaling, massage, music therapy, pet therapy, relaxation, spirituality, and touch. For each complementary therapy an explanation of the therapy is provided, along with potential benefits of the activity, and quotes from other patients who have enhanced their coping and healing with the therapy (Mayo Foundation, 1998). The nurse discusses the described complementary therapies, answers questions, and assists the patient in selecting one or two therapies to begin using.

To reinforce patient education, another brochure given to patients by nurses in many specialties is the *Introduction to Relaxation Skills*

(Mayo Foundation for Medical Education and Research, 2008). The booklet focuses on the importance of relaxation to eliminate tension in the body and mind. It describes the complementary therapies of relaxed breathing, progressive muscle relaxation, autogenic relaxation, imagery, and other activities such as Tai Chi, self-hypnosis, yoga, and meditation. The nurse uses this resource to introduce complementary therapies that will assist a patient to use holistic healing. Emphasis is placed on learning relaxation skills that may improve overall health and quality of life.

Other ways nurses integrate complementary therapies into patient care include a closed circuit television channel with continuous relaxing music available in each patient's room. Compact disk (CD) players and CDs are available for patient use. Other resources include CDs with audio guided imagery, a chaplain service available on request to provide spiritual support, and ongoing therapies of nursing presence, touch, and humor.

Specialty Programs Featuring Complementary/Alternative Therapies

Healing Enhancement

At Mayo Clinic a Healing Enhancement Program was initiated based on patient feedback and review of the patient experience for cardiovascular surgery patients. A team that includes nurses was formed to address the needs of patients, including managing pain, anxiety, tension, stress, sleeplessness, and nausea that can occur with and after cardiac surgery. When the team realized that an initial order focusing on pain medications was not enough, a trial of massage and music therapies aimed at reducing patients' complaints of musculoskeletal pain and decreasing anxiety and tension after surgery was initiated. Studies have confirmed positive findings (Cutshall et al., 2007).

Nurses educate patients and their families about complementary/alternative resources and coordinate the delivery of services. Enthusiastic nurses promote patient use of a wide array of therapies. A full-time massage therapist is available to provide treatment for back, neck, and shoulder pain. CD players are available in each of the cardiac surgical rooms for music therapy, with a small CD library available on each unit and additional CDs located in the patient library. The Patient Education Section facilitates guided imagery CD's specific to *Successful Surgery* (Naparsteck, 1992), and an audiotaped program entitled *Healthful Sleep* (Naparsteck, 2000) can be accessed on each patient's television. CD resources for passive muscle relaxation, stress management, and additional imageries are also available. Patient education classes on *Stress and Wellness* and *Healing Movement* are offered on an ongoing basis. Live soothing music is sometimes available in clinical areas. Patients are able to select art for their hospital room. Some hospital volunteers are trained to offer hand massage to patients, family members, and staff (Cutshall et al., 2007).

The success of the Healing Enhancement Program has led to its replication in other surgical areas at Mayo Clinic, including the colorectal surgery and transplant surgery specialties. Recognizing the benefits to patients, nurses continue to collaborate with other health care providers and the outpatient Complementary and Integrative Medicine Program to expand resources and opportunities for additional services and to other patient populations.

Pain Rehabilitation Center

The Mayo Comprehensive Pain Rehabilitation Center (PRC) is an exemplary model in which nurses integrate complementary/alternative therapies into their practice. It was among the first pain rehabilitation programs in the nation, being established in 1974. It is now one of the largest pain rehabilitation programs in the nation. The PRC is focused on functional restoration with a cognitive-behavioral basis and extensive use of complementary therapies (Mayo Foundation for Medical Education and Research, 2006).

A team of health care professionals, with nurses being integral members of the team, delivers care to patients in the program. Patients are provided education on medication management, chemical health education, complementary therapies, education and group therapy, stress management and relaxation, physical therapy, occupational therapy, biofeedback, sleep hygiene, and lifestyle management. Complementary therapies included have been carefully researched and demonstrated to be helpful, including biofeedback, meditation, and specific relaxation techniques. Additional complementary therapies are explained and discussed so as to provide the patient with options to use in managing pain.

Many patients who have lived with chronic pain for much of their lifetime inform the nurses that they are skeptical that if large dosages of medication have not helped their pain, nonpharmacological methods such as complementary therapies are unlikely to be effective. Program outcome data support not only overwhelming patient satisfaction with the program (94%), but also a reduction in depressive symptoms (79%), a gain in activity level (75%), and a reduction in pain severity (73%)(Mayo Foundation, 2006). Most of the patients leave the program having a positive response to complementary therapies and viewing them as an effective part of their pain rehabilitation program and improved quality of life.

NURSES' USE OF COMPLEMENTARY THERAPIES

Nurses are in a key position to help integrate use of complementary and alternative therapies into practice. Because they are available "24/7," they can play a unique role in guiding the growth and use of complementary therapies in hospitals. Nurses have the philosophical background and educational preparation that focuses on holistic care. The nursing profession has long been a strong advocate of integrated care (O'Connell & Russel, 2003).

A national survey explored the use of complementary therapies by critical care nurses (Tracy et al., 2005). The study sought to determine these nurses' attitudes, knowledge, perspectives, and use of complementary and alternative therapies. A random sample of 726 members of the American Association of Critical Care Nurses was surveyed. Most of the respondents indicated they were using one or more complementary and alternative therapies in their practice. The most common therapies noted were diet, exercise, relaxation techniques, and prayer. A majority of the nurses had some knowledge of more than half of the 28 therapies listed on the survey and a majority desired additional training for 25 therapies. The participants generally required more evidence to use or recommend conventional therapy than to use or recommend complementary and alternative therapies. Overall, the respondents viewed complementary and alternative therapies positively and were open to use of these therapies. They perceived these therapies as legitimate and beneficial to patients for managing a variety of symptoms.

A majority of the respondents desired an increase in the availability of therapies for patients, families, and nursing staff. Respondents' professional use of the therapies was related to having more knowledge of them, perceiving benefits of them, total number of therapies they recommended to patients, personal use, and affiliation with a mainstream religion. This study concluded that there would be benefit to having educational programs for nurses that provide information about complementary and alternative therapies. Evidence for usefulness of these therapies would increase their use by critical care nurses (Tracy et al., 2005).

Nursing as a profession is well grounded in understanding the need to reduce stress in patients and thus promote healing. Nurses are exposed to stress in their own lives and in the work environment. Nurses can personally benefit from using complementary and integrative therapies in self-care to reduce stress and prevent professional burnout. There is a great potential for turmoil, stress, and burnout among new nurses (Boychuk Duchscher, & Cowin, 2006). In a recent study of new nurses with less than 2 years tenure, 66% were found to have symptoms of burnout, mental exhaustion, and depression (Cho, Laschinger, & Wong, 2006). Instruction about complementary therapies aimed at stress reduction and relaxation should be included in orientation programs and staff development offerings to help nurses to manage ongoing stressful activities and events.

Nurses have an influence on standards and guidelines for clinical nursing and complementary/alternative therapies polices. Examples in this chapter illustrate incorporation of nursing guidelines related to complementary and alternative therapies to promote a culture of holistic nursing care. Nursing standards and guidelines also promote safety in nurses' use of complementary and alternative therapies. Standards and guidelines such as those developed by the American Holistic Nurses Association and the New York Nurses' Association may be helpful to institutions in developing standards and guidelines that are specific to their health care setting. Ongoing nursing staff development is related to the standards and guidelines that integrate the use of complementary and alternative therapies safely and effectively into practice.

Serving as an advocate for patients and their family members and communicating individual needs and preferences to the interdisciplinary team are responsibilities of the nursing professional. Nurses are the coordinators of daily care and recognize that each patient's needs oftentimes can be optimally met by combining the best of conventional medical care with complementary strategies. Patient-centered care provides information and choices combined with active participation and collaboration between the interdisciplinary team and the patient and his/her family.

Nurses are essential in helping to develop and sustain frameworks and practice models for complementary alternative services. Woodwinds Health Center, Abbott Northwestern, and Mayo Clinic illustrate examples of individualized care in which nurses and their multidisciplinary colleagues truly focus on a healing environment that includes complementary and alternative therapies. Because of the emphasis being placed on evidence-based practice and cost-effectiveness, ongoing research and evaluation studies are needed to provide support for these holistic models of care delivery.

REFERENCES

Allina Hospitals & Clinics. (2008). *Abbott Northwestern Hospital—The Penny George Insitute for Health and Healing.* Retrieved November 1, 2008, from http://www.allina. com/ahs/anw.nsf/page/ihh_home

Boychuk Duchscher, J. E., & Cowin, L. S. (2006). The new graduates' professional inheritance. *Nursing Outlook, 54*(3), 152–158.

Clapesattle, H. (1990). *The Doctors Mayo.* Rochester, MN: Mayo Foundation for Medical Education & Research.

Cho, J., Laschinger, H. K. S., & Wong, C. (2006). Workplace empowerment, work engagement and organizational commitment of new graduate nurses. *Canadian Journal of Nursing Leadership, 19*(3), 43–60.

Cutshall, S., Fenske, L., Kelly, R., Phillips, B., Sundt, T., & Bauer, B. (2007) Creation of a Healing Enhancement Program at an academic medical center. *Complementary Therapies in Clinical Practice, 13,* 217–223.

Libster, M. (2001). *Demonstrating care: The art of integrative nursing.* New York: Thomson Learning.

Lincoln, V. (2003) Creating an integrated hospital: Woodwinds Health Campus. *Integrative Nursing, 2*(1), 12–13.

Mayo Clinic. (2007). *Nursing at Mayo: Guidelines and manuals—Procedure guideline I-3.2: Mayo nursing care model.* (2007). Retrieved November 1, 2008, from http:// mayoweb.mayo.edu/nurs-pro/gi03-02.htm

Mayo Clinic. (2008). *Nursing at Mayo: Guidelines and manuals—Procedure guideline G-32: Pain management.* Retrieved November 1, 2008, from http://mayoweb.mayo.edu/ nurs-pro/gg32-00.html

Mayo Clinic. (2009). *Mayo's mission: primary value.* Retrieved November 1, 2008, from http://www.mayoclinic.org/about/missionvalues.html

Mayo Foundation for Medical Education and Research. (1998). *Coping strategies: Exploring complementary therapies.* (Brochure). Rochester, MN: Mayo Foundation for Medical Education and Research.

Mayo Foundation for Medical Education and Research. (2006). *Comprehensive Pain Rehabilitation Center: Program guide.* (Brochure). Rochester, MN: Mayo Foundation for Medical Education and Research.

Mayo Foundation for Medical Education and Research. (2008). *Introduction to relaxation skills.* (Brochure). Rochester, MN: Mayo Foundation for Medical Education and Research.

Naparsteck, B. (1992). *Mediations to promote successful surgery.* (Compact disk). Akron, OH: Health Journeys.

Naparsteck, B. (2000). *A mediation to help you with healthful sleep.* (Compact disk). Akron, OH: Health Journeys.

O'Connell, E., & Russel, G., (2003). Federal CAM policy: Politics and practice. *Critical Care Nursing Clinics of North America. 15,* 381–386.

Sendelbach, S., Carole, L., Lapensky, J., & Kshettry, V. (2003). Developing an integrative therapies program in a tertiary care cardiovascular hospital. *Critical Care Nursing Clinics of North America, 15,* 363–372.

Tracy, M. F., Linquist, R., Savik, K., Watanuki, S., Sendelbach, S., Kreitzer, M. M., et al. (2005). Use of complementary and alternative therapies: A national survey of critical care nurses. *American Journal of Critical Care, 14*(5), 404–415.

Woodwinds Health Campus. (2008a). *About us.* Retrieved November 1, 2008, from http://www.woodwinds.org/About/index.cfm

Woodwinds Health Campus. (2008b). *Programs and services.* Retrieved November 1, 2008, from http://www.woodwinds.org/Careservice/4_Healing_Arts/index.cfm

30 Integrating Complementary Therapies into Education

CARIE A. BRAUN

Nursing curricula are constantly evolving to improve patient care and keep pace with the ever-changing health care environment. The integration of complementary therapies in the nursing curriculum is no exception. The rationale for this integration includes: the proliferation of the use of complementary/alternative therapy by the public; various governmental, legislative, and other mandates; safety issues with the combining of conventional and alternative modalities; cultural competency and the need to provide patient-centered care; and increasing evidence of the positive impact of integrative health care systems on health care outcomes (Gaylord & Mann, 2007). These influences have permeated the practice of nursing and, as a result, nursing standards and guidelines have evolved to include complementary therapies. For example, the National Council Licensure Examination (NCLEX-RN®), a reflection of actual nursing practice and an important indicator of nursing program quality, has expected a knowledge base in complementary therapies for entry-level registered nurses (RNs) since 2004 (Stratton, Benn, Lie, Zeller, & Nedrow, 2007). In 2007, the detailed test plan for the NCLEX-RN® (found at https://www.ncsbn.org/1287.htm) again required the ability to incorporate complementary therapies into the client's plan of care.

Other documents have been equally influential. The *AACN Essentials of Baccalaureate Education for Professional Nursing Practice* (2008) specifically identified baccalaureate generalist practice to include a beginning understanding of complementary and alternative modalities. For graduate education, the *AACN Essentials of Master's Education for Advanced Practice Nursing* (2004) directed master's-level nurses to deliver health care services within integrated care systems. Similarly, the *AACN Essentials of Doctoral Education for Advanced Practice Nursing* (2006) directs DNP programs to prepare graduates to synthesize concepts related to clinical prevention and population health, including psychosocial dimensions and cultural diversity.

The initial discourse in the 1990s about whether or not complementary therapies *should* be taught in nursing and other health care programs has now been replaced with discussion and debate about *what* should be included and *how* to most effectively evaluate student learning (Stratton et al., 2007). This chapter will address those "what" and "how" questions to provide a framework to guide nurse educators in the implementation of a curriculum inclusive of complementary and alternative therapies.

DEFINING COMPLEMENTARY THERAPY CORE COMPETENCIES

At present, there is no complementary therapy core curriculum to guide generalist nursing practice. Nurse educators must rely on the current scope and standards of practice and ethical directives to guide actual performance of complementary therapies by pre-licensure students (Reed, Pettigrew, & King, 2000). The American Nurses Association (ANA), in the book *Nursing: Scope and Standards of Practice* (ANA, 2004), spells out the practice parameters and responsibilities for all RNs in the United States. The practice standards of assessment, diagnosis, outcome identification, planning, implementation, and evaluation allow for an individualized plan of care that is sensitive to diverse health care practices for all patients. The professional performance standards of quality of practice, practice evaluation, education, collegiality, collaboration, ethics, research, resource utilization, and leadership commit nurses to constantly improve knowledge, skills, and competencies appropriate to the nursing role.

The ANA's *Scope and Standards of Practice* (2004) indicates that nurses must be knowledgeable about and sensitive to a range of health practices so that holistic nursing care can be provided. The document does not identify specific therapies that nurses may or may not incorporate into nursing practice. The *Nursing Interventions Classification* (Bulechek, Butcher, & McCloskey Dochterman, 2008), however, provides a comprehensive listing of treatments that nurses can perform. This list includes the following complementary therapies, which are within the realm of nursing given the appropriate training or certification: acupressure, animal-assisted therapy, aromatherapy, art therapy, biofeedback, massage, music therapy, self-hypnosis facilitation, and therapeutic touch. Although the knowledge base for many complementary therapies may be part of the educational program, performance proficiency is often not achieved during an undergraduate or even graduate nursing education. Therefore, even though nurses *can* perform these therapies, they *should* perform them only with the appropriate training and certification.

Complementary therapy implementation patterns are also in evidence in various Boards of Nursing (BON) within the U.S. states and territories, which regulate nursing practice to ensure patient safety. Of the 53 BONs surveyed, 47% had statements or positions that included specific complementary therapies or examples of these practices, 13% had them under discussion, and 40% had not formally addressed the topic but did not necessarily discourage these practices (Sparber, 2001). BONs are increasingly aware of and supportive of the integration of complementary therapies into nursing practice. The BONs are continuously clarifying what is within the scope of nursing practice and identifying basic education and competencies required for nursing practice. Because the interpretation of the nursing scope of practice can vary based on the different state or territorial BONs, nurses must be aware of their own state's position regarding complementary therapies, must have the documented knowledge and competencies to perform the therapy, and must adhere to licensure and credentialing regulations.

Internationally, BON equivalents have also articulated the role of the nurse in understanding and practicing complementary therapies. The Nurses Board of Western Australia has designated *Guidelines for the Use of Complementary Therapies in Nursing Practice* (2003). The guidelines indicate that "nurses are responsible for acquiring and maintaining their complementary therapy knowledge and competence and for being aware of the limitations of their knowledge and competence in relation to complementary therapies" (p. 1). Selection of the educational program in the specific complementary therapy is the responsibility of the nurse. The Nurses Board of Western Australia cautions that the course must be of adequate quality, be accredited or approved as appropriate, confer the appropriate qualifications and level of practice, and build upon the prior learning of the nurse.

Similarly, the College and Association of Registered Nurses of Alberta published the *Alternative and/or Complementary Therapy Standards for Registered Nurses* (2006) to provide "guidance to registered nurses in making decisions about providing care that involves complementary or alternative health-care therapies and natural health products as an adjunct within their nursing practice" (p. 2). These standards require adequate knowledge, skills, and licensure when appropriate to provide the specified alternative/complementary therapy through relevant educational or certificate programs. The provision of such therapies must fall within the current scope of nursing practice for Canadian RNs if the RN is providing the therapy under his/her RN license.

Specialty organizations have also weighed in on the debate about what nurses with specialty certifications can and should perform. The American Holistic Nurses' Association (AHNA) and the American Nurses' Association (ANA) have jointly developed the *Scope and Standards of Practice for Holistic Nursing* (2007), which includes a core curriculum for integrative health care practice infused with the principles of complementary and alternative therapies and competencies consistent with holistic nursing practice. The examination to determine certification in holistic nursing was developed based on an accepted inventory of professional activities and knowledge of a holistic nurse (Dossey, Frisch, Forker, & Lavin, 1998). The certification is not routinely required as part of the nurse's pre-licensure or advanced education, but offers important insights as to the expectations of holistic nursing practice.

The specialized training required to safely and effectively practice specific complementary therapies is not typically found in general nurse education programs. There is, however, in such programs, a major emphasis on helping student nurses to better understand the role of complementary therapies in patient health. Multiple authors have suggested required knowledge content applicable to the undergraduate and graduate nursing curriculum (Cuellar, Cahill, Ford, & Aycock, 2003;

Gaster, Unterborn, Scott, & Schneeweiss, 2007; Kligler et al., 2004; Lee et al., 2007; Reed et al., 2000). The following is a compilation of suggested student learning outcomes that address the necessary dimensions for educating students within general nursing practice:

- Describe the prevalence and patterns of complementary therapy use by the public.
- Compare and contrast the underlying principles and beliefs in Western belief systems and alternative health belief systems.
- Communicate effectively with patients and families about complementary and alternative therapies.
- Critique the scientific evidence available for the most commonly used complementary and alternative therapies.
- Identify reputable sources of information to support continued learning about complementary and alternative therapies.
- Explore the roles, training, and credentialing of complementary and alternative therapy practitioners.
- Reflect upon and improve self-care measures and wellness to incorporate complementary therapies for self, where applicable.

CURRENT STATE OF COMPLEMENTARY THERAPIES IN NURSING EDUCATION

Lee and colleagues (2007) recognized that in nursing programs the integration of complementary therapies requires little or no shift in philosophical paradigm because issues like wellness, prevention, and holistic health have long been at the core of nursing practice. There is ample evidence to suggest that nursing education programs are already attending to the knowledge base needed to understand the role of complementary therapies in health care. For example, multiple studies have confirmed that nursing faculty and students believe that complementary therapies must be integrated into the nursing curriculum and that nurses must be prepared to advise patients regarding best practices in integrative health care (Halcón, Chlan, Kreitzer, & Leonard, 2003; Keimig & Braun, 2004; Kim, Erlen, Kim, & Sok, 2006; Kreitzer, Mitten, Harris, & Shandeling, 2002; Kreitzer, Mann, & Lumpkin, 2008; Melland & Clayburgh, 2000; Nedrow, Istvan, et al., 2007; Öztekin, Ucuzal., Öztekin, & Issever, 2007; Uzun & Tan, 2004). A few of these studies also determined that nursing students, upon graduation, did not feel prepared to integrate complementary therapies and that more education was desired (Keimig & Braun, 2004; Kim et al., 2006; Melland & Clayburgh, 2000; Uzun & Tan, 2004).

Fenton and Morris (2003), Dutta and colleagues (2003), and Richardson (2003) sampled nursing schools across the United States to determine the extent to which the schools integrated complementary and alternative modalities into their curricula. For all three studies, a large percentage already included complementary therapies in the curriculum (49–85%) and almost all of the programs were planning to incorporate additional complementary therapies in the future. The same appears to be true for family nurse practitioner programs (Burman, 2003). Very few of the responding schools had a separate required course on complementary therapies (11–15%); whereas most offered a separate elective course (37–84%) and about one third of schools offered a continuing education option. The most commonly included therapies were spirituality/prayer/meditation, relaxation, guided imagery, herbals, acupuncture, massage, and therapeutic touch.

Internationally, nursing education programs are also addressing the need to integrate complementary therapies. In the United Kingdom (UK), 73% of nursing schools included complementary therapies (Morgan, Glanville, Mars, & Nathanson, 1998). In 2004, Sok, Erlen, and Kim reported that more than 10 universities in the UK offered students full-time degree programs in complementary and alternative therapies, such as osteopathy, chiropractic medicine, herbal medicines, acupuncture, and homeopathy. Hon and colleagues (2006) reported that the regulatory body for nursing in Hong Kong now requires that the nursing curriculum contain 20 hours devoted to Traditional Chinese Medicine (TCM). Similarly, Yeh and Chung (2007) investigated the current and expected levels of competence in TCM that baccalaureate nurses should possess in Taiwan, where Western nursing education is considered mainstream and the expectations that nurses possess skills in TCM have been met with disappointment by consumers. In Korea, one College of Nursing Science now has a 1-year program that leads to a certificate in complementary and alternative therapies for clinical nurses and researchers (Sok et al., 2004).

FACULTY QUALIFICATIONS AND DEVELOPMENT

Although the majority of nursing programs integrate complementary therapies in some way, the greatest challenges included the need for qualified faculty, a crowded and changing curriculum, lack of definition for "best practices" in integrative care, and sustainability (Lee et al., 2007). Family nurse practitioner programs reported that most faculty used self-study to gain complementary therapy expertise, with very few faculty being certified in holistic nursing practice (Burman, 2003).

Stratton and colleagues (2007) identified essential faculty development indicators needed to facilitate learning in integrative health care. First and foremost, a critical mass of knowledgeable faculty is essential to the successful integration and sustainability of complementary therapies into a nursing curriculum. Viewing complementary therapy information through the discovery lens of evidence-based practice is a suggested way of gaining faculty acceptance and providing an opportunity for faculty to become more familiar with complementary therapy principles and research (Stratton et al., 2007). Faculty development requires time and resources, access to scholarly writings, reference and research resources, reassigned time, consultations, collaboration, continuing education, and support. Ideally, continuing education workshops or conferences should be structured using a collaborative approach representing the varying perspectives of complementary and alternative therapy practitioners. Encouraging and supporting faculty research in the area of complementary therapies is another mechanism of generating a team of qualified faculty.

CAM EDUCATION PROJECT

The exploration of best practices in integrative health care education has been an ongoing focus of the National Center for Complementary and Alternative Medicine (NCCAM). The Complementary and Alternative Medicine (CAM) Education Project funded by NCCAM was designed to incorporate CAM information into the curricula of selected health profession schools (Pearson & Chesney, 2007). Competitive NCCAM grants were awarded to 15 health profession schools in the United States; of these, two were awarded exclusively to nursing programs (Rush University Medical Center and the University of Washington). The University of Minnesota also engaged the School of Nursing through this project along with other programs. The work of the CAM Education Project has been highly influential in bringing forward the concept of integrative health care systems (Nedrow et al., 2007). Integrative medicine or health care is that which combines conventional treatments and complementary/alternative therapies proven to be safe and effective (Nedrow et al.). Currently, the Consortium for Academic Health Centers for Integrative Medicine (www.imconsortium.org) meets twice per year to coordinate efforts to promote integrative health systems, including integrative education, research, policy, and patient care. Through this consortium's education subcommittee, core competences in integrative medicine have been developed and disseminated to U.S. medical schools (Kligler et al., 2004). Additional outcomes of these projects were documented in the October 2007 issue of *Academic Medicine* and are summarized below.

IMPLEMENTATION MODELS: INTEGRATIVE CURRICULA

Building upon the Center for Spirituality and Healing, established in 1997, the School of Nursing at the University of Minnesota initiated curricular revisions to incorporate complementary and alternative health philosophies and practices into baccalaureate, master's, and doctoral programs (Halcón, Leonard, Snyder, Garwick, & Kreitzer, 2001). The curriculum was revised to strengthen didactic and experiential learning to encompass complementary therapies theory and research, support interdisciplinary courses as part of the graduate minor in complementary therapies and healing practices, and incorporate self-care concepts.

Rush University was awarded an NIH/NCCAM grant to integrate complementary therapies into the baccalaureate and master's curricula and to develop a continuing education program for nurses and other health care providers (Fenton & Morris, 2003). All students in the undergraduate (currently phasing out and taking no new students) and graduate (including an entry-level generalist master's and advanced specialty practice) programs are exposed to complementary therapy content through required courses such as pharmacology, health assessment, nutrition, research, and community health nursing. Curricular competencies have been outlined involving assessment, therapy indications and contraindications, safety, evidence-based practice, and collaboration. Much of the coursework was designed through Web-based modules for use in the curriculum and as continuing education offerings. Four foundational modules and seven case-based modules are currently offered.

The University of Washington School of Nursing, in partnership with Bastyr University (a leader in the natural health sciences and natural medicine), provided faculty development and improved faculty knowledge of complementary therapies through a summer educational program (Fenton & Morris, 2003; Nedrow, Heitkemper, et al., 2007). Faculty then brought back what they learned to support integration of complementary therapies into the nursing curriculum. In addition, the University of Washington developed an international center for complementary therapies and women's health research in collaboration with Ewha Womans' University School of Nursing and School of Oriental Medicine of Wonkang University in Iksan, South Korea, and developed a complementary therapy certificate program in nursing.

Other nursing programs throughout the world are also implementing integrative educational models to build the complementary therapy knowledge base of generalist nurses. Helms (2006) articulated the need for integration of complementary therapy concepts into every course of the nursing curriculum, with course objectives that reflect the expectations of performing (or referrals for) complementary and alternative therapies in patient care. The integration of complementary therapies is a natural fit with the nursing curriculum. Nurse educators can readily infuse already existing nursing courses with complementary therapy topics. For example, health care system or policy courses could include the history of and philosophical basis for complementary and alternative therapies and health systems. Health assessment courses should include a history-taking expectation inclusive of complementary and alternative therapies. Pharmacology courses are a logical placement for herbal medicines, essential oils, and homeopathic preparations. Nutrition courses could add a component of dietary/biologically-based therapies. Psychiatric nursing courses could emphasize cognitive-behavioral therapy or meditation. And nursing research courses could discuss all aspects of complementary therapy efficacy through the lens of evidence-based practice. Wetzel, Kaptchuk, Haramati, and Eisenberg (2003) recommend the use of carefully placed case studies as a strategy to integrate complementary therapies throughout the curriculum.

Chlan and Halcón (2003) have also advocated for an integrated curriculum grounded in holistic, patient-centered care beginning at the baccalaureate level. The same authors identified six core competencies used to determine whether or not complementary therapies have been effectively integrated into the nursing curriculum:

1. An environment is created where patients openly discuss their use of complementary and alternative therapies;
2. The safety and efficacy of selected therapies are frequently evaluated;
3. Patients are consistently advised regarding their use of complementary and alternative therapies from an evidence-based perspective;
4. Students work within interdisciplinary teams that include complementary and alternative therapy practitioners;
5. Appropriate complementary therapies are incorporated into nursing practice or appropriate referrals are provided; and
6. Self-reflection and self-care are included in the personal wellness plan.

IMPLEMENTATION MODELS: A COURSE IN COMPLEMENTARY THERAPIES

Lee and colleagues (2007) surveyed the CAM Education Project schools discussed above to gauge how complementary therapies were integrated into the various medical and nursing programs. Elective courses were commonly offered and were determined to be an effective format for introducing complementary and alternative therapies. Eventually, however, these institutions pushed for the integration of successful elective materials into one or more required courses. These institutions utilized other strategies as well, such as collaborating with and offering these courses to students in other disciplines, such as Anthropology, Pharmacy, and Social Work.

Groft and Kalischuk (2005) described a 13-week, 3-hour undergraduate elective course on health and healing. Students explored a range of complementary and alternative therapies commonly used by patients. The course was determined to be highly effective in aiding students to understand a new dimension of health and healing and wholeness. Similar elective courses have been developed at the degree-completion and graduate level. Breda (1998) reported on a required capstone project for last-semester RNs in an RN-to-BSN program where students explored and experienced a complementary healing therapy through a literature search and analysis as well as an experiential component. Stephenson, Brown, Handron, and Faser (2007) described a 3-semester-hour elective graduate-level online nursing course designed to: (a) evaluate the theoretical bases and empirical evidence for various complementary/alternative therapies; (b) explore strategies for integrating evidence-based complementary/alternative therapies; and (c) synthesize advanced knowledge, theory, and research on complementary/alternative therapies into nursing.

IMPLEMENTATION MODELS: MINOR AND MAJOR FIELDS OF STUDY

Similar to the graduate minor in Complementary Therapies and Healing offered at the University of Minnesota, Sofhauser (2002) described the development of a 15-credit-hour minor in complementary health at the Indiana University South Bend. Graduate programs with a major in nursing have also been established in integrative health practices for advanced practice clinical nurse specialists (Jossens & Ganley, 2006). This graduate program emphasized both Western and CAM practices with two overall goals: (a) to generate nursing leaders with advanced knowledge of, and appreciation for, the diversity of approaches and philosophies concerning health; and (b) to graduate nurses with expertise in the assessment, use, and systematic evaluation of both Western and non-Western practices, contributing to the enhanced health of the community by facilitating the integration of health practices.

IMPLEMENTATION MODEL: EXPERIENTIAL LEARNING

An experiential component is highly recommended for any students learning about complementary therapies to promote a greater depth of understanding (Wetzel et al., 2003). Chlan, Halcón, Kreitzer, and Leonard (2005) studied the influence of skills lab practice on nursing student confidence levels in performing select complementary therapy skills. Student confidence in the performance of the five therapies (hand massage, imagery, music interventions, reflexology, and breathing/mindfulness) increased after the lab session. The greatest increases in confidence were seen with hand massage, reflexology, and imagery. This exercise demonstrated a first step in bringing practical application of CAM into undergraduate nursing education. Similarly, Cook and

Robinson (2006) implemented an intensive massage therapy experience to promote nursing student competence. The vast majority of student participants indicated that the experience was valuable in their development as nurses by contributing to the nurse-patient relationship and holism in patient care.

IMPLEMENTATION MODEL: CONTINUING EDUCATION OFFERINGS

Effective continuing education opportunities are needed to advance knowledge and skills in complementary therapies for nurses. Nurse practitioners responding to one survey indicated complementary therapy continuing education needed to include information on scientific principles, evidence of efficacy, potential interactions with conventional medicine, and pharmacology. The preferred mechanism for advancing this knowledge was online continuing nursing education (67%), conferences (60%), workshops (60%), and newsletters (51%) (Patterson, Kaczorowski, Arthur, Smith, & Mills, 2003). Given that, the following Web site provides a useful summary of a multitude of online and conference opportunities that can assist practicing nurses in improving complementary therapy knowledge and skills: http://www.healthandhealingny.org/professionals/nurse.asp. In addition, the University of Minnesota modules developed through the CAM Education Project grant can be found at: http://www.csh.umn.edu/modules/index.html.

FACILITATING AND EVALUATING STUDENT LEARNING

Creative pedagogies are needed to facilitate student learning and support effective teaching of complementary therapies. According to Lee and colleagues (2007), CAM Education Project schools used a variety of instructional delivery strategies to help students learn about complementary therapies, including classroom-based programs, online modules, and experiential learning. These authors also recognized that personal reflection and self-care are critical components of student learning. Oliver and Hill (1992) described a learning activity designed to assist students to integrate holistic and traditional nursing interventions in which students design care measures for a comatose male, focusing on providing nutritional support through a tube feeding. The interventions incorporate guided imagery and aromatherapy to elicit a more pleasant meal-time experience for the simulated patient. Forjuoh, Rascoe, Symm, and Edwards (2003) effectively taught complementary therapies using evidence-based medicine principles.

Effective teaching and student learning must be facilitated through access to appropriate research databases and other resources (Ezzo et al., 2002; Gaster, Unterborn, Scott, & Schneeweiss, 2007). Following is a listing of such resources that can facilitate learning about complementary and alternative therapies:

- NCCAM (http://nccam.nih.gov)
- The Cochrane Database (http://www.cochrane.org)
- Medline Plus: Herbs and Supplements (www.medlineplus.gov)
- Natural Medicine Comprehensive Database (www.naturaldatabase.com)
- CINAHL: Cumulative Index to Nursing & Allied Health Literature (http://www.cinahl.com)
- Medline: PubMed (http://www.ncbi.nlm.nih.gov/entrez/query.fcgi)
- BMJ Clinical Evidence (www.clinicalevidence.com)
- FDA Center for Food Safety (www.cfsan.fda.gov/dms/supplmnt.html)

The effective assessment and evaluation of student learning in the realm of complementary therapies must also occur to facilitate program improvement. At the course level, traditional student learning evaluation methods, such as written papers, exams, and other projects must be accompanied by explorative methods to gain course evaluation information for course improvement such as through interviews, focus groups, or one-minute feedback papers. An analysis of the CAM Education Project schools demonstrated a wide range of methods were used to determine student learning and program effectiveness (Stratton, Benn, Lie, Zeller, & Nedrow, 2007). As Stratton and colleagues (2007) indicated:

> In the absence of a single, established set of approved CAM education or competency standards, an array of curricula exist....Consequently, the approaches to evaluating curricular efforts were equally diverse and in-

volved the development and refinement of assessment tools to measure a wide variety of attitudes, beliefs, motivations, knowledge bases, and skills (p. 959).

CONCLUSIONS

In 2000, Lindeman predicted the future of nursing education would include "greater diversity in clinical experiences to provide contact with people from different cultures, ethnic groups, economic levels, and with alternatives to western medicine" (p. 11). This certainly has been the case, accompanied, of course, by the requisite fears of adding to an already overcrowded curriculum. Lee and colleagues (2007) attempted to ease this anxiety by refocusing successful curriculum integration as an enjoyable opportunity to cultivate relationships and the excitement of discovery inherent in student learning. Wetzel and colleagues (2003) outlined a viable mechanism to avoid adding to an already packed curriculum, using a theme that embraces the essence of both nursing care and complementary therapies, such as holistic or integrative health care. Whether or not advancing complementary therapy knowledge or attitudes translates into effective or improved patient outcomes remains a question (Stratton et al., 2007). However, all nursing programs can contribute to the advancement of complementary therapy linkages to health care outcomes through the implementation of clear student learning and program outcomes, rigorous research design, and precise measurement (Stratton et al.).

The future of nursing education inclusive of complementary therapies requires attention to a set of accepted knowledge and performance core competencies for entry-level and graduate-level nurses (Halcón et al., 2003). Stratton and colleagues (2007), however, recognize that this task represents a moving target, complicated by ever-changing educational and health care environments. Only through thoughtful reflection on the current curriculum, adherence to the scope and standards of practice for nurses, and attention to educational and health care influences can we continue to move forward.

REFERENCES

American Association of Colleges of Nursing. (2004). *The essentials of Master's education for advanced practice nursing.* Retrieved November 1, 2008, from www.aacn.nche.edu

American Association of Colleges of Nursing. (2006). *The essentials of doctoral education for advanced practice nursing.* Retrieved November 1, 2008, from www.aacn.nche.edu

American Association of Colleges of Nursing. (2008). *The essentials of baccalaureate education for professional nursing practice.* Retrieved November 1, 2008, from www.aacn.nche.edu

American Holistic Nurses Association & American Nurses Association. (2007). *Holistic nursing: Scope and standards of practice.* Silver Spring, MD: American Holistic Nurses Association/American Nurses Association.

American Nurses Association. (2004). *Nursing: Scope and standards of practice.* Washington, DC: American Nurses Association.

Breda, K. (1998). Teaching complementary healing therapies to nurses. *Journal of Nursing Education, 37,* 394–397.

Bulechek, G., Butcher, H., & McCloskey Dochterman, J. (Eds.) (2008). *Nursing Interventions Classification (NIC).* St. Louis, MO: Mosby Elsevier.

Burman, M. (2003). Complementary and alternative medicine: Core competencies for family nurse practitioners. *Journal of Nursing Education, 42,* 28–34.

Chlan, L., & Halcón, L. (2003). Developing an integrated baccalaureate nursing education program: Infusing complementary/alternative therapies into critical care curricula. *Critical Care Nursing Clinics of North America, 15,* 373–379.

Chlan, L., Halcón, L., Kreitzer, M., & Leonard, B. (2005). Influence of an experiential education session on nursing students' confidence levels in performing selected complementary therapy skills. *Complementary Health Practice Review, 10,* 189–201.

College & Association of Registered Nurses of Alberta. (2006). *Alternative and/or Complementary Therapy Standards for Registered Nurses.* Retrieved November 1, 2008, from www.nurses.ab.ca

Cook, N., & Robinson, J. (2006). Effectiveness and value of massage skills training during pre-registration nurse education. *Nurse Education Today, 26,* 555–563.

Cuellar, N., Cahill, B., Ford, J., & Aycock, T. (2003). The development of an educational workshop on complementary and alternative medicine: What every nurse should know. *The Journal of Continuing Education in Nursing, 34,* 128–135.

Dossey, B., Frisch, N., Forker, J., & Lavin, J. (1998). Evolving a blueprint for certification: Inventory of professional activities and knowledge of a holistic nurse. *Journal of Holistic Nursing, 16,* 33–56.

Dutta, A., Dutta, A., Bwayo, S., Xue, Z., Akiyode, O., Ayuk-Egbe, P., et al. (2003). Complementary and alternative medicine instruction in nursing curricula. *Journal of National Black Nurses Association, 14,* 30–33.

Ezzo, J., Wright, K., Hadhazy, V., Bahr-Robertson, M., Beckner, W., Covington, M., et al. (2002). Use of the Cochrane electronic library in complementary and alternative medicine courses in medical schools: Is the giant lost in cyberspace? *Journal of Alternative and Complementary Medicine, 8,* 681–686.

Fenton, M., & Morris, D. (2003). The integration of holistic nursing practices and complementary and alternative modalities into curricula of schools of nursing. *Alternative Therapies, 9,* 62–67.

Forjuoh, S., Rascoe, T., Symm, B., & Edwards, J. (2003). Teaching medical students complementary and alternative medicine using evidence-based principles. *Journal of Alternative and Complementary Medicine, 9,* 429–439.

Gaster, B., Unterborn, J., Scott, R., & Schneeweiss, R. (2007). What should students learn about complementary and alternative medicine? *Academic Medicine, 82,* 934–938.

Gaylord, S., & Mann, D. (2007). Rationales for CAM education in health professions training programs. *Academic Medicine, 82,* 927–933.

Groft, J., & Kalischuk, R. (2005). Nursing students learn about complementary and alternative health care practices. *Complementary Health Practice Review, 10,* 133–146.

Halcón, L., Chlan, L., Kreitzer, M., & Leonard, B. (2003). Complementary therapies and healing practices: Faculty/student beliefs and attitudes and the implications for nursing education. *Journal of Professional Nursing, 19,* 387–397.

Halcón, L., Leonard, B., Snyder, M., Garwick, A., & Kreitzer, M. (2001). Incorporating alternative and complementary health practices within university-based nursing education. *Complementary Health Practice Review, 6,* 127–135.

Helms, J. (2006). Complementary and alternative therapies: A new frontier for nursing education? *Journal of Nursing Education, 45,* 117–123.

Hon, K., Twinn, S., Leung, T., Thompson, D., Wong, Y., & Fok, T. (2006). Chinese nursing students' attitudes toward traditional Chinese medicine. *Journal of Nursing Education, 45,* 182–185.

Jossens, M., & Ganley, B. (2006). Integrated health practices: Development of a graduate nursing program. *Journal of Nursing Education, 45,* 16–24.

Keimig, T., & Braun, C. (2004). Student nurses' knowledge and perceptions of alternative and complementary therapies. *Journal of Undergraduate Nursing Scholarship, 6,* 1–9.

Kim, S., Erlen, J., Kim, K., & Sok, S. (2006). Nursing students' and faculty members' knowledge of, experience with, and attitudes towards complementary and alternative therapies. *Journal of Nursing Education, 45,* 375–378.

Kligler, B., Maizes, V., Schachter, S., Park, C., Gaudet, T., Benn, R., et al. (2004). Core competencies in integrative medicine for medical school curricula: A proposal. *Academic Medicine, 79,* 521–531.

Kreitzer, M., Mitten, D., Harris, I., & Shandeling, J. (2002). Attitudes toward CAM among medical, nursing, and pharmacy faculty and students: A comparative analysis. *Alternative Therapies in Health and Medicine, 8*(6), 44–53.

Kreitzer, M., Mann, D., & Lumpkin, M. (2008). CAM competencies for the health professions. *Complementary Health Practices Review, 13,* 63–72.

Lee, M., Benn, R., Wimstatt, L., Cornman, J., Hedgecock, J., Gerick, S., et al. (2007). Integrating complementary and alternative medicine instruction into health professions education: Organizational and instructional strategies. *Academic Medicine, 82,* 939–945.

Lindeman, C. (2000). The future of nursing education. *Journal of Nursing Education, 39,* 5–12.

Melland, H., & Clayburgh, T. (2000). Complementary therapies: Introduction into a nursing curriculum. *Nurse Educator, 25,* 247–250.

Morgan, D., Glanville, H., Mars, S., & Nathanson, V. (1998). Education and training in complementary and alternative medicine: A postal survey of UK universities, medical schools, and faculties of nurse education. *Complementary Therapies in Medicine, 6,* 64–70.

Nedrow, A., Heitkemper, M., Frenkel, M., Mann, D., Wayne, P., & Hughes, E. (2007). Collaborations between allopathic and complementary and alternative medicine health professionals: Four initiatives. *Academic Medicine, 82,* 962–966.

Nedrow, A., Istvan, J., Haas, M., Barrett, R., Salveson, C., Moore, G., et al. (2007). Implications for education in complementary and alternative medicine: A survey of entry attitudes in students at five health professional schools. *Journal of Alternative and Complementary Medicine, 13,* 381–386.

Nurses Board of Western Australia. (2003). *Guidelines for the use of complementary therapies in nursing practice.* Retrieved November 1, 2008, from www.nbwa.org.au

Oliver, N., & Hill, L. (1992). Teaching complex nursing interventions: Integrating holistic and traditional behavior. *Journal of Nursing Education, 31,* 185–185.

Öztekin, D., Ucuzal., M., Öztekin, I., & Issever, H. (2007). Nursing students' willingness to use complementary and alternative therapies for cancer patients: Istanbul survey. *Tohoku Journal of Exp Medicine, 211,* 49–61.

Patterson, C., Kaczorowski, J., Arthur, H., Smith, K., & Mills, D. (2003). Complementary therapy practice: Defining the role of advanced nurse practitioners. *Journal of Clinical Nursing, 12,* 816–823.

Pearson, N., & Chesney, M. (2007). The CAM education program of the National Center for Complementary and Alternative Medicine: An overview. *Academic Medicine, 82,* 921–926.

Reed, F., Pettigrew, A., & King, M. (2000). Alternative and complementary therapies in nursing curricula. *Journal of Nursing Education, 39,* 133–139.

Richardson, S. (2003). Complementary health and healing in nursing education. *Journal of Holistic Nursing, 21,* 20–35.

Sofhauser, C. (2002). Development of a minor in complementary health. *Nurse Educator, 27,* 118–122.

Sok, S., Erlen, J., & Kim, K. (2004). Complementary and alternative therapies in nursing curricula: A new direction for nurse educators. *Journal of Nursing Education, 43,* 401–405.

Sparber, A. (2001). State boards of nursing and scope of practice of registered nurses performing complementary therapies. *Online Journal of Issues in Nursing, 6.* Available at: *www.nursingworld.org/MainMenuCategories/ANAMarketplace/ANAPeriodicals/ OJIN/Tableofcontents/Volume62001/No3Sept01/ArticlePreviou sTopic/complementary TherapiesReport.aspx*

Stephenson, N., Brown, S., Handron, D., & Faser, K. (2007). Offering an online course: Complementary and alternative therapies in nursing practice. *Holistic Nursing Practice, 21,* 299–302.

Stratton, T., Benn, R., Lie, D., Zeller, J., & Nedrow, A. (2007). Evaluating CAM education in health professions programs. *Academic Medicine, 82,* 956–961.

Uzun, Ö., & Tan, M. (2004). Nursing students' opinions and knowledge about complementary and alternative medicine therapies. *Complementary Therapies in Nursing & Midwifery, 10,* 239–244.

Wetzel, M., Kaptchuk, T., Haramati, A., & Eisenberg, D. (2003). Complementary and alternative medical therapies: Implications for medical education. *Annals of Internal Medicine, 138,* 191–196.

Yeh, Y., & Chung, U. (2007). An investigation into competence in TCM of BSN graduates from technological universities in Taiwan. *Journal of Nursing Research, 15,* 310–317.

31 Perspectives on Future Research

RUTH LINDQUIST
MARIAH SNYDER
YEOUNGSUK SONG

Nursing's commitment to the generation of high-quality, cost-effective patient outcomes requires that a sound scientific basis for practice be established. Previous chapters have identified existing research related to the therapies reviewed; however, most chapters end with statements that more research is needed. The need for more evidence related to the safety, efficacy, timing, "dose," and specific indications for most therapies is clearly evident. As previously noted, there is a large and growing interest in and use of complementary therapies by the public. In fact, the number of annual visits to providers of complementary and alternative therapies outnumbers visits to primary care physicians (Institute of Medicine [IOM], 2002). The 2007 annual National Health Survey, a comprehensive in-person survey of Americans regarding their health, found that 38.8% of adults and 11.8% of children surveyed in the United States reported use of a form of complementary and alternative medicine in the preceding 12 months (Barnes, Bloom, & Nahin, 2008; NCCAM, 2008). Interest in complementary therapies is encountered in a broad range of health care practice settings. Along with public and patient interest, there is a concomitant interest on the part of providers who not only want to deliver these therapies to patients but also have an interest in the same therapies for their own personal use (Lindquist,

Tracy, & Savik, 2003). As a result of the significant demand and common use of complementary and alternative therapies, there is a heightened urgency to expand the evidence base to support their use.

Health providers and researchers are challenged to create and employ a solid evidence base to undergird the broad range of complementary therapies used by substantial segments of the U.S. population and persons throughout the world. There is an acute need to know and understand benefits of therapies and whether they work according to the purpose for which they are used; there is also a need to ensure the safety and efficacy of complementary therapies and to understand their effects and interactions when used in combination with other complementary and allopathic therapies (NCCAM, 2008). In this chapter, the need for more evidence to support the expanding use of complementary therapies in practice is presented; research designs appropriate for the study of complementary therapies are explored; the overall state of research on complementary therapies is described; and implications that the state of evidence and expanded use of complementary therapies have for future nursing research are identified.

NEED TO EXPAND THE EVIDENCE BASE

The documented growing interest in and use of alternative and complementary therapies and alternative systems of care have caused health care providers to consider the appeal of these therapies to consumers as well as the consideration of their safety and efficacy. Concomitantly, questions regarding costs and cost-effectiveness for third-party payment and for individuals paying out-of-pocket need to be answered (NCCAM, 2009a). Questions need to be answered through research related to which therapies and how many treatment sessions should be covered, and what results from the treatment can be expected. The optimal mix and relative cost of the complementary or alternative therapies versus traditional Western treatments need to be determined.

With the widespread use of complementary and alternative therapies, there is reason for concern regarding the safety of their use and about their potential interactions with Western medicine. An example is the interaction of herbal remedies such as St. John's wort with prescribed pharmacotherapy, including psychotropic agents, in the family of selective serotonin reuptake inhibitors. Contributing to the difficulty is the lack of regulation of complementary and alternative therapies such as herbal products (Klepser & Klepser, 1999), although increasing attention is being paid to this in an effort to provide guidance for the creation of national policies (World Health Organization, 2005). Scientific data are needed by providers, so as to inform their practice. Accurate and reliable knowledge is also needed by consumers who wish to make informed decisions regarding their own health practices.

There is a rising interest in and indeed a mandate for evidence-based practice. Evidence-based practice integrates the best scientific evidence with clinical expertise and patient preferences. Evidence-based practice (EBP) has been defined by McKibbon (1998) as:

> an approach to health care wherein health professionals use the best evidence possible, i.e., the most appropriate information available, to make clinical decisions for individual patients. EBP values, enhances and builds on clinical expertise, knowledge of disease mechanisms, and pathophysiology. It involves complex and conscientious decision-making based not only on the available evidence but also on patient characteristics, situations, and preferences. It recognizes that health care is individualized and ever-changing and involves uncertainties and probabilities. Ultimately EBP is the formalization of the care process that the best clinicians have practiced for generations. (p. 396)

Nurses and other providers practicing in the context of conventional allopathic care rely on an evidence base. So, too, nurses and other health professionals are relying on or requiring similar evidence in their use of complementary therapies (IOM, 2002); however, in a national survey, critical care nurses generally reported that they needed more evidence for conventional allopathic remedies than they did for complementary and alternative therapies (Tracy et al., 2005).

It is important that resources to access knowledge about complementary and alternative therapies be identified, made available, and used by providers. Research findings regarding the safety and efficacy of therapies must be disseminated broadly to practitioners, who need to be informed so that the safety of patients can be protected and the potential benefits of therapies realized. A number of personal data assistants (PDA)–based resources provide access to authoritative information as a resource to professional practice. Databases of research findings (e.g., the Cochrane Database of Systematic Reviews) are good resources for synthesized research findings (www.cochrane.org/reviews/). As of 2004, this online source contained 145 reviews related to complementary and alternative therapies, and more reviews have been added since. Web sites of government agencies, such as the National Institutes of Health's (NIH) National Center for Complementary and Alternative Medicine (NCCAM), provide other sources of information on a wide range of complementary and alternative therapies (http://nccam.nih.gov/health/ bytreatment.htm).

NCCAM's growing funding of investigator-initiated research and other programmatic initiatives (NCCAM, 2009a) has begun building a solid foundation from which therapies can be selected and delivered with growing confidence as to their safety and efficacy. However, there is, of course, much work to be done. The ideal evidence base for complementary therapies would support decision making in a broad range of complex patient situations. It would differentiate effects on and appropriateness for persons with diverse characteristics (e.g., age, gender, body mass) and from various cultures (accounting for dietary practices, social acceptability, and cultural traditions, etc.) and would outline the potential differing effects and indications for persons suffering the full range of pathologies and comorbidities.

There are legitimate safety concerns related to therapy selection, quality of the product (the purity or technique of delivery), dose, timing, duration, and other considerations related to specific therapies such as herbal therapies, nutraceuticals, and supplements. For example, more research is needed to identify potentially adverse drug–herbal interactions, to answer questions related to whether particular drugs and herbs can be ingested simultaneously; if not, the half-life of herbs in the body, or their "wash-out" times, need to be determined. Research is also needed to provide data to document the relative risks and benefits of therapies such as the use of diet therapy for hypertension (as opposed to standard allopathic pharmacologic therapies), or to consider the potential reduction of the side effects of an allopathic agent if used at a reduced dose in combination with a complementary therapy.

The growing evidence base provides much needed information for the consumer and provider. However, additional research is needed to determine the potential beneficial outcomes of complementary therapies. Likewise, studies are needed to generate findings that protect the public from harm or from needless, costly therapies that have no evidence to support them, or evidence that clearly shows no benefit. For example, therapies such as the use of laetrile to combat cancer caused concern among allopathic providers who feared that the false hope of cure would dissuade patients from seeking legitimate forms of cancer therapy while bleeding fortunes from desperate families, despite the fact that there was no basis for its claims of beneficial effects (Pinn, 2001). Extramural funding opportunities and the peer review system of NIH ensure the continued accumulation of high-quality evidence and encourage investigators who have the ideas, curiosity, and scientific expertise to explore potential therapies for human use.

RESEARCH DESIGNS FOR COMPLEMENTARY THERAPIES

Most scientists would agree that the most rigorous design to test complementary and alternative therapies is the randomized, placebo-controlled, double-blind design which has long been the standard for testing therapies and advancing fields of inquiry (Duley & Farrell, 2002; Fogg & Gross, 2000; IOM, 2002). However, this design is not the only one that provides useful information, and data that are generated from quantitative studies are not the only available evidence base for practice. Other designs and sources of evidence are also important and contribute to our knowledge and understanding of patients' responses to therapies, both allopathic and nonallopathic.

Consumers may be increasingly reluctant to enroll in clinical trials; hence, alternative study designs and strategies for the conduct of clinical research to advance the field may be necessary (Gross & Fogg, 2001). The Committee on the Use of Complementary and Alternative Medicine by the American Public was commissioned by the Institute of Medicine, the Agency for Health Care Quality & Research, NCCAM, and 15 other agencies and institutes of NIH to study and provide specific recommendations regarding complementary and alternative therapies. As part of their report (IOM, 2002), innovative designs that could be used to provide information about the effectiveness of therapies were identified, including:

- **Preference RCTs**—trials that include randomized and nonrandomized arms, which then permit comparisons between patients who chose a particular treatment and those who were randomly assigned to it

- **Observational and cohort studies**—studies that involve the iden- tification of patients who are eligible for study and who may receive a specified treatment as part of the study
- **Case-control studies**—studies that involve identifying patients who have good or bad outcomes, then "working back" to find aspects of treatment associated with those differing outcomes
- **Studies of bundles of therapies**—analyses of the effectiveness, as a whole, of particular packages of treatments
- **Studies that specifically incorporate, measure, or account for placebo or expectation effects**—patients' hopes, emotional states, energies, and other self-healing processes are not considered ex- traneous, but are included as part of the therapy's main "mecha- nism of action"
- **Attribute-treatment interaction analyses**—a way of accounting for differences in effectiveness outcomes among patients within a study and among different studies of varying design (p. 3).

In an effort to identify major issues in research design in funding proposals submitted to a specific funding program for clinical trials of complementary and alternative medicine for cancer symptom manage- ment, a number of problems with scientific methodology were found (Buchanan et al., 2005). Common issues included "unwarranted as- sumptions about the consistency and standardization of CAM interven- tions, the need for data-based justifications for the study hypothesis, and the need to implement appropriate quality control and monitoring procedures during the course of the trial" (Buchanan et al., p. 6682). Such problems need to be addressed and resolved, to ensure the rigor and merit of studies of therapies for cancer symptom management as well as the study of a broader array of therapies.

Another important area that continues to challenge investigators involves the placebo effect and placebo/attention control groups (Gross, 2005). The placebo effect has been studied with respect to pain and analgesia, neuroimmunology, fear, anxiety, and pharmacotherapy and may have the capacity to stimulate dramatic healing (Harrington, 1997). The power of the placebo effect should not be underestimated (Turner, Deyo, Loesser, Von Korff, & Fordyce, 1994). Placebo effects may lead to improvements in well over 50% of subjects in trials of medical therapies. There is evidence that the placebo effect in clinical trials of CAM is similar to the placebo effect observed in clinical trials of conventional medicine (Dorn et al., 2007). Methods to manage placebo effects must be carefully considered in research on complementary therapies. In addition, when assessing the overall effects of a therapy, the potential added impact of the healer and the therapeutic relationship on the outcome must be considered (Quinn, Smith, Ritenbaugh, Swanson, & Watson, 2003).

Complementary therapies are often administered in the context of other therapies. This makes it challenging to differentiate the effects of the complementary therapies from those of other therapies given simultaneously, while dissecting out effects of other concomitant disease processes and their treatments. Therapies may have both direct and indirect effects as well as salutary and adverse effects. These must be determined through systematic observation and research. The mechanism of action of many therapies remains elusive. It is hard to understand the effects without framing the therapy within the culture or practice of the healing tradition. Also the terms and measures of outcomes across cultures may not be the same, resulting in barriers for transglobal communication and learning from a commonly held and supported evidence base.

Simply knowing that a therapy may be beneficial is not enough. Questions need to be answered; for example: What are the conditions under which it is effective? What is the dose needed? What dose is too much? How often must a therapy be delivered to achieve a benefit? How long does the effect last? How much therapy should insurers cover? There is a need for studies on the cost-effectiveness of complementary therapies and for research that compares and contrasts complementary therapies with other conventional therapies (IOM, 2002).

Cultural Considerations

Studies of therapies relevant to aging populations, populations at varied developmental stages, and those having varied cultural backgrounds are also needed. These populations present challenges for the design, recruitment, and implementation of studies. Elderly subjects often have multiple comorbidities and may be taking multiple medications. Language and lack of cultural understanding may pose barriers to the inclusion of new immigrants. Access to young children, adolescents, vulnerable adults, and the unique ethical issues surrounding their recruitment and participation may also be perceived as barriers to the inclusion of these groups.

There are other outcomes sought by health care consumers. That a therapy is shown to have beneficial health effects is not the only legitimate reason for its use. Immigrants tend to use complementary and alternative therapies first and then seek conventional medical help if these are not effective (Garcés, Scarinici, & Harrison, 2006). Therapies may have cultural significance or be intricately tied with healing traditions; therapies may lead to patients' peace of mind; they may meet patient and family expectations, or lead to their increased satisfaction. If they have come to the United States from other countries, the cultural belief in alternative or complementary medicine is not changed. In considering the use of complementary therapies, the costs, risks, and value to recipients must be carefully weighed.

Longitudinal Studies

Many studies have employed small samples and short-term effects of therapies. If we want to know the real risks and benefits of complementary and alternative therapies, we need longitudinal studies because, with some complementary and alternative therapies, we can determine the severity and occurrence of adverse events only when they are applied on a long-term basis. Although similar longitudinal studies using the same design are done, different results may be obtained from persons from different cultures. Therefore, it is important that we study complementary and alternative therapy using the same or similar design in other countries and different cultures.

NCCAM's strategic plan has created two interrelated offices to address ethnic and cultural issues: The Office of Special Populations (to eliminate racial and ethnic disparities), and the Office of International Health Research (to identify promising international CAM practices, foster rigorous scientific study, and develop effective CAM applications through productive international scientific collaborations while embracing the heritage and practices of indigenous peoples; NCCAM, 2002). NCCAM program initiatives are further described in the next section.

CURRENT STATE OF RESEARCH ON COMPLEMENTARY THERAPIES

As previously noted, chapter authors have included the most recent research and have identified where more research is needed to provide knowledge to guide practice. Specific research challenges include the need for data-based decision support resources for the combination of therapies. Such resources would include data related to potential adverse interactions or potentiating of effects when combining therapies. There is a need for research to be conducted with special populations, including children, frail elders, and the critically ill. Research is needed to study the effects of complementary therapies in specific health conditions or disease states. Clearly, research lags behind the public's appetite for complementary therapies; knowledge of the putative mechanisms of action, the qualities of therapies, and the predictability of outcomes is uneven across therapies. The IOM report, *Complementary and Alternative Therapies in the United States* (IOM, 2004), provides perhaps the most comprehensive, authoritative summary of the research and knowledge base in the field. The report provides an assessment of what is known about complementary and alternative therapies and their use; it also proposes research methods and priorities for research and product evaluation.

Insistence on the use of standard conventions of scientific inquiry has been helpful in increasing the amount of evidence that has been systematically obtained to provide information for decision making in complementary therapies. However, information is lacking on the appropriate dose and timing of interventions and on those for whom the interventions may have the most beneficial effects. A solid evidence base for complementary therapies would support decision making in broad and complex patient situations. Complementary therapies may have different effects on people of diverse ethnic backgrounds and demographic characteristics. So, too, they may have potentially different indications and effects in persons suffering differing pathologies or medical conditions. The lack of such information is limiting to practitioners who rely on a more fully developed evidence base, and this may hinder the full integration of the use of complementary therapies in practice.

Often, studies have been done that have relatively small sample sizes; meta-analyses can be conducted on such studies to synthesize findings to estimate "effect size" of therapies when examined across studies. More of this type of work is also needed in addition to basic research. Synthesis and review articles would also contribute to the availability of well-organized, available information.

The NCCAM, established by Congress in 1999, has as its mission the exploration of "complementary and alternative healing practices in the context of rigorous science, training CAM researchers, and disseminating authoritative information to the public and professional community" (NCCAM, 2005, p. 2). As previously mentioned, the NCCAM Web site (http://nccam.nih.gov) provides updated online information about the research conducted in the area of these therapies. It also provides a listing of clinical trials that are alphabetized by the name of the therapies and further organized by the five domains of complementary and alternative therapies (the same NCCAM domains used to organize chapters in the intervention sections of this book). The work of this NIH center promises to increase the scientific evidence base and improve the context and delivery of therapies in years to come.

NCCAM has played a vital role in promoting the generation, organization, and dissemination of data for practice and research. It has fostered a standard language and is a source for arguably the most definitive information, and for funding. Fortunately, there has been increasing funding for NCCAM over the years, resulting in substantial investigative activity in the area of complementary/alternative medicine (NCCAM, 2009a).

NCCAM has created and funded centers to foster more rapid development of the knowledge base for the use of complementary and alternative therapies (NCCAM, 2009b). These include the Centers of Excellence for Research on CAM; Centers for Dietary Supplements Research on Botanicals; Developmental Centers for Research on CAM; Centers for CAM Research; and International Centers for Research on CAM. The work within the Centers of Excellence comprises 3 to 4 synergistic research projects that focus on elucidating the mechanisms of action of CAM. The Centers of Excellence focus on research in the areas of major health problems, including, for example, HIV/AIDS, arthritis, asthma, and pain. The Developmental Centers for Research on CAM support developmental CAM research in the context of collaborations between CAM schools and biomedical research institutions. The International Centers for Research on CAM conduct both basic and clinical studies with the United States and international partners that focus on traditional medicine that is indigenous to the locations of the partners.

IMPLICATIONS FOR NURSING RESEARCH

There is a great need for nurses and scientists in other disciplines to develop ongoing programs of research related to specific complementary therapies. As primary care providers, nurses are in an excellent position to address patients' need for complementary therapies. Nurses have a vested interest in generating information that can be used to build the knowledge database underlying the use of specific therapies that may benefit patients. They may also generate data that refute the use of therapies or reveal adverse risk/benefit ratios. Nurses have conducted research on a number of complementary therapies. Most nurse scientists are educated in both qualitative and quantitative designs. This gives them an understanding of multiple ways to construct research studies to determine effects of complementary therapies. The need for the expansion and dissemination of evidence and access to it has particular significance for the discipline of nursing and underlies recommendations for future directions in nursing research.

The need to generate information that can be used to build the evidence base for complementary therapies is compelling for nurse scientists. Specialized clinical expertise of nurse researchers can be used to select therapies to test and to target outcomes of importance to their patient populations. Specialized clinical knowledge has the potential to enhance the identification of instruments that are sensitive enough to assess potential effects of therapies (subjective, objective, or behavioral). Nurses play important roles in generating, disseminating, and utilizing the evidence base for practice.

The *Research Teams of the Future* program of the NIH is an initiative to harness and extend advances in science through interdisciplinary research (NIH, 2004). Interdisciplinary collaborations between nurse investigators and investigators from other disciplines who bring complementary strengths from basic science, genetics, complementary therapies, or clinical practice may lead to growth of the knowledge base and its breadth, depth, and relevance, which should ultimately improve the quality of care for patients. Collaborations between scientists who are capable of conducting research across disciplines may lead to new breakthroughs in regard to CAM therapies.

Broadening frames of reference of nurse scientists to include global perspectives and information from around the world will ensure an appropriate and comprehensive view of the field. The World Health Organization (2002) has launched a global strategic initiative to assist countries in blending complementary therapies with the countries' established health care systems. Such global initiatives should serve as catalysts in making information available to practitioners worldwide and should advance the field of complementary/alternative medicine.

Electronic means of posting new knowledge, warnings, or updated information on clinical trials speeds the availability of information and literally has the potential to bring a world of information to bear on practice—but only if utilized. Electronic publishing speeds the transfer of research findings to practice settings. The mandate set by medical publishers (DeAngelis et al., 2004) to enroll in a registry of clinical trials if investigators desire to publish the results of their clinical trials in highly distinguished medical journals is also a step in the right direction.

Clinical research is costly. Advanced research training may help to hone nurse-investigators' grant-writing skills to pursue needed funds for investigative work to generate new knowledge in the field. Design skills that permit nurse investigators to rigorously test interventions and advance clinical knowledge about the use of complementary therapies are critical. However, studies conducted in nonclinical settings, including surveys of public use of complementary therapies, are also important. Nursing research is also needed to focus on the costs, relative cost-versus-benefits ratio, and ethical issues surrounding access to and delivery of therapies.

Nurses and other providers have responsibilities to provide the public with guidance in the use of complementary therapies; to interpret and share scientific information; and to contribute to the development of the knowledge base through investigation and research dissemination. Guidelines that are founded in the evidence are clearly needed to set standards for appropriate use of complementary therapies (IOM, 2004).

Making optimal use of available knowledge and methods to disseminate research electronically and making information available at the point of care are important. However, many questions remain to be answered for the application of therapies in general and also for gender, culture, age, and comorbidities. More research is needed and it is increasingly recognized that interdisciplinary, multicultural, and transglobal partnerships may be the most fruitful in answering these questions.

Imagine the future with a new culture of care: one that is open and that offers patient-centered care grounded in a well-established evidence base; a future world in which care is viewed through the lens of the patient experience and integrates the best of Western medicine with the best of available nonallopathic remedies. The exploration of therapeutic

options includes the consideration of allopathic and nonallopathic remedies by patients and their providers, followed by the evaluation of the
outcomes of the therapies selected. With the exploding increase in the
use of complementary therapies, there will be new and interesting
therapies explored and adopted based on evidence that supports their
efficacy. Imagination aside, new information regarding the health practices of immigrant groups, increased global sharing of healing practices,
and the public's appetite for new ways to achieve better health, to effect
cures, or to forestall aging, all guarantee that the future of the use of
complementary therapies by nurses, health care providers, and the
public will always be fresh and interesting.

REFERENCES

Barnes, P. M., Bloom, B., & Nahin, R. (2008, December). *National Health Statistics Report #12*. Complementary and alternative medicine use among adults and children in the United States, 2007.

Buchanan, D. R., White, J. D., O'Mara, A. M., Kelaghan, J. W., Smith, W. B., & Minasian, L. M. (2005). Research-design issues in cancer-symptom-management trials using complementary and alternative medicine: Lessons from the National Cancer Institute Community Clinical Oncology Program experience. *Journal of Clinical Oncology, 23*(27), 6682–6689.

DeAngelis, C. D., Drazen, J. M., Frizelle, F. A., Haug, C., Hoey, J., Horton, R., et al. (2004). Clinical trial registration: A statement from the International Committee of Medical Journal Editors. *Journal of the American Medical Association, 292*(11), 1363–1364.

Dorn, S. D., Kaptchuk, T. J., Park, J. B., Nguyen, L. T., Canenguez, K., Nam, B. H., et al. (2007). A meta-analysis of the placebo response in complementary and alternative medicine trials of irritable bowel syndrome. *Neurogastroenterology & Motility, 19*(8), 630–637.

Duley, L., & Farrell, B. (Eds.). (2002). *Clinical trials*. London: BMJ Books.

Fogg, L., & Gross, D. (2000). Threats to validity in randomized clinical trials. *Research in Nursing & Health, 23,* 79–87.

Garces, I. C., Scarinici, I. C., & Harrison, L. (2006). An examination of sociocultural factors associated with health and health care seeking among Latina immigrants. *Journal of Immigrant Health, 8,* 377–385.

Gross, D. (2005). On the merits of attention-control groups. *Research in Nursing & Health, 28,* 93–94.

Gross, D., & Fogg, L. (2001). Clinical trials in the 21st century: The case for participant-centered research. *Research in Nursing & Health, 24,* 530–539.

Harrington, A. (1997). Introduction. In A. Harrington (Ed.), *The placebo effect: An interdisciplinary exploration* (pp. 1–11). Cambridge, MA: Harvard University Press.

Institute of Medicine. (2004). *Complementary and alternative medicine (CAM) in the United States* (Executive Summary, pp. 1–11). Washington, DC: The National Academies Press.

Institute of Medicine, Committee on the Use of Complementary and Alternative Medicine by the American Public. (2002). *Executive summary: Complementary and alternative medicine in the United States.* Washington, DC: National Academy Press. Retrieved August 5, 2009, from http://books.nap.edu/catalog/11182.html

Klepser, T. B., & Klepser, M. E. (1999). Unsafe and potentially safe herbal therapies. *American Journal of Health Systems Pharmacy, 56*(2), 125–38.

Lindquist, R., Tracy, M. F., & Savik, K. (2003). Personal use of complementary and alternative therapies by critical care nurses. *Critical Care Nursing Clinics of North America, 15*(3), 393–399.

McKibbon, K. A. (1998). Evidence based practice. *Bulletin of the Medical Library Association, 86*(3), 396–401.

National Center for Complementary and Alternative Medicine. (2002, June). *Office of International Health Research expanding global horizons of health care 5-year strategic plan* (June 2002). Retrieved April 26, 2009, from http://nccam.nih.gov/about/plans/oihr/#jump3

National Center for Complementary and Alternative Medicine. (2005). *Executive summary: Our mission.* Retrieved May 29, 2005, from http://nccam.nih.gov/about/plans/2005/page2.htm

National Center for Complementary and Alternative Medicine. (2008, December). *The use of complementary and alternative medicine in the United States.* Retrieved April 27, 2009, from http://nccam.nih.gov/news/camstats/2007/camsurvey_fs1.htm#use

National Center for Complementary and Alternative Medicine. (2009a). *Paying for CAM treatment.* Retrieved April 27, 2009, from http://nccam.nih.gov/health/financial/

National Center for Complementary and Alternative Medicine. (2009b). *Research sponsored by NCCAM.* Retrieved April 26, 2009, from http://nccam.nih.gov/research

National Institutes of Health. (2004, February). *NIH roadmap for medical research: A briefing by the NIH director and senior staff, February 27, 2004.* Retrieved May 29, 2005, from http://nihroadmap.nih.gov/briefing/executive summary.asp

Pinn, G. (2001). Herbal medicine in oncology. *Australian Family Physician, 30*(6), 575–580.

Quinn, J. F., Smith, M., Ritenbaugh, C., Swanson, K., & Watson, M. J. (2003). Research guidelines for assessing the impact of the healing relationship in clinical nursing. *Alternative Therapies in Health and Medicine, 9*(3), SuppA, 65–79.

Tracy, M. F., Lindquist, R., Savik, K., Watanuki, S., Sendelbach, S., Kreitzer, M. J., & Berman, B. (2005). Use of complementary and alternative therapies: A national survey of critical care nurses. *American Journal of Critical Care, 14*(5), 404–414.

Turner, J., Deyo, R., Loesser, J., Von Korff, J., & Fordyce, W. E. (1994). The importance of placebo effects in pain treatment and research. *Journal of the American Medical Association, 271*(10), 1609–1614.

World Health Organization. (2002). *WHO traditional medicine strategy: 2002–2005.* Geneva: World Health Organization. Retrieved May 29, 2005, from www.who.int/medicines/library/trm/trm_strat_eng.pdf

World Health Organization (2005). National policy on traditional medicines and regulation of herbal medicines—A report of a WHO global survey. Retrieved April 26, 2009, from http://ww w.who.int/medicinedocs/en/d/Js7916e/

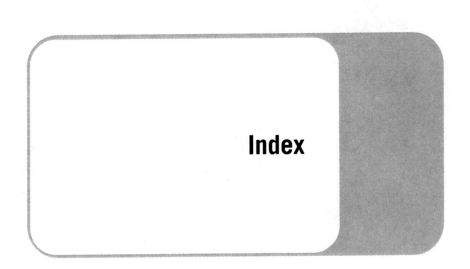

Index